Practical **MRI** of the Foot and Ankle

Edited by
Alison R. Spouge, M.D.
Thomas L. Pope, M.D.

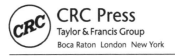

CRC Press
Taylor & Francis Group
Boca Raton London New York

CRC Press is an imprint of the
Taylor & Francis Group, an **informa** business

CRC Press
Taylor & Francis Group
6000 Broken Sound Parkway NW, Suite 300
Boca Raton, FL 33487-2742

First issued in paperback 2019

© 2007 by Taylor & Francis Group, LLC
CRC Press is an imprint of Taylor & Francis Group, an Informa business

No claim to original U.S. Government works

ISBN-13: 978-0-8493-0281-7 (hbk)
ISBN-13: 978-0-367-39815-6 (pbk)

Library of Congress Cataloging-in-Publication Data

Practical MRI of the foot and ankle / edited by Alison R. Spouge and Thomas L. Pope.
p. ; cm.
Includes bibliographical references and index.
ISBN-13: 978-0-8493-0281-7 (hardcover : alk. paper); ISBN-10: 0-8493-0281-1 (hardcover : alk. paper)
1. Foot--Magnetic resonance imaging. 2. Ankle--Magnetic resonance imaging. 3.
Foot--Diseases--Diagnosis. 4. Ankle--Diseases--Diagnosis. I. Spouge, Alison R. II.
Pope, Thomas Lee.
[DNLM: 1. Foot--pathology. 2. Ankle--pathology. 3. Foot Diseases--diagnosis. 4.
Magnetic Resonance Imaging--methods. WE 880 P895 2000]

RC951.P73 2000
617.5'8507548--dc21   00-039845 CIP

Visit the Informa Web site at
www.informa.com

and the Informa Healthcare Web site at
www.informahealthcare.com

Preface

Imaging of the foot and ankle presents considerable challenges. The complex and diminutive anatomy coupled with the diverse pathology affecting the anatomic region can be daunting. Technical advances in MR imaging have significantly improved the ability to image the foot and ankle and higher strength gradients, now standard on current imaging units, enable detailed depiction of the anatomy and pathology in this region. When combined with the high inherent contrast discrimination, images of superior diagnostic quality unsurpassed by any other modality are produced. With improvement in the technology and increased experience, our understanding of the MR imaging appearance of many pathologic conditions has advanced over the past 10 years.

Practical MRI of the Foot and Ankle provides an up-to-date guide to MR imaging of the foot and ankle. The reader is initially presented with background information regarding MR imaging techniques appropriate for this anatomic region, followed by a brief discussion of the normal anatomy of the foot and ankle in Chapters 1 and 2. Subsequent chapters encompass a spectrum of topics including pediatric pathology and normal variants, tendon and ligament injuries, neoplastic and traumatic osseous conditions, arthropathies, inflammatory pathology, the diabetic foot, unique conditions of the foot and ankle, and the value of magnetic resonance imaging from the orthopedist's perspective.

The authors hope that this book will become a standard part of the reference material that imagers have close at hand on a day-to-day basis. The authors are optimistic that referring physicians will consider this book a welcome and practical guide to MR imaging of foot and ankle disorders.

Editors

Alison R. Spouge, M.D., FRCPC, received her undergraduate and medical education at the University of British Columbia in Vancouver, British Columbia, Canada. She earned her Doctor of Medicine degree in 1983 and completed a rotating internship in Toronto, Ontario, Canada. She subsequently undertook specialty training in diagnostic radiology followed by fellowships in both cross-sectional imaging at the University of Toronto, and musculoskeletal and body MR imaging at the University of Western Ontario in Ontario, Canada. In 1990 Dr. Spouge was on staff at the Humana Hospital affiliated with the University of Louisville in Louisville, Kentucky. She is currently an assistant professor in the Faculty of Medicine at the University of Western Ontario in London, Ontario, and teaches radiology residents and medical students body and musculoskeletal MR imaging. She is the director of body and musculoskeletal MR imaging in the department of diagnostic radiology at the University Campus of the London Health Sciences Centre.

Dr. Spouge holds memberships in several societies including the Canadian Association of Radiologists, the American Roentgen Ray Society, Radiological Society of North America, and the International Society of Magnetic Resonance in Medicine. She has published scientific papers, review articles, and book chapters on MR imaging of the foot and ankle. Her major clinical interests include musculoskeletal and body imaging.

Thomas L. Pope Jr., M.D., FACR, received his Bachelor of Arts degree in religion in 1973 from the University of North Carolina at Chapel Hill and his Doctor of Medicine degree from the same institution in 1978. Following a flexible internship and diagnostic radiology residency at the University of Virginia (UVA) School of Medicine in Charlottesville, Virginia, he entered academic radiology and spent 6 years at UVA. From 1989 to 1997 he was professor of radiology and orthopedics at Wake Forest University Baptist Medical Center and moved to Charleston, South Carolina, to become professor of radiology and orthopedics at the Medical University of South Carolina in 1999 after a brief stint in private practice at Roper Hospital in the same city.

Dr. Pope is a member of numerous professional organizations including the American College of Radiology, AMA, American Roentgen Ray Society, International Skeletal Society, and the Radiological Society of North America. He has served a Duke endowment foreign fellowship to study the British National Health Service and was awarded an endowed professorship, the "Boerhaave Professor of Radiology" at the University of Leiden, in Leiden, the Netherlands, in 1994. He has served as an oral boards examiner for the American Board of Radiology in bone and joint radiology, chest radiology, and breast imaging, and has served as the American Roentgen Ray Visiting Scientist at the Armed Forces Institute of Pathology at which he still lectures as part of their faculty.

Dr. Pope has co-edited the following books: *Arthroscopy of the Wrist and Elbow, Basic Radiology, Aunt Minnie's Atlas and Imaging Specific Diagnosis* and *Practical Atlas of Musculoskeletal Imaging.* He is author and co-author of more than 140 research articles and 26 book chapters as well as multiple abstracts, editorials, book reviews, and letters to the editor.

Dr. Pope is currently professor and chair of radiology at the Medical University of South Carolina in Charleston. His major clinical interests are musculoskeletal radiology, breast imaging, and outreach imaging.

Contributors

Annunziato Amendola, M.D.
Assistant Professor
Department of Orthopedic Surgery
Fowler Kennedy Sports Medical Clinic
University of Western Ontario
London, Ontario, Canada

E. Michel Azouz, M.D., FRCPC
Professor of Radiology
McGill University
Montreal Children's Hospital and Shriners
  Hospital for Children
Montreal, Quebec, Canada

Joseph G. Craig, M.B., Ch.B.
Staff Radiologist
Henry Ford Hospital
Detroit, Michigan

Joshua M. Farber, M.D.
Department of Radiology
Medical University of South Carolina
Charleston, South Carolina

Donald J. Flemming, M.D.
Head Orthopedic Radiology Division
National Naval Medical Center
and
Assistant Professor
Department of Radiology and Nuclear
  Medicine
Uniformed Services School of the Health
  Sciences
Bethesda, Maryland

Clyde A. Helms, M.D.
Department of Radiology
Duke University Medical Center
Durham, North Carolina

Mark J. Lee, B.Sc.
Department of Radiology
Vancouver General Hospital
Vancouver, British Columbia, Canada

Nancy M. Major, M.D.
Department of Radiology
Duke University Medical Center
Durham, North Carolina

Cindy R. Miller, M.D.
Assistant Professor
Duke University Medical Center
Durham, North Carolina

Peter L. Munk, M.D.
Department of Radiology
Vancouver General Hospital
Vancouver, British Columbia, Canada

Kamaldine Oudjhane, M.D., M.Sc.
Associate Professor
McGill University
Montreal Children's Hospital and Shriners
  Hospital for Children
Montreal, Quebec, Canada

Thomas L. Pope, M.D., FACR
Professor of Radiology
Department of Radiology
Medical University of South Carolina
Charleston, South Carolina

David A. Rubin, M.D.
Assistant Professor of Radiology
Mallinckrodt Institute of Radiology
St. Louis, Missouri

Joel Rubenstein, M.D.
Department of Medical Imaging
Sunnybrook Women's College Health Sciences
  Center
University of Toronto
Toronto, Ontario, Canada

Steven Shankman, M.D.
Vice Chairman
Department of Radiology
Maimonides Medical Center
Brooklyn, New York

David F. Sitler, M.D.
Clinical Fellow
Department of Orthopedic Surgery
Fowler Kennedy Sports Medicine Clinic
University of Western Ontario
London, Ontario, Canada

Alison R. Spouge, M.D., FRCPC
Assistant Professor
Department of Diagnostic Radiology
London Health Sciences Centre
London, Ontario, Canada

Monique Starok, M.D.
Department of Medical Imaging
Sunnybrook Women's College Health Sciences
  Centre
University of Toronto
Toronto, Ontario

Marnix T. van Holsbeeck, M.D.
Director
Musculoskeletal and Emergency Radiology
Henry Ford Hospital
Detroit, Michigan

Contents

1 MR Imaging Technique and Principles

David A. Rubin

CONTENTS

INTRODUCTION

Magnetic resonance (MR) imaging has revolutionized imaging of the entire musculoskeletal system. Using commercially available machines, the physician can generate a strikingly detailed picture of virtually any part of a patient's anatomy, displayed in any orientation, without the risks of ionizing radiation. The physical principles governing MR imaging are quite complex; fortunately, the practitioner who performs clinical imaging does not need to understand all of them fully. Nevertheless, a knowledge of some basic principles is invaluable when designing imaging studies to ensure patient comfort and safety, as well to generate high-quality images, which in turn will improve diagnostic accuracy. The same information will influence decisions regarding equipment purchases. This chapter reviews these principles, stressing those that are unique to the foot and ankle. Readers interested in a more rigorous discussion of the detailed physics of MR imaging can consult one of several comprehensive texts dedicated to the subject.[1,2]

BASIC PRINCIPLES

To produce an MR image, the anatomic part to be examined is placed within a powerful, directional, relatively homogeneous magnetic field. This large, static magnetic field, called B_0, is oriented along the patient's head-to-foot axis (the z-axis) on most high-field-strength systems. The protons in the body (chiefly those in water and lipid species) generate their own smaller magnetic fields and align themselves with the B_0 field. The portion of the collective magnetization of the protons that is aligned with the B_0 field is called longitudinal magnetization. The magnitude of this longitudinal magnetization ultimately determines how much a given tissue can contribute to the final MR image. Tissues that start with no longitudinal magnetization will not show up in the image, and are said to be "suppressed." In reality, protons precess along the z-axis in a wobbling, spinning motion like a top. The precessional frequency is proportional to the resonant frequency for each proton, which is uniquely determined by its chemical environment, and is proportional to the strength of the magnetic field in the immediate vicinity of the proton. This local field varies slightly because of imperfections in the B_0 field and the effect of neighboring structures. The net result of placing a patient in the scanner is that, initially, the body's protons will precess around the same axis, each with minimally different frequencies. As an example, in a 1.5-tesla (T) magnetic field, protons precess at approximately 63 megahertz (MHz), with the resonant frequencies of fat and water protons differing by a mere 220 Hz (less than 1/1000 of 1%).

The resonant frequencies fall within the radiofrequency (RF) range. Thus, pulses of radio waves (RF energy) can be intermittently applied to disrupt the alignment of some of the protons temporarily. One of the more common strategies is to use enough RF energy to realign the protons from the z-axis into a perpendicular plane, converting longitudinal magnetization in the z-axis into transverse magnetization in the xy-plane. Such an RF pulse is called a 90° pulse (90 is called the flip angle) because the motion from the z-axis to the xy-plane is geometrically a change of 90°. Once the RF energy is turned off, the protons begin to realign with the B_0 axis. The process of changing and reestablishing the proton alignment also produces small bursts of RF energy, which are detected as small induced voltages by a receiver coil. A coil is basically a wire antenna that is tuned to pick up this signal, much like a radio antenna picks up radio signals. It is important to note that the coil can only detect transverse magnetization (in the plane orthogonal to the main magnetic field). The MR machine converts the received voltage changes into digital data by an analog-to-digital converter, and then deciphers the digital data to produce the final images.

Protons in different tissues (e.g., in water or in fat) have different magnetic properties which dictate how they will react to the magnetic field and RF pulses. The first critical property, proton density, represents the number of protons present in a given tissue volume. Higher proton density results in a larger generated signal. The second property is how quickly the protons realign with the static magnetic field following an RF excitation pulse, described by a time constant called T1. A second time constant, T2, describes how quickly the transverse magnetization decays over time, reflecting the tendency of different protons, which are initially aligned together after a 90° pulse, to precess quickly out-of-sync with each other. This process is called dephasing. Each tissue in the body has a characteristic T1, T2, and proton density. MR imaging exploits these differences to generate images in which unique tissues can be distinguished from each other. The MR scanner accomplishes this task by applying combinations of RF pulses in a pulse sequence.

Many different MR pulse sequences have been described. They differ in the number, strength, and timing of the applied RF pulses. Each sequence is designed so that the strength of the signal (sometimes called an echo) peaks at a specific time after the start of the sequence. This time is called the TE (time to echo) and is measured in milliseconds (msec). TEs less than 30 msec are considered "short"; those greater than 60 msec are relatively "long." Sequences using ultrashort (<10 msec) or very long (>140 msec) TEs are not commonly used for musculoskeletal imaging. A finite block of time is set aside around the TE for reception of the signal. Pulse sequences may also be designed to generate more than one peak of signal after times TE_1, TE_2, and so on, and the signal received at each TE can contribute to different images (as is typically done in multiecho spin-echo sequences) or can contribute to the same image (as is the case for fast spin-echo imaging). The combination of RF pulses is transmitted repeatedly at an interval called TR (time of repetition), each time generating echoes after the designated TE time(s).

Typical TRs range from below 100 msec (useful for three-dimensional pulse sequences, as described below) to several thousand milliseconds. Usually, TR is much longer than TE; this allows time for some of the protons (those with the shortest T1s) to realign themselves with the B_0 field before subsequent RF pulses are transmitted. Thus, during the TR period, the majority of time is not spent gathering the signal, but rather waiting for T1 relaxation to occur before delivery of the next RF pulses, which will re-excite those protons that have undergone some T1-relaxation. This time is not wasted, however. Most pulse sequences are designed to use this time to image other slices.[3,4] After the signal is received from one slice but before the end of the TR period, RF energy is delivered to protons in another slice and their signal is gathered after the TE time(s). Thus, data from multiple slices are gathered nearly simultaneously, in a slightly staggered fashion. The longer the TR, the more slices can be acquired because there is more "waiting" time between the end of the last TE period and the beginning of the next TR period.[4]

The selected TR/TE combination is a major factor determining the appearance of the final image. The effect is easiest to appreciate for spin-echo pulse sequences, one of the most common types employed in musculoskeletal MR imaging. In a spin-echo sequence, a 180° RF pulse is applied at time TE/2 after the initial 90° pulse, to correct for dephasing that results from imperfections in the magnetic field. Spin-echo images acquired with a short TR and short TE are relatively "T1-weighted," meaning that differences in proton T1 values in large part determine the strength of their emitted signals. Tissues with relatively *short T1s* (e.g., fat, melanin, met-hemoglobin, and tissues containing gadolinium-based contrast agents) recover most of their longitudinal magnetization by the end of the TR period, so that they are mostly realigned with the B_0 field before the next RF pulses are delivered. Thus, a relatively large proportion of these protons participate in each subsequent signal-gathering period, producing a large amount of signal. Tissues containing these protons appear relatively *bright* in the final images. Tissues with *long T1s* (muscle, water, and inflammation, for example) only have enough time to recover a small amount of their longitudinal magnetization before the next RF pulse, so the protons in these tissues generate less signal, and will appear *dark*. As TR becomes longer, the images become less T1 weighted.

Conversely, in a long TR, long TE sequence, most of the tissues, regardless of their T1s, have time to regain their longitudinal magnetization before subsequent RF pulses, so differences in T1 values are less important. The long TE also means that the protons will have time to dephase with respect to each other before the echo is collected. When many protons are precessing out of phase, the echoes that they generate are destructive when summed (their signals cancel out), resulting in lower overall signal intensity in the images. Because tissues with very long T2s will be less dephased (i.e., more in-phase) by time TE, they will contribute disproportionately more signal. Such an image is "T2-weighted" since chemical species with *long T2s* (such as water and edema) will be *bright*. A pulse sequence with a long TR but short TE will minimize the contributions from differences in both T1 and T2 values. This sequence would then be "proton density-weighted" as the number of protons in each volume of tissue, not their T1 or T2 values, would be the main determinant of the generated signal. Tissues with *few protons* (like cortical bone and air) would appear *dark*, while most other tissues would have fairly uniform intermediate-to-high signal intensity. Of course, structures with low proton density would be low signal (dark) on any pulse sequence since they contain few overall protons to generate signal. Other features of the protons, such as the ease with which they diffuse or whether they are in static tissue or flowing blood, also change the relative strength of their emitted signals, and hence their relative brightness in the final image. The brightness and darkness of the MR image is called contrast, and the ability to distinguish different tissue types based on their signal is referred to as contrast resolution.

To make sense of the received signal, the MR imaging system must also determine the location in the body from where the signal originated. For most physicians the way in which a signal is localized is probably the most confusing part of MR imaging. In general, the detailed physics and mathematics underlying this procedure need not be fully understood to protocol and interpret clinical studies. Familiarity with the general concepts, however, may be useful. Periodically during MR imaging, the static magnetic field is systematically varied. Gradient coils are rapidly turned on and off (which produces the characteristic tapping noise of an operating MR machine) to make some parts of the field temporarily slightly stronger and other parts temporarily slightly weaker. In turn, the protons within different areas of the field (and hence, within different regions of the patient's body) are briefly exposed to different magnetic fields. They react by precessing at different frequencies. Because of these differences, collecting signal during the application of a gradient yields localizing information in one linear dimension (one imaging axis). This process is called frequency encoding. If, before collecting the signal, a gradient in another direction were applied and then turned off, the protons located along different parts of that axis would end up precessing out-of-sync, because those that were located in a stronger part of the field while the gradient was on would have moved faster than other protons. This last property is called phase and it too can be used to localize the received signal in one axis. However, to locate the source of a signal unambiguously using phase information, the procedure must be repeated many times, each time applying a different strength gradient and collecting a different echo. Later, the signal is mathematically manipulated to reconstruct the spatial relationships, a process called phase encoding. In clinical MR imaging, repeating the phase-encoding process accounts for the majority of imaging time.

Both frequency encoding and phase encoding are used to generate the final image. A common strategy in MR imaging, called two-dimensional encoding, is to use a third orthogonal gradient applied while the RF pulse is given. Applying a gradient during RF excitation increases the precessional frequency of the protons on one side of the patient and decreases the frequencies on the other side. As the RF pulse will only influence or "excite" protons that are precessing with a given frequency, only a portion of the protons in the middle of the patient will have the correct frequency to be excited by the RF pulse. In this way, a slice of the area of interest is selected, and the location of the slice can be varied by changing the gradient. The locations within this slice are then frequency-encoded in one direction and phase-encoded in the perpendicular direction. The potential thinness of a slice is limited by the strength of the applied gradient. Alternatively, a three-dimensional technique can be used whereby phase encoding is performed in two dimensions, and frequency encoding is done in the third, allowing the acquisition of much thinner, contiguous slices. The main disadvantage of this approach is the time needed for complete phase encoding in two directions, as the procedure needs to be repeated many more times. With either technique, the final image consists of an area called the field-of-view (FOV) divided into many small picture elements called pixels, which have a length and width. The total number of pixels in an image is the matrix. An image composed of 256 pixels in one dimension, localized by frequency encoding, and 192 pixels in the perpendicular phase-encoded axis would thus have a 256×192 matrix, and would be composed of 49,152 separate pixels. In reality, each pixel belongs to a slice of anatomy, which has a given thickness, so each represents a small volume of tissue, or voxel. The brightness of each voxel represents the signal received from that volume of tissue. Images with small FOVs, small pixels (larger matrices), and thin slices will have high spatial resolution; that is, they will be capable of distinguishing small structures that are located close together. A factor limiting the matrix size is the prolonged acquisition time needed to complete a large number of phase-encoding steps.[5]

The entire process of image acquisition may be repeated any number of times, with the signal generated from each acquisition averaged to make one final image. The number of repetitions is called the NEX (number of excitations), or on some machines the NSA (number of signals averaged). The total time required for a complete pulse sequence is approximately equal to the TR multiplied by the number of phase encoding steps, then multiplied by the NEX. In clinical practice, the time required for a single pulse sequence can range from less than 1 min to upward of 10 min. However, it becomes very difficult for even the most motivated patient to remain still for more than 10 min. Ideal imaging times are 2 to 6 min/sequence. As a complete study typically encompasses 4 to 8 sequences, allotting 25 to 45 min for each examination, including patient positioning and setup time, is reasonable.

A critical concept that encompasses all the trade-offs involved in MR imaging is the signal-to-noise ratio (SNR).[6,7] In addition to the useful data (signal) generated from the patient's body, random and pseudorandom signal is also received by the coil. In part, this noise originates in tissues outside the area of interest that are affected by the RF pulses and gradients. These tissues also generate signal, which may be picked up by the receiver coil.[8] Within the region of interest, the random motion of charge carriers such as electrolytes also contributes to noise. A second component of the noise comes from the random fluctuations of electrons within the MR equipment itself, and this effect is proportionally larger at lower field strengths.[9] This background noise is superimposed on the useful signal, and if the noise is large enough compared with the signal (i.e., the SNR is low) the images will appear grainy and may be nondiagnostic. Conversely, when the SNR is high, the images will appear clear and crisp. More importantly, many variables including the choice of scanner and coil, and the selection of pulse sequence parameters, increase or decrease the SNR.[10]

In this way, SNR can be thought of as the "currency" of MR imaging. When adequate SNR is present, it can be used to "purchase" other desirable features, such as high contrast resolution, high spatial resolution, faster imaging times, or artifact reduction.[6] Conversely, at times, increasing the SNR will be necessary (e.g., by increasing the FOV) to allow other imaging options that require a high SNR. SNR is directly related to the size of the voxels and the number of protons within each voxel.[5] Thus, increasing FOV, decreasing matrix size, and/or increasing slice thickness will increase SNR. Conversely, high-resolution imaging with a small FOV, large matrix, or thin slices will require relatively high SNR, which may necessitate other imaging trade-offs, such as decreasing the TE (which would decrease the relative T2-weighting of the image). All else being equal, a shorter TE increases SNR because it allows less time for signal loss due to proton dephasing (T2 decay).

In reality, the effect of TE on SNR is more complex. Receiving the echo takes a finite amount of time. To some extent, the operator can vary the sampling (frequency) bandwidth (the rate that the received signal is digitized), which is inversely proportional to the sampling time. When TE is short, little time exists between the delivery of the RF pulses and the production of the echo. The signal acquisition is usually arranged so that the center of the echo falls near the center of the sampling interval. Thus, the sampling time must be reduced (bandwidth increased) to obtain images with very short TEs. The shorter sampling time translates into increased noise and lower SNR.[6,7,11,12] Conversely, decreasing the bandwidth is a valuable way to increase SNR at longer TEs, where the penalty of increased minimum TE is not a problem[13]; however, as discussed later, an increase in imaging artifacts may occur when the bandwidth is decreased.

Increasing the NEX will also increase SNR, but this method is relatively inefficient. To double the SNR, the number of acquisitions would need to be multiplied by four,[14,15] and the sequence would take four times as long to complete. Lengthening the examination also increases the risk of image degradation through patient motion, and decreases overall efficiency of the MR scanner as fewer patients can be examined in a given time. The remainder of this chapter discusses other trade-offs that hinge on SNR, but, as will be seen, one of the most efficient ways of increasing overall SNR in musculoskeletal imaging is the use of specialized local coils.

INSTRUMENTATION

Commercial MR systems are available in several configurations. Systems vary in the strength of the static magnetic field, measured in tesla, in the size and shape of the opening for the patient, in the available gradients and coils, in the available pulse sequence options, and of course in size and cost. Each system has advantages and disadvantages for MR imaging of the foot and ankle.

The magnetic field strength of clinical MR imaging machines falls into three broad categories: high-field (typified by a 1.5-T), mid-field (approximately 0.5-T), and low-field (0.2-T) scanners. On high-field machines, the B_0 field is produced by a supercooled, superconducting electromagnetic. Typically, the configuration is a cylindrical tube, which consists of the main magnet, the gradient coils, and a large receiver coil (frequently called the body coil). The patient lies on a bed within the bore, with the part to be examined as close to the center of the tube as possible, where the field is most homogeneous. Positioning the patient in the bore of the magnet can be problematic in those patients who experience severe claustrophobia as the diameter of the cylinder is relatively small, often leaving less than a meter between the patient's face and the top of the tube. The superconducting magnet requires a surrounding shell of liquid gases (cryogens) to keep the temperature a few degrees above absolute zero. The cryogens must be replenished periodically. If the temperature of the magnet rises, the field rapidly drops to zero. Thus, once started, the magnetic field is always kept "on," and care must be taken to keep loose metallic instruments and devices out of the room, as they can quickly become lethal projectiles. Additionally, the proper functioning of certain biomedical implants, such as heart pacemakers, cochlear implants, and neurostimulators are affected by the strong magnetic field. Patients and personnel with such devices must be kept a safe distance from the machine. Standard references listing safe and contraindicated devices are continually updated,[16,17] and at least one should be available for consultation at all MR imaging facilities. Additionally, ferromagnetic materials in critical regions of the body (such as aneurysm clips in the brain or metal shavings close to the retina) can become displaced and potentially injure adjacent sensitive structures.[18] Even if only the foot is to be examined, in a high-field scanner the rest of the patient's body lies within the strong magnetic field, and metallic objects in critical anatomic locations constitute a contraindication to MR imaging.

High-field MR systems are large and heavy. The main disadvantage of a high-field system is the cost of purchasing, siting, and maintaining the equipment. That said, high-field systems are probably the most popular for clinical imaging because of their versatility. The size of the bore means that all body parts can be examined (with different receiver coils) using the same scanner. Manufacturers and third-party providers offer many hardware and software options for these units. From the image quality standpoint, the chief advantage of a high-field system is that it provides inherently higher SNR compared with low-field systems.[19,20] Thus, a high-field system will require fewer imaging trade-offs and will provide more pulse sequence options than a low-field system. There is also a wider separation between the precessional frequencies of different chemical species at higher field strengths, which makes selective imaging of certain tissues easier. This fact is especially important in the musculoskeletal system where it is often advantageous to suppress the signal from fat. Additionally, differences in tissue T1 values decrease as field strength diminishes,[21] making distinction between species based on their T1 values easier at high field strengths.

Mid-field magnets represent a compromise between high-field and low-field systems. They are physically smaller and less expensive than high-field units, and they have less stringent siting requirements since the magnetic field surrounding the unit (the fringe field) is smaller. Additionally, mid-field systems can be designed in configurations other than a cylindrical tube, including "open" systems that do not completely surround the patient. These machines may be useful for imaging large patients who will not fit within the bore of a high-field system, and for patients with severe claustrophobia. SNR is lower than for high-field systems, and the static magnetic field tends to be less homogeneous. However, high-quality MR imaging of the foot and ankle can be performed using mid-field systems with choice of an appropriate receiver coil, careful attention to patient positioning, and the selection of proper pulse sequences (Figure 1.1).

Low-field MR imaging units are smaller and less expensive than mid-field and high-field systems, but they suffer from lower SNR, necessitating more acquisitions (higher NEX), and thus longer imaging times, to produce diagnostic images. Low-field systems can be built with permanent magnets instead of supercooled electromagnets, greatly simplifying maintenance and siting of the units. A recent development has been the introduction of dedicated extremity-only MR imaging systems.[22] These machines use a shielded, small-bore magnet with a very small footprint, and so can be set up in a relatively small space. Only the part to be examined is introduced through the opening in the scanner. Thus, these systems can only image the peripheral extremities, lacking the versatility of larger machines, which can image other body parts. A limited number and configuration of receiver coils are available, and on some systems the usable FOV is quite small (12 cm), limiting overall anatomic coverage. While the ankle and hind foot can be examined with a dedicated extremity system (Figure 1.2), it is difficult to position a patient comfortably to image the mid-foot or forefoot. Even for the ankle, patient positioning may be difficult, and motion due to patient discomfort is an issue. The problem is exacerbated at low field strength since the inherently low SNR means that imaging sessions of an hour or more are not uncommon. The adverse effect of motion artifacts cannot be overstated: Any techniques used to increase SNR or spatial resolution will be futile if patient motion degrades the images.[5] Additionally, as of this writing, there are no published studies evaluating diagnostic accuracy using extremity-only magnets for foot and ankle pathology. Nevertheless, these small

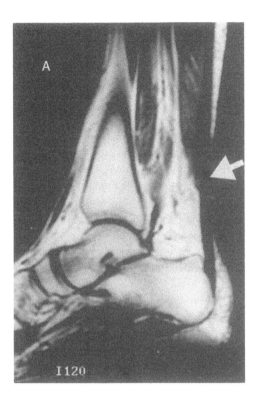
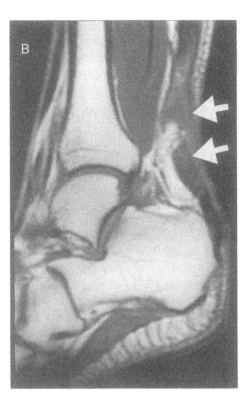

FIGURE 1.1 Comparison of high-field and mid-field MR systems. (A) Sagittal spin-echo (TR/TE = 450/15) image of a lacerated Achilles tendon (arrow) obtained with a 1.5-T system. Imaging time = 2:29 min. (B) Sagittal (SE 500/21) image of a high-grade Achilles tendon tear (arrows) in another patient obtained with a 0.5-T system. Note that comparable image quality was obtained in part by increasing the NEX, necessitating a longer imaging time (4:56 min).

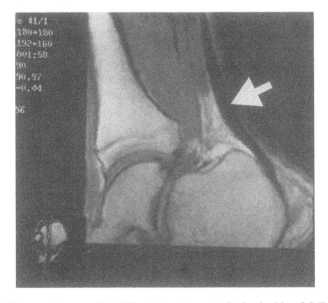

FIGURE 1.2 Sagittal image of a normal Achilles tendon (arrow) obtained with a 0.2-T dedicated extremity MR system. The image appears "grainy" compared with those shown in Figure 1.1 due to the lower SNR. Also note the smaller usable FOV (11 cm) compared with the images in Figure 1.1 (22 to 24 cm). (Courtesy of M. Tuite, Madison, WI.)

scanners may provide MR imaging capabilities in areas where a larger, more expensive scanner would be impractical. Additionally, because the majority of the patient's body is outside the main magnetic field, bioimplants such as pacemakers and aneurysm clips will likely not be affected and it should be safe to image patients with such devices.[23,24]

RECEIVER COILS AND PATIENT POSITIONING

The choice of receiver coil critically impacts the quality of musculoskeletal MR images. Noise tends to be distributed fairly uniformly, and a coil detects noise within its entire receptive field. Thus, while the body coil can be used to receive the MR signal, this strategy would result in SNR that is much too low to produce high-resolution MR images of the foot and ankle. The body coil would receive the signal from the small area of interest (e.g., the foot), but would receive noise from the entire body. A better strategy would be the use of a local coil, a small receiver placed near the examined part. The chief advantage of a local coil is that it is highly sensitive to only a small volume of tissue (the region of sensitivity of the coil). As long as the anatomy of interest is within the receptive field, the coil will receive the signal to create the MR image, but will be less sensitive to noise generated outside of this area, resulting in higher SNR.[25,26] The smaller the coil, the greater the increase in SNR, at the expense of less anatomic coverage.[9] The use of a properly selected local coil is perhaps the most important factor for generating high-quality foot and ankle MR images.

Local coils can be easily built in a variety of shapes.[9,26] Several broad categories exist, and each can play a role in foot and ankle MR imaging. Whole-volume coils are cylindrical, similar in design but much smaller than the body coil.[9] Examples include the tubular coils used for head and knee imaging. Their advantage is relatively homogeneous sensitivity for the signal within a volume of tissue. The disadvantage is that the entire area to be examined must fit within the coil. Some of these coils can be used both to transmit the RF energy that excites the protons and to receive the subsequent echo. Different configurations of the conductor material within the coil yield different performance characteristics, and may require that the coil be positioned in a specific orientation to the static magnetic field.[9] For example, coils built with a solenoid design have an intrinsically higher SNR than those with a birdcage design,[10] but the bore of a solenoid coil must be placed perpendicular to the B_0 field (e.g., they cannot be oriented along the z-axis in a superconducting tubular magnet).

Another type of local coil is the surface coil. These are flat or slightly contoured, and are designed to lie along one side of the body part.[9] They have very high sensitivity near the surface of the coil, which drops off rapidly with distance from the coil face.[25] This signal drop-off is frequently advantageous when signal generated farther from the coil is responsible for artifacts that degrade the image. Thus, these coils are ideal for high-resolution imaging of relatively superficial structures. Typical surface coil designs consist of one or two turns of wire packaged in a circular or rectangular shape. Compared with whole-volume designs, surface coils provide more versatile positioning options, since they do not completely surround the body part. Their main drawback is the nonuniformity of the receptive field (Figure 1.3).[27]

Because the signal is much more intense near the coil surface, it may be necessary to view or photograph the images at more than one window and level setting to see relevant anatomic structures accurately. Alternatively, the final image can be digitally filtered to compress or "smooth out" the range of signal intensities that are displayed.[28,29] Last, surface coils cannot produce homogeneous RF pulses across their fields.[25] Thus, these coils are only used to receive signal; RF energy is still transmitted by a whole-volume coil (typically the body coil).

Partial-volume coils represent a compromise between whole-volume and surface coils. Partial-volume coils partly surround the area of interest, usually lying on two or three sides of the body part.[30] Thus, they can be used in some anatomic areas that cannot be completely encircled by a whole-volume coil. Like surface coils, they are most sensitive near the coil face(s), but their homogeneity lies between that of surface and whole-volume coils. Signal drop-off at a distance

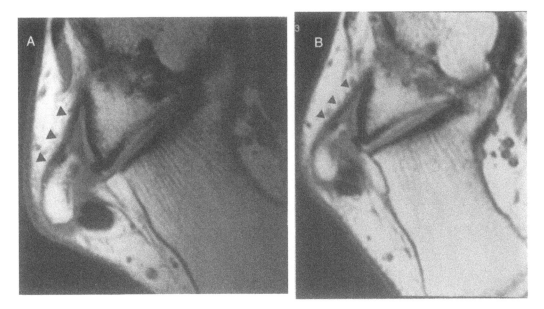

FIGURE 1.3 Comparison of surface and whole-volume coils. (A) Single 3-in. circular surface coil placed over lateral malleolus shows very high SNR in the near field, but severe signal drop-out farther from coil. Arrowheads = anterior talofibular ligament. (B) Whole-volume cylindrical extremity coil placed around same patient's hind foot has lower spatial resolution laterally (compare distinctness of anterior talofibular ligament, arrowheads), but homogeneous signal throughout the entire receptive field.

from the coil is less severe with a partial-volume coil compared with a surface coil, allowing imaging at greater depths within the patient. The signal from several surface coils can be combined to create a partial-volume coil if there is enough of a gap between the coils to prevent one coil from inducing a current and magnetic field within the other.[30] Two circular surface coils placed facing each other (a Helmholtz pair) is one example of this technique.[10]

Last, multiple coils can be combined as an array. With this approach, the coils gather signal simultaneously but independently; the data are then combined to create the final image.[31] If the coils receive signal from separate regions of the patient, as with a spine array that has rectangular coils in a row, the effect is to increase the area of coverage while maintaining the high SNR of a small coil.[9] When the coils receive signal from the same area, the result is an increase in SNR with no change in coverage. An example of this latter design is a quadrature extremity coil where two coils are packaged together within a cylindrical casing, both oriented along the same axis but rotated 90° with respect to each other.[6,9] Arrays require separate data pathways for each receiver component, adding to the expense and complexity of the system.

For foot and ankle MR imaging, selection of a coil starts with an understanding of what area needs to be imaged, which determines the amount of coverage needed. Then a consideration of the size and shape of the extremity, the coils available, and the desired resolution will suggest possible coil–patient position combinations. A useful rule of thumb is that the size of the receptive field of the coil should closely match the size of the area to be imaged.[6,26] Fortunately, many choices are available, and some creativity will suggest new possibilities. Figure 1.4 illustrates several easily implemented approaches.

For the ankle and hind foot, a whole-volume coil works well. While both ankles may be imaged simultaneously by placing them in a head coil (Figure 1.4A), the resultant SNR (and hence attainable resolution) suffers compared with placing one ankle in a smaller coil, and then repeating the study with the other ankle if a bilateral study is requested.[8] A better approach is to lay the patient supine and place the ankle in a smaller extremity coil (i.e., a "knee" coil) with the toes pointing straight

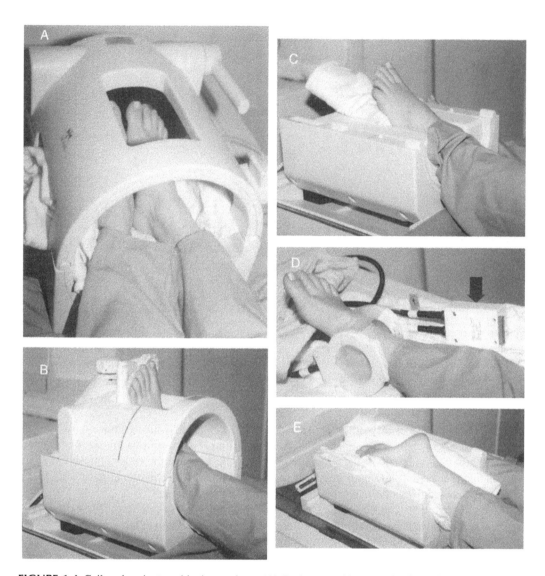

FIGURE 1.4 Coil and patient positioning options. (A) Both extremities examined together in a head coil. The spatial resolution of this approach is inferior to the other options. In all examples, the padding that is typically placed around the foot and ankle to augment immobilization has been removed for clarity. (B) Ankle and hind foot examined in an extremity coil. The patient is supine, the ankle is in neutral position, and the toes extend through the opening in the top of the coil. (C) Mild plantar flexion of the ankle allows more coverage distally and alleviates the problem of wraparound artifact on the sagittal images. The cover of the extremity coil has been removed for illustrative purposes. (D) Two circular surface coils placed on either side of the ankle. In this example the signal from both coils is combined via a connector box (arrow). This setup allows more freedom for ankle flexion and extension. (E) With the patient prone and the ankle fully plantar-flexed, cross-sectional imaging of the ankle tendons is simplified (see text). This position can be used for the forefoot and mid-foot as well as for the ankle and hind foot. The top of the extremity coil has been removed to show the orientation of the foot.   (*continued*)

up (Figure 1.4B). Most extremity coils have an opening in the top that facilitates the toes. The ankle and hind foot are then imaged in neutral position, which simplifies image interpretation. For an average-sized patient, the coverage will typically include the myotendinous junction of the Achilles tendon superiorly, and the metatarsal bases distally. One disadvantage of this position is

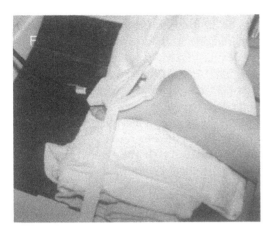
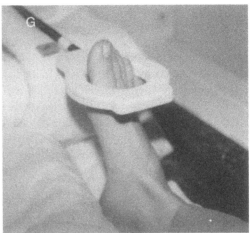

FIGURE 1.4 (continued) (F) A flat surface coil applied to the bottom of the foot (or the dorsum in a supine patient) can be used to image the mid-foot and metatarsals. (G) A loop surface coil placed encircling the toes for high-resolution imaging of the forefoot.

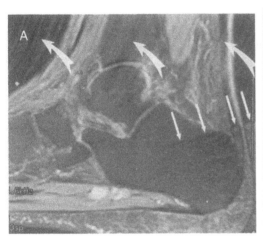
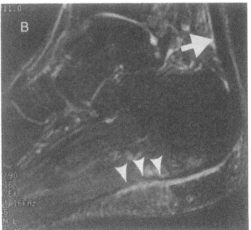

FIGURE 1.5 Effect of positioning on wraparound artifact. (A) On a fat-suppressed sagittal (FSE 3000/16) image with the ankle in neutral position (Figure 1.4B), signal from the toes is superimposed on the distal Achilles tendon and calcaneus (straight arrows) and may either mimic or obscure pathology. Note also artifact characterized by alternating dark and bright stripes in the lower leg (curved arrows) due to pulsatile flow in the dorsalis pedis artery. This artifact, which also obscures part of the Achilles tendon, could have been reduced by using a saturation band above the ankle, or through gradient moment nulling ("flow compensation"). The phase-encoding direction is the heel-to-toe axis. (B) In a different patient, slight plantar flexion of the ankle (Figure 1.4C) allows signal from the toes to wrap outside the field of view, permitting a confident diagnosis of a normal Achilles tendon (arrow) but a high-grade plantar fascia injury (arrowheads). Patient is a professional football placekicker. STIR image (3116/68, TI = 155).

that signal from the forefoot may alias ("wraparound") and become superimposed on the calcaneous and Achilles tendon on sagittal images (Figure 1.5A), potentially obscuring pathology. This appearance is an artifact of the phase-encoding scheme and can be eliminated by phase oversampling, a software option often called "no phase wrap." The penalty of this software solution is that more data are acquired and then discarded, resulting in a longer acquisition, or in decreased SNR if the imaging time is kept constant (in which case the effect is analogous to a decrease in NEX).

A positioning solution to the problem of aliasing is to plantar-flex the ankle mildly (Figure 1.4C), so that any aliased signal from the toes projects below the heel (Figure 1.5B). This position also allows more of the forefoot to be included in the images, at the expense of coverage in the distal leg. Patients must be cooperative and somewhat flexible to achieve this position comfortably. A disadvantage of this position is that it places the hind foot in a position that is no longer perpendicular to the leg. With the hind foot in this nonstandard position it may become difficult to identify matching areas of cartilage abnormality on the talus and tibia, or to identify confidently certain anatomic structures such as the anterior talofibular ligament and anterolateral gutter.

If an extremity coil is not available, a partial-volume coil can be constructed easily by placing two circular coils along the medial and lateral malleoli (Figure 1.4D). The cables from the two coils can be joined through a connector box, or each can be plugged into an array input. Before using this technique, mark the faces of each coil (for example, "A" and "B"). Image a volunteer or phantom, trying all combinations of coil orientation (both "A" sides facing each other, one "A" side facing one "B" side, etc.) and record which orientation produces the best signal. Use this orientation when imaging subsequent patients. More setup time, padding, and taping is required with this approach, compared with the use of an extremity coil, which is nearly form-fitting to the ankle. However, one advantage of using paired coils is that the ankle may be dorsiflexed and plantar-flexed without removing the coils, allowing supplemental imaging in different ankle positions.

With the ankle in neutral position or mildly plantar-flexed, the medial tendons (posterior tibialis, flexor digitorum longus, and flexor hallucis longus) and lateral tendons (peroneus brevis and longus) curve around the malleoli, while the anterior tendons (anterior tibialis, extensor hallucis longus, and extensor digitorum longus) curve anterior to the ankle joint. This change in orientation has two important implications for MR imaging. Images oriented transversely to the distal leg will be perpendicular only to the proximal portion of each tendon. To image the distal portions of the tendons in cross section, additional images in the coronal plane will be needed. Even then, there will be no images that show a true cross section along the curved parts without volume averaging. The second problem relates to an artifact called the magic angle phenomenon. On images acquired with a short TE (approximately 30 msec or less at 1.5 T), structures whose orientation approximates a 55° angle (the "magic" angle) to the B_0 field will appear artifactually brighter than those at other orientations.[32] This artifact relates to loss of dipole–dipole interactions, which normally contribute to the low signal intensity of primarily collagenous and fibrous structures, such as tendons and ligaments. At the magic angle, the contribution of these interactions becomes minimal, so less signal is lost and the structures appear brighter.[32] The apparent increase in signal intensity can mimic or obscure pathology. Because of the trajectory of the ankle tendons, they frequently pass through the magic angle. The effect is especially prominent in the peroneus brevis tendon (Figure 1.6). Note that the magic angle artifact is independent of the imaging plane; its occurrence only depends on the orientation of the structure to the static magnetic field.

One way to avoid problems due to tendon orientation in the foot and ankle is to plantar-flex the ankle fully. In this position, the course the tendons is now a straight line from the distal leg to the mid-foot, and transverse images will show the true cross-sectional appearance of each tendon along its entire extent. Furthermore, the tendons will now be reoriented with respect to the B_0 field, reducing or eliminating the magic angle phenomenon (Figure 1.7). However, it is very difficult for a supine patient to maintain full plantar flexion. The solution is to place the patient prone, still using an extremity coil (Figure 1.4E). This position also places more of the mid-foot and forefoot in the coil, often permitting one examination of the entire ankle and foot. Most patients find this position surprisingly comfortable, leading to fewer problems with involuntary motion.[33] Additionally, some patients who are very claustrophobic may be able to complete the examination when placed prone.[34] The likely explanation is that a prone subject can lift his chin and see out of the magnetic bore, but a supine subject will always be looking upward, seeing and sensing the close

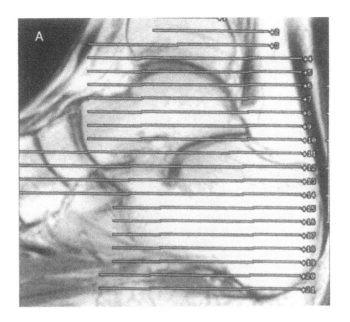

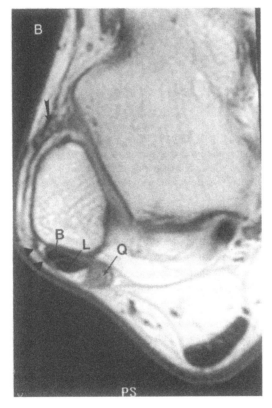

FIGURE 1.6 Effect of neutral ankle position on tendon appearance. (A) Sagittal examination in a supine patient with the ankle in neutral position (Figure 1.4B) shows prescription for subsequent axial images. (B) Axial (SE 450/17) image above the malleolar tips (corresponding to level 8 in A) shows lateral tendons in cross section. B = peroneus brevis tendon, L = peroneus longus tendon, Q = peroneus quartus muscle (normal variant). Arrowheads indicate superior peroneal retinaculum. Note scar (straight arrow) from prior surgery on the anterior talofibular ligament.   (*continued*)

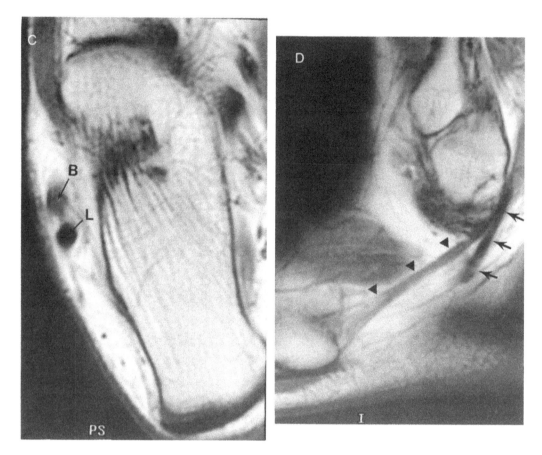

FIGURE 1.6 (continued) (C) Axial (SE 450/17) image below the malleoli (level 14 in A) is no longer perpendicular to tendons. Artifactually increased signal intensity occurs in the peroneus brevis tendon (B) due to magic angle phenomenon. L = peroneus longus tendon. (D) Sagittal (SE 466/17) image shows the trajectories of the distal peroneus longus (arrows) and peroneus brevis (arrowheads) tendons, with the latter oriented approximately 55° to main magnetic field.

proximity of the top of the tube. Disadvantages of the prone position include distortion and severe foreshortening of the Achilles tendon, and reorientation of the ankle joint structures, including the supporting ligaments, so they no longer lie in their expected anatomic planes.

The mid-foot and forefoot can also be examined with an extremity coil with the patient prone, sliding the coil downward if the foot is especially large and the tips of the toes need to be seen (Figure 1.4E). Alternatively, since the structures in the mid-foot and forefoot are relatively superficial, a surface coil may be a logical choice. Taping a flat coil (either rectangular or circular) along the plantar aspect of the foot in a prone patient (Figure 1.4F) works well in cases of suspected metatarsal stress fracture, intermetatarsal bursitis, Morton neuroma, and abnormalities of the tarsometatarsal or metatarsophalangeal joints. If the patient cannot tolerate the prone position, a surface coil can be taped to either the plantar or dorsal aspect of the forefoot with the patient lying on his or her back. Alternatively, on systems where the main magnetic field lies along the axis from the patient's head to feet (typical for high-field, tubular-bore magnets) a solenoid-type coil may be placed around the forefoot when the ankle is in neutral position and the toes are pointed up.[35] This arrangement orients the coil perpendicular to the B_0 field, which is necessary for solenoid coil operation. If a dedicated solenoid coil is not available, encircling the toes with a circular surface coil (Figure 1.4G) works nearly as well and provides excellent SNR.[35]

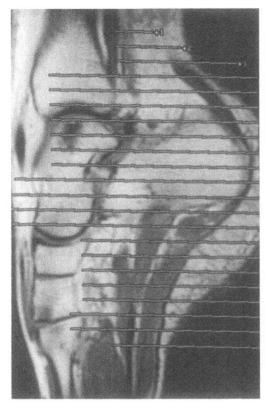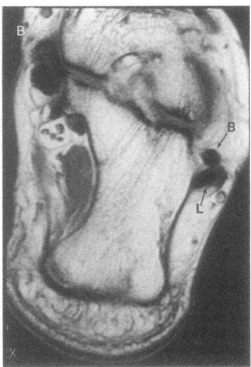

FIGURE 1.7 Effect of ankle plantar flexion on tendon appearance. (A) Sagittal image of prone patient with ankle in maximal plantar flexion shows prescription of transverse images. This position reorients the major foot and ankle tendons so they follow a relatively straight path from the distal leg through the mid-foot. (B) Oblique (SE 500/18) image of hind foot distal to the fibular tip (corresponding to level 12 in A) shows peroneus longus (L) and brevis (B) tendons in cross section without increased signal from magic angle phenomenon. Contrast to Figure 1.6C. In this position, other structures, such as Achilles tendon, will be distorted and foreshortened.

When the extremity is placed in a nonstandard position, an issue arises regarding correct terminology for the anatomic planes of the foot and ankle.[36,37] An approach that will minimize ambiguity is to distinguish imaging planes, which are described with respect to the MR machine, from anatomic planes, which refer to the patient's body.[38] The former do not change with different patient positions and provide a convenient common language for communication between the physician prescribing the imaging routine and the technical staff who interact with the scanner and actually perform the imaging. Thus, the transverse (or "transaxial" or "axial") imaging plane will always be perpendicular to the axis of a tubular MR machine, even though images in this orientation will be in the short axis of the foot (the anatomic coronal plane) when the ankle is plantar-flexed (Figure 1.7A), and parallel to the sole of the foot (the anatomic axial plane) when the ankle is in neutral position (Figure 1.6A).

A second issue is choosing and generating images in the optimal orientation to depict pathology, especially for the mid-foot and forefoot. Frequently images in a plane along the course of a metatarsal, phalanx, forefoot joint, or tendon will yield the most useful diagnostic information. However, these structures need not lie in orthogonal planes.[39] In fact, even the structures within a single ray (the metatarsal bone with its associated phalanges) need not be colinear if a deformity such as a hammer toe or joint subluxation is present. One solution would be to orient the extremity forcibly and then immobilize it so that the part of interest lies within one of the standard imaging very few slices are needed for the preliminary images, meaning they can be obtained with a short TR. For the mid-foot, oblique coronal images that display the metatarsal bases and mid-foot bones are typically most useful (Figure 1.9), while many forefoot structures are best examined in an oblique sagittal plane that parallels the long axis of either the metatarsals (Figure 1.8) or the

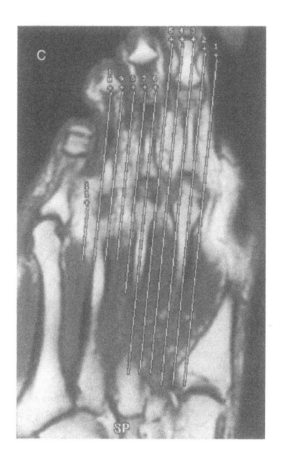

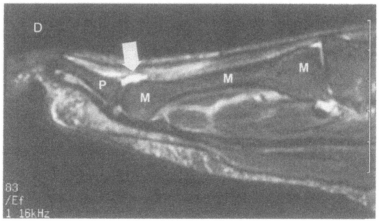

FIGURE 1.8 (continued) (C) In turn, the resultant oblique axial (SE 316/16) image is used to prescribe images along the axes of the desired metatarsals. (D) The final oblique sagittal, fat-suppressed (FSE 2703/96) image displays the entire third metatarsal (M), metatarsophalangeal joint effusion (arrow), and third proximal phalanx (P). Entire process from coronal images through final images took less than 10 min.

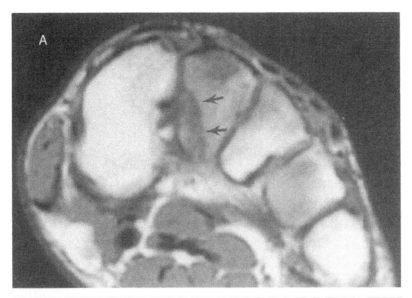

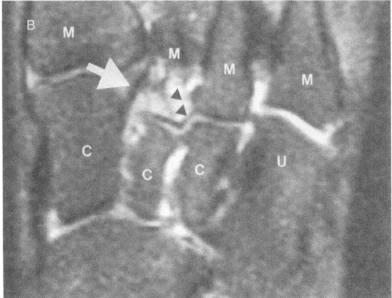

FIGURE 1.9 Imaging plane for mid-foot. (A) Patient is prone with foot in an extremity coil (Figure 1.4E). Coronal (SE 516/17) image through metatarsal bases shows fracture (arrows) through medial aspect of second metatarsal. (B) Fat-suppressed, oblique axial (FSE 2600/69) image prescribed from (A) shows relationship of Lisfranc ligament (arrow) to fracture line (arrowheads). C = cuneiforms, M = metatarsal bases, U = cuboid.

phalanges (Figure 1.10). For any pathology, however, at least two imaging planes should always be obtained: while long-axis images often give the best overview of the anatomic relationships, cross-sectional images frequently show better the extent of diseased tissue (Figure 1.11).

One final word about positioning: when possible, the examined part should be placed as close to the center of the magnet as possible. The field becomes less homogeneous near the sides of the bore, increasing artifacts and making procedures such as fat suppression more difficult. Additionally, there is a drop-off in signal and SNR moving away from isocenter (toward the head or foot of the bed for a cylindrical magnet).[41]

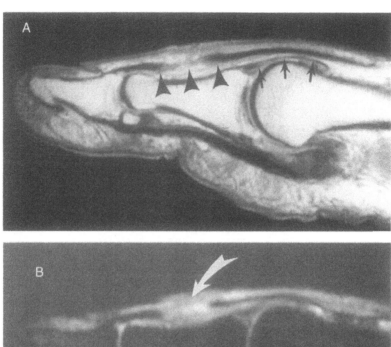

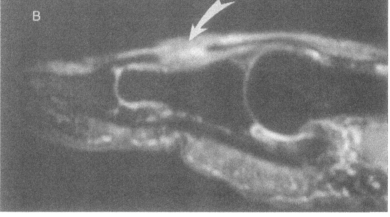

FIGURE 1.10 Imaging plane for toes. (A) Oblique sagittal (SE 685/20) image of great toe, obtained with same technique as shown in Figure 1.8, but with images centered over the proximal phalanx. Note ruptured extensor hallucis longus tendon (arrowheads) and intact extensor hallucis brevis tendon (arrows). (B) Oblique sagittal (STIR 3180/30, TI = 150) image confirms extensor hallucis longus tendon laceration (arrow). Patient had dropped a chef's knife on his foot.

PULSE SEQUENCES AND IMAGING OPTIONS

Once the physician purchases the instrumentation, selects the coil, positions the patient, and determines the imaging planes, it is time to choose the pulse sequences that will constitute the MR imaging study. Each sequence also offers some variability in the specific imaging parameters and available options. Although not every combination of parameters will be available on every machine, most manufacturers offer a large number. Different sequences are chosen to balance the desired contrast and/or spatial resolution of the images with the requirements of maintaining reasonable examination times and minimizing imaging artifacts.

Conventional spin-echo imaging is available on all MR systems. As described in the Basic Principles section above, the addition of a 180° RF pulse after the initial 90° excitation corrects for the interproton dephasing that occurs because of magnetic field heterogeneity. Spin-echo sequences with a short TR and short TE result in T1-weighted images. Because these parameters produce images with high SNR in relatively short imaging times,[15] high-spatial-resolution (small FOV, large matrix, or thin slices), T1-weighted images can be acquired easily. Fat, which appears planes. The drawback to this approach is that it is frequently uncomfortable, and patient motion soon becomes a problem.

A better approach is to allow the patient to assume the most comfortable position within the confines of the magnet and coil, and then gently immobilize the foot and ankle with foam cushions and tape. The system software is then used to obtain the desired oblique imaging planes.[40] Fortunately, all major MR manufacturers offer relatively simple ways to prescribe images in any plane, including those that are oblique to all three standard imaging planes.[39] The technique involves first obtaining images in the short axis of the foot (Figure 1.7A). From these images, an oblique plane can be described to isolate the structures in question. Then using the resultant oblique plane as a new frame of reference, a new set of images can be prescribed in virtually any orientation (Figure 1.8). The entire process can usually be accomplished in less than 10 min of imaging time,[39] since

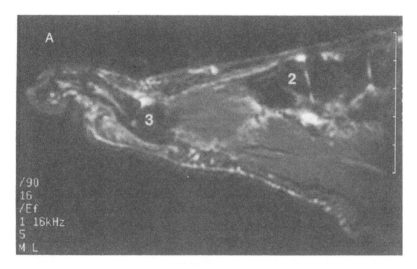

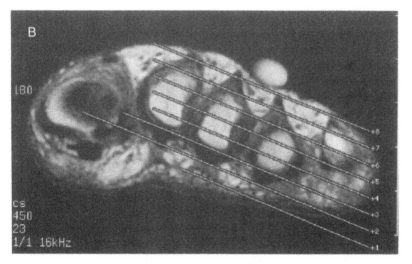

FIGURE 1.8 Imaging plane for metatarsals and metatarsophalangeal joints. (A) With the patient prone and the foot plantar-flexed (Figure 1.4F), a standard sagittal STIR (4216/76, TI = 155) image does not show a single ray, but instead shows portions of the second metatarsal base (2) and third metatarsal head (3). (B) Coronal (SE 450/23) image centered at the metatarsal heads, obtained as shown in Figure 1.7A, is used to prescribe oblique axial images that encompass the lesser metatarsals. Note use of a rectangular FOV for this coronal image (the phase-encoding direction is along the dorsoplantar axis of the foot), which reduces imaging time since fewer phase steps are acquired in the reduced dimension. *(continued)*

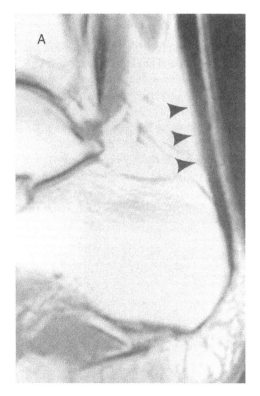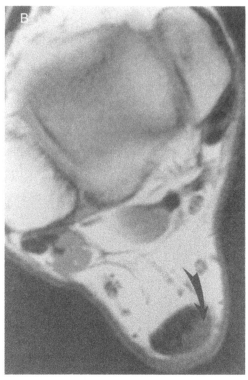

FIGURE 1.11 Importance of multiplanar imaging. (A) Sagittal (SE 733/16) image shows indistinctness of Achilles tendon (arrowheads), which does not appear focally enlarged. Area of mildly increased signal intensity might be misinterpreted as volume-averaging artifact. (B) Axial (SE 600/16) image clearly shows that tendon is hypertrophic, with replacement of approximately 40% of cross-sectional diameter by high-signal-intensity tear, scar, or granulation tissue (arrow).

bright on T1-weighted images, is a natural contrast in musculoskeletal MR imaging, separating and outlining individual muscles, tendons, ligaments, joint capsules, fascia, and neurovascular bundles. T1-weighted images also nicely depict bone marrow abnormalities like osteomyelitis and fractures (Figure 1.9). Spin-echo T1-weighted images therefore are quite valuable in musculoskeletal imaging; every foot-and-ankle protocol should probably include these images in at least one imaging plane.

One disadvantage of a T1-weighted spin-echo sequence is the limited number of slices that can be acquired, due to the short TR. Lengthening the TR does allow acquisition of more slices, but at the expense of increased imaging time and decreased T1 weighting. Fortunately, only a few slices are required to cover the entire foot or ankle in the sagittal plane. If many slices are needed in the coronal or transverse planes, it is often more efficient to prescribe two separate sequences with short TRs, with each prescription acquiring half the required number of slices, rather than prescribing one acquisition that acquires all the slices using a longer TR. For example, if a TR of 800 msec were needed to image 20 slices, then 10 slices could be obtained with a TR of 400 msec, and a second set of 10 slices could be obtained with a second acquisition, again with a TR of 400 msec. Imaging time would be the same (800 = 400 × 2 acquisitions), but the images acquired with the 400 msec TR would be more T1 weighted. Furthermore, if the slices are acquired in an interleaved order (the first acquisition collects data from slices numbered 1, 3, 5, etc., and the second, from slices numbered 2, 4, 6, etc.), there is an additional gain in SNR due to reduced cross talk between slices, as discussed below. Most standard MR software offers simple ways to automate this process.

While T1-weighted images are important for showing anatomic detail, most pathology is characterized by an increase in tissue T2 values, necessitating T2-weighted images for depiction. Conventional spin-echo images with a long TR and long TE can produce such images. However, the long TR translates into prolonged imaging times with the inherent risk of patient motion, and the disadvantage of decreased patient throughput. Furthermore, T2-weighted spin-echo images have inherently lower SNR compared with T1-weighted images, often necessitating other compromises such as decreased spatial resolution, or increased NEX (which would further prolong the acquisition time). Thus there is a need for pulse sequences that can generate T2-weighted images faster than is possible with spin-echo imaging.

One approach is the use of gradient-echo pulse sequences. These use an RF pulse with a "partial" flip angle of less than 90°. The received signal (echo) is generated through reversal of the readout (frequency) gradient, not by a 180° refocusing pulse, as is the case for spin-echo imaging.[42] The partial flip angle and lack of 180° pulses allows use of shorter TRs, and thus imaging time can be reduced.[43] Reducing the TR to the range of 20 to 60 msec also makes three-dimensional imaging (with phase encoding in two directions) feasible. Three-dimensional gradient-echo images can be acquired with thin, contiguous sections to decreased partial-volume artifacts. The resultant high-spatial-resolution images are useful for detecting very small structures and small lesions, for example, in articular cartilage (Figure 1.12). Additionally, if the voxel size is chosen to be nearly isotropic (equal in size in the slice and in-plane dimensions), the images can be reformatted into any desired plane.[5,44] One artifact unique to three-dimensional sequences is aliasing in slice selection direction (called slab wrap), whereby tissues near the ends of the imaging volume will appear superimposed.[5,45]

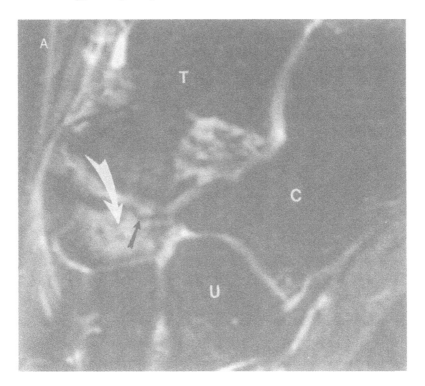

FIGURE 1.12 Comparison of pulse sequences. (A) Sagittal FSE inversion recovery (IR-FSE 4000/60, TI = 155) image shows large amount of marrow edema within tarsal navicular bone (white arrow) overlying a small chondral defect in the proximal articular surface (black arrow). Slice thickness is 4 mm. C = calcaneus, T = talus, U = cuboid.   (*continued*)

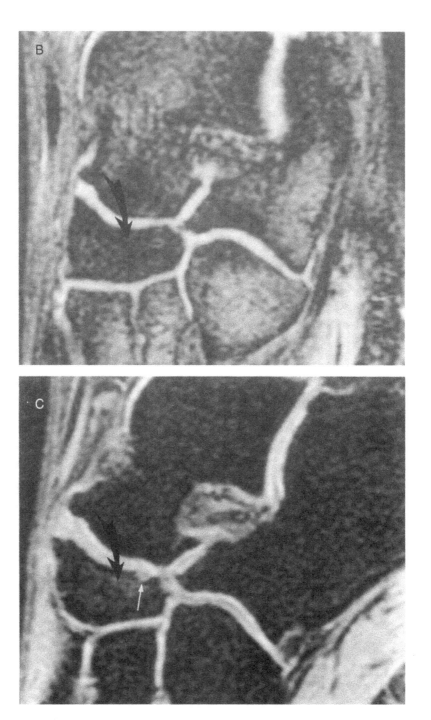

FIGURE 1.12 (continued) (B) Sagittal two-dimensional gradient-recalled (GRASS 216/11, flip angle = 10°) image is T2* weighted, but does not show marrow edema (black arrow) because of signal loss due to dephasing within trabecular bone. Cartilage defect is also not seen on this 3-mm-thick section. (C) Sagittal three-dimensional spoiled gradient-recalled (SPGR 53/7, flip angle = 35°) image allows reconstruction into thin sections (1.5 mm) and shows cartilage defect (white arrow). However, marrow edema is underestimated (black arrow), despite use of fat suppression, since the image is relatively T1 weighted. Also note brightness of surrounding muscles on both gradient-recalled images compared with STIR image, making detection of muscle abnormalities more difficult on the gradient-recalled images.

Contrast weighting in gradient-echo sequences is accomplished through manipulation of the flip angle and other imaging parameters. T1-weighted images can be obtained by using a relatively large flip angle (usually greater than 30°) and adding a spoiler gradient after each excitation to remove residual transverse magnetization, reducing the contribution from long T2 species.[46] Commercially available examples include FLASH (fast low-angle shot) and SPGR (spoiled gradient-recalled) sequences; unfortunately, each manufacturer uses different acronyms to describe similar sequences.[47,48] One musculoskeletal imaging application of fast T1-weighted gradient-echo sequences is the demonstration of dynamic enhancement following intravenous contrast administration.[49,50]

Nonspoiled gradient-echo sequences use rewinder gradients, which are applied after the echo is generated, to undo the phase changes that result from the phase-encoding gradients, thus preserving transverse magnetization.[51] An equilibrium then develops between transverse and longitudinal magnetization. Common sequences that use this technique include FISP (fast imaging with steady-state precession) and GRASS (gradient-recalled acquisition in the steady state). The images become more T2 weighted as the flip angle is decreased. Technically, the weighting is based on a property called T2*, which is shorter than T2. Transverse magnetization is lost both from inherent T2 decay in the tissues and from dephasing due to distortions of the local magnetic field. (In spin-echo imaging, the 180° pulse corrects for the signal loss due to magnetic field heterogeneity.) The end result is that there is a more rapid signal loss at given TE in gradient-echo pulse sequences compared with spin-echo sequences.[47] The gradient-recalled sequences are especially susceptible to areas of local field heterogeneity,[42,43] such as at the heel where the curved interface between the soft tissues and surrounding air creates local imperfections in the magnetic field. Additionally, gradient-echo sequences do not show marrow edema reliably (Figure 1.12) because the bony trabeculae within cancellous bone create local field disturbances, which result in signal loss.[52,53]

A more versatile approach to fast imaging is the use of turbo or fast spin-echo (FSE) sequences. In conventional spin-echo imaging only one phase-encoding step is acquired during each TR period. (If more than one 180° refocusing pulse is used, the additional signal is used to generate an image with a different TE but does not reduce the total number of excitations needed to collect all the phase-encoded echoes.) In FSE imaging, a train of several 180° RF pulses follows each 90° excitation, with the echo generated after each 180° pulse encoded with a different phase shift. Typically between 3 and 32 (the number is called the echo train length or turbo factor) 180° pulses are used. Each generated echo contributes to the same image. Thus, the number of times the excitation is repeated is reduced by the echo train length. For example, if 256 phase steps are needed, to collect all the required data with spin-echo imaging would mean repeating the TR period 256 times. If, instead, an FSE sequence with an echo train of 8 were employed, all the data could be collected with just 32 repetitions of the TR cycle (256 divided by 8), each time collecting 8 different phase-encoded echoes. With a long TR, the time savings would be substantial. Of course, the savings in imaging time can be traded back for higher SNR (by increasing the NEX), which in turn can be used to obtain higher-resolution images (by decreasing the FOV or slice thickness or by increasing the matrix).

For an FSE sequence, the software determines the effective TE of the image by acquiring the phase-encoding steps in a specific order.[5,54,55] Dual-echo FSE imaging can also be performed to produce two differently weighted images during the same acquisition.[55] However, unlike the case for conventional spin-echo imaging where adding a proton density-weighted acquisition to a T2-weighted sequence does not cost anything in terms of time or signal, doing the same with an FSE sequence is not "free." If an FSE sequence with an echo train length of 8 is designed to obtain both short effective TE (proton density-weighted) and long TE (T2-weighted) images, during each TR interval, 4 echoes will contribute to each of the two images and the time savings over a spin-echo sequence will only be a factor of 4, not 8.

There are other important differences between FSE and conventional spin-echo imaging. The signal from fat tends to be much higher on FSE images compared with spin-echo images acquired with comparable TEs. On long TE images, the brighter appearance of fat decreases the contrast between fat and most pathologic processes, which are also bright because of increased water content.[56,57] Thus, T2-weighted FSE images are often accompanied by some form of fat suppression, at a cost of fewer slices or longer imaging times, as discussed below. The second major difference between FSE and conventional spin-echo imaging occurs when a short effective TE and a long echo train length are used together. Because of the method of ordering the phase-encoding steps, FSE images acquired with these parameters appear blurred, and this lack of sharpness can decrease the conspicuity of subtle abnormalities that are best seen on proton-density-weighted images.[5,55,57,58] Additionally, although in general SNR per unit time is higher for FSE images compared with conventional spin-echo images,[59] this is not true for proton-density-weighted FSE images.[57] Thus, FSE sequences provide substantial time savings over spin-echo sequences for acquiring T2-weighted images (where a long echo train length can be used), but FSE sequences have a much smaller advantage for proton-density-weighted and T1-weighted images (where a shorter echo train length must be used to avoid image blurring).

There are two other circumstances where an FSE sequence may be preferable to a conventional spin-echo sequence. Spectral fat suppression (see below) can be applied with less of a time penalty in FSE sequences compared with conventional spin-echo sequences, because the fat suppression pulse only needs to be delivered once for each echo train. Additionally, FSE sequences that employ long echo train lengths are less prone to susceptibility and chemical shift artifacts.[56,59] This property makes FSE sequences useful for visualizing soft tissue structures adjacent to metallic orthopedic instrumentation, where a "blooming" artifact due to extreme distortion of the local magnetic field may obscure detail.[60] On the other hand, artifacts such as ghosting and ringing may be more prevalent in FSE compared with conventional spin-echo ones, because of discontinuities within the data set that is used to reconstruct the final images.[55]

Although the choice of pulse sequence and timing parameters (TR, TE, flip angle) dictate the contrast of the image, spatial resolution is determined by the choice of FOV, matrix, and slice thickness. Each of these is intricately linked to SNR. The FOV should approximate the size of the area of interest. Decreasing the FOV improves spatial resolution, but with a severe SNR penalty. Because the FOV is two dimensional, any changes in FOV affect the SNR as the square of the change. Thus, halving the FOV decreases SNR by factor of 4. Doubling the matrix size while keeping the FOV unchanged would result in the same in-plane resolution (same pixel size) as halving the FOV, while again reducing the SNR to 1/4 of its original value. The difference would be that a smaller area would be imaged by changing the FOV, while a time penalty would be incurred by changing the matrix (doubling the matrix doubles the imaging time because twice as many phase-encoding steps are needed).

A standard option to reduce imaging time is the use of a rectangular FOV. Decreasing the FOV dimension in the phase-encoding direction means that fewer phase-encoding steps will be necessary to cover the area, while maintaining pixel size (in contrast to keeping the same FOV but decreasing the number of phase-encoding steps, which would save time but increase the pixel size and decrease the spatial resolution). In the foot and ankle, a rectangular FOV is most advantageous for short-axis images of the forefoot, whose width is generally greater than its height. If the phase direction is in the dorsoplantar direction, reducing the FOV in this dimension decreases the number of phase steps and imaging time, while maintaining the in-plane resolution (Figure 1.8B). Since there are no tissues above or below the foot, there are no disadvantages to this technique. When a rectangular FOV is used in a region where there are tissues excluded from the FOV, problems can arise from aliasing (wrap) of these structures into the image. If the anatomy of interest is in the center of a rectangular FOV, the aliasing, while unaesthetic, can be ignored as it should not obscure the relevant pathology; otherwise, aliasing can be reduced by application of saturation pulses outside the FOV.[61]

Slice thickness also impacts spatial resolution and SNR. Halving the slice thickness halves the SNR. Thicker slices, while providing better SNR, also result in more partial-volume artifacts, which can decrease the detectability of small structures and lesions.[62] Using thicker slices also means that fewer slices overall will be needed to cover the area of interest. The maximum number of slices obtainable in one acquisition depends on the TR, the TE (or the longest TE in a multiecho acquisition), and, to a much lesser extent, the sampling time.[4] Typically, if more slices are needed, the TR can be increased (with a concomitant prolongation of imaging time) only up to a point. Changing the TR too drastically will change the contrast weighting of the images. After that point, more coverage would require more than one acquisition (increasing imaging time), an increase in slice thickness (decreasing spatial resolution), or an increase in interslice gap (the spacing or "skip" between slices). This last approach has advantages from the SNR standpoint.

The RF pulses do not excite perfect slice profiles; that is, some excitation of the protons in neighboring slices occurs. This phenomenon is called cross talk.[63] The problem is more severe for 180° pulses compared with 90° pulses, since the 180° pulses last twice as long. The effect on neighboring slices is a decrease in T1 values, because protons in those slices have their magnetization partly saturated by the RF pulses from adjacent slices. Thus, there is less net longitudinal magnetization in these slices when it comes time to excite them. Additionally, for short TE sequences, there is a decrease in T1 weighting as the signal from water protons increases with respect to the signal from fat protons, decreasing fat–water contrast. The opposite is true for long TE sequences where the same effect (increased water signal compared with fat) increases contrast.[41] Cross talk is reduced by increasing the interslice gap, and reaches a minimum when the gap equals 75% of the slice thickness.[41,63] Large interslice spacing increases the risk that some pertinent anatomy or pathology will be missed (i.e., it will be hidden "between" the slices), so imaging is usually performed with gaps of 10 to 30% of the slice thickness, which represents a reasonable compromise between signal loss due to cross talk and anatomic coverage. An alternative to the use of an interslice gap is to excite the slices in a nonsequential order.[63] This approach gives neighboring slices more time to recover magnetization that is lost from cross talk before they are excited. Some manufacturers automatically use nonsequential excitation as the default for all multislice pulse sequences. On other systems, selection of an interleaved option forces the software to acquire every other slice in a first acquisition, and then fill in the remaining slices in a second acquisition. This approach increases imaging time unless the number of slices needed is already large enough to warrant two acquisitions.

In addition to increasing spatial resolution, it is often desirable to increase contrast resolution, i.e., to increase the conspicuity of an abnormality. In musculoskeletal MR imaging, fat suppression is frequently used to this end. By decreasing the signal intensity of fat, high-signal-intensity objects adjacent to or within primarily fatty areas (such as the subcutaneous tissues or the bone marrow) are seen more easily.[64] Such entities include gadolinium-enhanced tissues on T1-weighted images,[65] or areas of edema on T2-weighted images.[66] Using fat suppression also improves the efficiency of analog-to-digital converter of the the scanner, because the dynamic range of the converter is less than that of the entire MR signal, when the very high signal from fat is left unaltered.[67] In turn, eliminating the high signal from fat allows the MR machine to use a higher receiver gain to bring out more contrast within the received signal from water.[13] Fat-suppressed images may also be easier to display and photograph, because of the decreased range of intensities that the monitor or film needs to show. Additionally, the fatty contents of some lesions, such as lipomas, can be confirmed by demonstrating that their internal signal is decreased when fat suppression is applied. Last, fat-suppression techniques are useful for eliminating chemical shift misregistration artifacts (see below) that may arise from fatty tissues.[13,61]

There are several approaches that can be used to achieve fat suppression in MR imaging, each with unique advantages and disadvantages. One technique, often referred to as "fat sat" is based on the frequency or spectral separation of fat and water species. The resonant frequencies of fat and water protons differ by about 3.5 parts per million or approximately 220 Hz in a 1.5-T magnetic field. Thus, if a selective RF presaturation pulse tuned to the resonant frequency of fat is applied to the imaging volume, it should only affect fat protons. A "spoiler" gradient is then applied to destroy the transverse magnetization of the excited spins (the fat protons). When this procedure is immediately followed by a pulse sequence, fat protons will not contribute to the subsequent echo.[68] The presaturation pulse must be repeated at the beginning of each TR period, and thus one cost of fat suppression is that fewer slices can be obtained for a given TR.[61] Alternatively, the TR can be increased (with a concomitant increase in imaging time) to maintain the same number of slices. The penalty is less severe for FSE compared with conventional spin-echo imaging, since only one fat suppression pulse is needed for each echo train in FSE imaging.

Because the difference in precessional frequencies between fat and water protons is slight, spectral fat suppression works best on relatively high-field systems, where the separation is more pronounced. On low-field systems, other methods of fat suppression are necessary. Even at high field strength, spectral fat suppression requires a uniform magnetic field. Thus, fat suppression is less effective with large FOVs,[61] and at the periphery or at either end of the magnet bore. Spectral fat suppression also suffers in regions where there is local field inhomogeneity, such as next to metallic implants, or at irregularly shaped soft tissue–air interfaces such as around the heel or toes. In these circumstances, the local field may vary enough so that the frequency of the fat excitation pulse differs from the local precessional frequency of fat protons.[68] At best, suppression of fatty tissues will fail; at worst, suppression of water species may occur,[13] obscuring pathology (Figure 1.13). One solution is to place partially filled bags of distilled water around the foot. This maneuver eliminates the air interface and improves the homogeneity of the local field, and so improves the quality of fat suppression.[69]

The phase-contrast method of fat suppression relies on the principle of chemical shift.[70] Two sets of spin-echo images are obtained, designed so that fat and water protons are in phase with each other in one set of images, and out of phase in the second set. Precisely chosen TEs for the two sequences, based on the resonant frequency difference between water and fat protons, determines whether they are in phase or out of phase. The two sets of images can then be combined on a workstation, effectively canceling the fat signal while preserving the water signal.[71] This technique has been used to provide fairly uniform fat suppression in the feet,[71] but the images are typically T1 weighted, which is valuable for showing areas of enhancement following gadolinium administration, but which are not useful for showing areas of edema. Additionally, two separate acquisitions are necessary (four, if precontrast and postcontrast images are obtained), which means longer examination times. Furthermore, if the patient moves between the two acquisitions, combining the

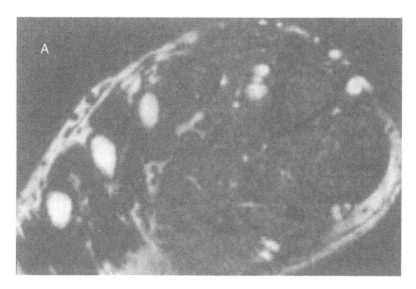

FIGURE 1.13 Heterogeneous fat suppression. (A) Coronal (FSE 3500/98) image with a frequency-selective fat-suppression pulse demonstrates fat suppression only in the medial half of the foot (contrast signal intensities within the metatarsals).   (*continued*)

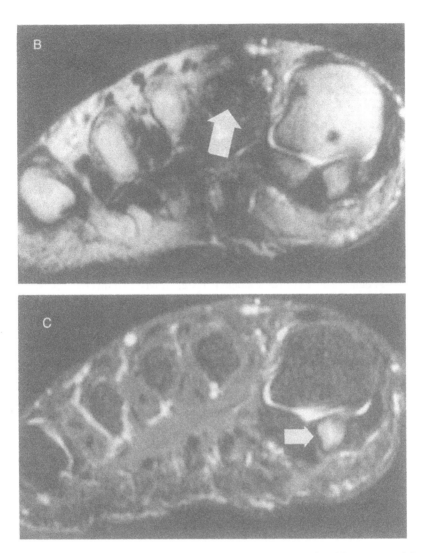

FIGURE 1.13 (continued) (B) Farther distal, only second metatarsal fat signal is suppressed (arrow). Not only will lack of suppression make some pathology more difficult to see, but also there may be suppression of water signal in other parts of the image. (C) Coronal inversion recovery (IR-FSE 5300/30, TI = 150) image in same patient demonstrates homogeneous suppression of fat signal making edema in medial sesamoid (arrow) obvious in this patient with sesamoiditis. Even in retrospect, sesamoid edema is not evident in (B).

data sets becomes problematic. And like spectral fat suppression, the phase-contrast method still relies on the presence of a relatively homogeneous magnetic field.[72] Variations of this technique have been described to overcome field inhomogeneity problems further,[73] and to eliminate the need for postprocessing.[72]

A third method of fat suppression, the short-TI-inversion recovery (STIR) sequence, is very useful for musculoskeletal MR imaging. STIR imaging is not based on the resonant frequency differences between water and fat protons. Instead, the sequence relies on the very short T1 of fat. A 180° RF pulse is delivered a set time (the inversion time, TI) before the first RF pulse of a spin-echo or gradient-echo sequence. The inversion pulse rotates the spins of all the protons so they lie in a direction directly opposite to the B_0 field (i.e., so that their net magnetization has a negative magnitude). The protons then begin to reestablish their longitudinal magnetization in the B_0 direction, with their net magnetization first becoming less negative, then zero, and finally positive. Fat protons, which have the shortest T1 values, recover the fastest. If the TI is set so that it equals the time for fat to undergo T1 decay to exactly zero, fat protons will have no longitudinal magnetization when the initial exciting RF pulse of the sequence occurs. Thus, these protons cannot contribute any signal when the remainder of the sequence is played out.[74] The TI to suppress fat is dependent on the field strength, equaling 150 to 160 msec at 1.5 T. There is also an interaction between TR and TI; when using a short TR (where the fat protons are already partly saturated and have less longitudinal magnetization to start with), the TI must be reduced.[75]

Because STIR imaging does not depend on the frequency separation of fat and water protons, it can be used at low field strength.[75] Additionally, there is no dependence on magnetic field homogeneity, so STIR imaging is useful for fat suppression over large anatomic areas or in regions where there is local field heterogeneity (Figure 1.13). However, the STIR sequence has inherently lower SNR compared with spin-echo images.[74] The low SNR usually means that thicker slices and/or a larger FOV are needed for STIR images. Additionally, the STIR sequence is relatively inefficient, providing fewer slices for a given TR compared with other sequences, because of the presence of the TI delay. This last disadvantage is lessened when an inversion pulse is added to an FSE sequence.[59] While the resultant IR-FSE sequence is more prone to blurring, especially when small matrices are used, it does provides similar lesion conspicuity compared with a conventional STIR sequence.[76] STIR (and IR-FSE) sequences differ from all other sequences in that both longer T2 and longer T1 values result in increased signal intensity,[74,77] which may be the reason the sequence is so sensitive to water and edema, which have relatively long T1 and T2 values. However, since gadolinium-based contrast agents work by shortening T1 values, STIR imaging should not be used after contrast administration, as enhancing tissues may paradoxically lose signal.[78] Last, at least theoretically, chemical species other than fat may coincidentally have the same T1 as fat and thus be suppressed on STIR images.[68]

While optimizing image contrast and spatial resolution are important, equally crucial to the generation of high-quality, diagnostic MR images is the elimination or reduction of MR imaging artifacts. Aliasing or wraparound artifact occurs when objects outside the FOV contribute a signal that is received by the coil. This signal is falsely mapped to a location inside the FOV, causing objects outside the FOV to appear "folded" into the image. Aliasing occurs in the phase-encoding direction in two-dimensional sequences and in the phase and slice directions in three-dimensional sequences. Several simple steps can reduce or eliminate this artifact. The first is the use of a coil matched to the size of the imaged part, as larger coils are more prone to aliasing.[6] Positioning adjacent parts so they will not wrap onto the area of interest will also help, as described above for sagittal imaging of the ankle. Careful selection of the frequency- and phase-encoding directions is also important. For example, the phase direction should be anterior-to-posterior, not left-to-right, for transaxial imaging of the ankle, to avoid wrap from the contralateral ankle. Sometimes, however, the phase direction cannot be altered. For coronal plane imaging of the ankle, if the phase-encoding direction is superior-to-inferior, the upper body will wrap onto the ankle. Conversely, if the phase-encoding direction is left-to-right, there is a risk of wrap from the other ankle. In this case, magnetically shielding the opposite ankle to prevent the RF pulses from exciting the protons can be easily accomplished by wrapping the contralateral ankle in aluminum foil.[79] Last, all the major MR equipment manufacturers provide a software solution to eliminate aliasing through an option called phase oversampling, whereby extra phase encoding steps are collected from outside the FOV. The signal from these additional excitations is then discarded so it does not contribute to the final image. Oversampling should only be used when there are no other alternatives, because the time needed to collect the additional phase-encoding steps prolongs the pulse sequence without generating data that will be used to reconstruct the image.

As previously emphasized, patient motion will distort MR images and can severely hamper diagnostic interpretation. The received signal from any structure that changes position during the pulse sequence will appear to the scanner as if its phase has changed. This unexpected phase difference results in incorrect mapping of the signal in the phase-encoding direction during image reconstruction. In fact, motion along any axis will produce artifacts in the phase-encoding direction.[80] The best way to avoid the problem is to ensure the patient's comfort and then gently immobilize the foot and ankle. However, even when the examined part remains still, motion can create artifacts. Similar to aliasing, ghosting can occur from moving structures outside the FOV. Additionally, flowing blood within an anatomic slice can propagate artifacts within the image. A simple way to reduce artifacts from inflow, ghosting, or even wrap is through the use of presaturation pulses.[81] Basically, a structure cannot lead to an artifact if it generates no signal.

Saturation bands are tailored RF pulses that are applied to a slab of tissue outside the FOV before the pulse sequence is initiated. The RF energy excites the region to be suppressed, a spoiler gradient is immediately applied, and then the desired pulse sequence is run. As in the case of spectral fat suppression, the volume(s) of tissue that experience the suppression pulses will contain no protons capable of generating signal. A saturation pulse placed over the nonimaged ankle would reduce aliasing in coronal images. Alternatively, a saturation pulse applied to the distal leg would reduce the signal contained in arterial blood as it enters the foot. A second method to decrease artifacts from moving structures is to reshape the gradients (other than the phase-encoding gradient) to rephase spins that have become displaced due to motion.[82] This method is called flow compensation or gradient moment nulling and can be used to counteract motion in either the frequency or slice direction. The disadvantage of this technique is that it takes a finite amount of time to apply these gradients before readout can occur. The penalty is an increase in the minimum obtainable TE, so flow compensation is typically only used with long TE sequences.

Another MR imaging artifact is chemical shift. Because fat and water protons differ slightly in their resonant frequencies, the position of pixels containing fat is misrepresented with respect to pixels containing water in the frequency-encoding axis, where frequency data are used to determine the location of the received signal.[83] This effect is most noticeable at fat–water interfaces. Chemical shift can artifactually increase or decrease the apparent thickness of cortical bone in the frequency-encoding direction, because of the juxtaposition of marrow fat and water.[84] Increased chemical shift occurs when the bandwidth is decreased because the strength of the frequency-encoding gradient must be decreased to maintain pixel size when bandwidth is decreased.[13] When bandwidth is held constant, the chemical shift effect becomes more pronounced as the field strength increases.[8] Steps to decrease this artifact include using a smaller FOV (which necessitates larger frequency-encoding gradients) or increasing the sampling bandwidth. In many circumstances, the best solution is the use of fat suppression to reduce chemical shift artifact, in which case a narrow bandwidth can be employed to improve SNR.[13,61]

The presence of ferromagnetic metal, common in orthopedic instrumentation, will severely distort the local magnetic field, creating artifact that can obscure the MR imaging appearance of nearby structures. Titanium implants are usually less problematic than steel ones.[85,86] The artifact is most severe in the slice and frequency-encoding directions, and less severe in the phase-encoding direction.[60] Thus, if a critical structure lies to one side of a metallic implant, it is probably best to orient the phase direction along the implant axis. Occasionally, reorienting the foot will decrease the artifact, which is most severe when the long axis of the metal implant is perpendicular to the main magnetic field.[86,87] Metal artifact is reduced by any change that reduces voxel size, such as a decrease in FOV or slice thickness, or an increase in matrix size.[86] Maintaining the same matrix but increasing bandwidth accomplishes the same thing by increasing the readout gradient strength.[88] The choice of pulse sequence is also important. Gradient-echo sequences, which do not utilize refocusing RF pulses, are most severely affected by metal artifact. On the other hand, the use of FSE sequences rather than conventional spin-echo sequences will diminish the artifact.[86] Especially with short interecho spacing, the closely spaced 180° pulses probably refocus the signal before there is too much signal loss from dephasing.[60]

Currently used contrast agents for musculoskeletal MR imaging are chelates of gadolinium, a paramagnetic substance.[89] These agents act by decreasing the T1 and T2 of tissue. Thus, enhancing tissues appear bright on short TR/short TE (T1-weighted) images.[90] Except at very high concentrations, the T2-shortening effect is minor and does not cause signal loss. Because fat also has high signal intensity on T1-weighted images, the enhancement of structures next to or within fat is easier to see if fat suppression is applied (Figures 1.14 and 1.15).[91] Either a frequency-selective or phase-sensitive technique of fat suppression should be used; as indicated above, gadolinium-enhanced tissues will lose signal on STIR images. Fat suppression added to a conventional spin-echo sequence may necessitate an increase in TR to maintain the required number of slices, thus prolonging the time of acquisition and decreasing the T1 weighting of the sequence. When very fast images are needed to investigate dynamic enhancement patterns,

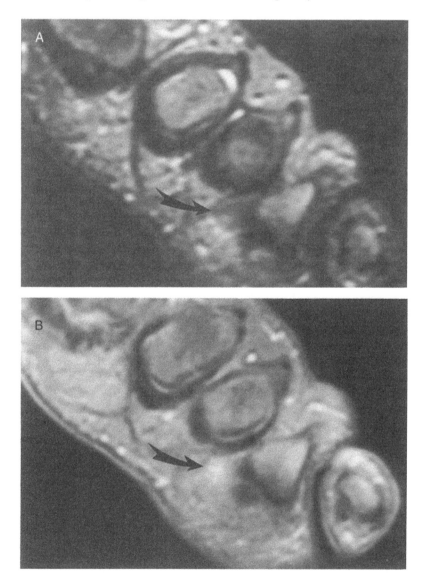

FIGURE 1.14 Value of intravenous contrast. (A) Small surgically proved Morton neuroma (arrow) is relatively subtle on coronal T2-weighted (SE 2500/80) image because its signal intensity is close to that of the surrounding tissues. (B) Fat-suppressed T1-weighted (SE 550/17) image following intravenous gadolinium administration shows enhancement within the lesion (arrow), increasing observer confidence.

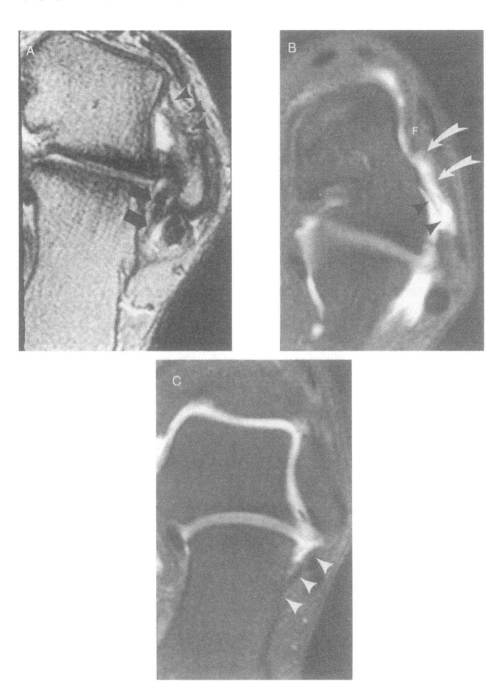

FIGURE 1.15 Value of intra-articular contrast. (A) Coronal T2-weighted (FSE 3000/104) image in prone patient who has had multiple prior ankle sprains, shows indistinct, thickened anterior talofibular (arrowheads) and calcaneofibular (arrows) ligaments. While both ligaments appear scarred, it is difficult to determine if they are intact. Both ligaments were torn at surgery. (B) In a patient with a similar history, an axial fat-suppressed, T1-weighted (SE 600/17) image made following intra-articular instillation of a dilute gadolinium solution shows contrast extravasation (arrows) through disrupted anterior talofibular ligament (arrowheads), which was confirmed and reconstructed at subsequent surgery. Suppressing usually bright fat (F) anterior to ligament makes identification of contrast extravasation easier. (C) Coronal MR arthrogram fat-suppressed (SE 600/17) image in same patient as (B) shows intact calcaneofibular ligament (arrowheads), which was also confirmed at surgery.

a T1-weighted spoiled gradient-recalled sequence can be substituted. A second approach is the use of a short-TE, FSE sequence. Even when an echo train length of two is used to reduce blurring, time savings will be substantial since only half the number of fat-suppression presaturation pulses are needed (one per echo train) compared with a spin-echo sequence.

In the foot and ankle, gadolinium-based intravenous contrast is most useful for identifying and characterizing soft tissue masses such as fibromas or Morton neuromas,[92] for investigating inflammatory processes, and for staging bone and soft tissue infections (Figure 1.14). Gadolinium chelates can also be used as intra-articular contrast agents. This route of administration is not specifically approved by the U.S. Food and Drug Administration and is considered an off-label use. However, extensive experience with large numbers of patients indicates that intra-articular use of gadolinium compounds is extremely safe.[93] The optimal intra-articular concentration is 0.5 to 2.0 mmol/l,[94,95] which for practical purposes is 0.1 ml diluted in 20 to 25 ml of normal saline. The injection is typically made with fluoroscopic guidance immediately before MR imaging. Arthrography can also be performed "indirectly": gadolinium-based compounds injected intravenously will slowly diffuse into joints, and the process is faster when the joints are exercised.[96] Compared with direct arthrography, the indirect method does not provide joint distension. Also there may be difficulty separating enhancing synovitis from para-articular contrast extravasation on indirect MR arthrograms. In the ankle, MR arthrography improves the assessment of lateral ligament injuries compared with conventional MR imaging (Figure 1.15), typically with shorter imaging times using relatively fast T1-weighted sequences.[97] In the knee, MR arthrography has also been shown to increase the conspicuity of articular cartilage defects,[98] osteochondritis dissecans,[99] and loose bodies,[100] and to aid in the assessment of postoperative joints.[101] While these applications have not been specifically researched in other joints, it is very likely that MR arthrography would perform similarly in the ankle.

REFERENCES

1. Edelman, R. R., Kleefield, J., Wentz, K. U., and Atkinson, D. J., Basic principles of magnetic resonance imaging, in *Clinical Magnetic Resonance Imaging*, Edelman, R. R. and Hesselink, J. R., Eds., Saunders, Philadelphia, 1990, chap. 1.
2. Mitchell, D. G., *MRI Principles*, Saunders, Philadelphia, 1999.
3. Crooks, L. E., Ortendahl, D. A., Kaufman, L., Hoenninger, J., Arakawa, M., Watts, J., Cannon, C. R., Brant-Zawadzki, M., Davis, P. L., and Margulis, A. R., Clinical efficiency of nuclear magnetic resonance imaging, *Radiology*, 146, 123, 1983.
4. Kneeland, J. B., Knowles, R. J., and Cahill, P. T., Multi-section multi-echo pulse magnetic resonance techniques: optimization in a clinical setting, *Radiology*, 155, 159, 1985.
5. Mezrich, R., A perspective on K-space, *Radiology*, 195, 297, 1995.
6. Bradley, W. G., Jr. and Tsuruda, J. S., MR sequence parameter optimization: an algorithmic approach, *AJR*, 149, 815, 1987.
7. Kaufman, L., Kramer, D. M., Crooks, L. E., and Ortendahl, D. A., Measuring signal-to-noise ratios in MR imaging, *Radiology*, 173, 265, 1989.
8. Rubin, D. A. and Kneeland, J. B., MR imaging of the musculoskeletal system: technical considerations for enhancing image quality and diagnostic yield, *AJR*, 163, 1155, 1994.
9. Kneeland, J. B. and Hyde, J. S., High-resolution MR imaging with local coils, *Radiology*, 171, 1, 1989.
10. Erickson, S. J., High-resolution imaging of the musculoskeletal system, *Radiology*, 205, 593, 1997.
11. Feinberg, D. A., Crooks, L. E., Hoenninger, J. C., Watts, J. C., Arakawa, M., Chang, H., and Kaufman, L., Contiguous thin multisection MR imaging by two-dimensional Fourier transform techniques, *Radiology*, 158, 811, 1986.
12. Vinitski, S., Griffey, R., Fuka, M., Matwiyoff, N., and Prost, R., Effect of the sampling rate on magnetic resonance imaging, *Magn. Reson. Med.*, 5, 278, 1987.
13. Mitchell, D. G., Vinitski, S., Rifkin, M. D., and Burk, D. L., Jr., Sampling bandwidth and fat suppression: effects of long TR/TE MR imaging of the abdomen and pelvis at 1.5 T, *AJR*, 153, 419, 1989.

14. Bradley, W. G., Jr., Kortman, K. E., and Crues, J. V., Central nervous system high-resolution magnetic resonance imaging: effect of increasing spatial resolution on resolving power, *Radiology*, 156, 93, 1985.

15. Stark, D. D., Hendrick, R. E., Hahn, P. F., and Ferucci, J. T., Jr., Motion artifact reduction with fast spin-echo imaging, *Radiology*, 164, 183, 1987.

16. Shellock, F. G., and Kanal, E., *Magnetic Resonance Bioeffects, Safety, and Patient Management*, Lippincott Raven, Philadelphia, 1996.

17. Shellock, F. G., *Pocket Guide to MR Procedures and Metallic Objects: Update 1997*, Lippincott Raven, Philadelphia, 1997.

18. Kelly, W. M., Paglen, P. G., Pearson, J. A., San Diego, A. G., and Soloman, M. A., Ferromagnetism of intraocular foreign body causes unilateral blindness after MR study, *AJNR*, 7, 243, 1986.

19. Crooks, L. E., Arakawa, M., Hoenninger, J., McCarten, B., Watts, J., and Kaufman, L., Magnetic resonance imaging: effects of magnetic field strength, *Radiology*, 151, 127, 1984.

20. Rothschild, P. A., Domesek, J. M., Kaufman, L., Kramer, D. M., Dye, S. F., Anderson, L. J., Lewis, J. L., and Gon, M. K., MR imaging of the knee with a 0.064-T permanent magnet, *Radiology*, 175, 775, 1990.

21. Johnson, G. A., Herfkens, R. J., and Brown, M. A., Tissue relaxation time: in vivo field dependence, *Radiology*, 156, 805, 1985.

22. Peterfy, C. G., Roberts, T., and Genant, H. K., Dedicated extremity MR imaging: an emerging technology, *Radiol. Clin. North Am.*, 35, 1, 1997.

23. Shellock, F. G. and Crues, J. V., Aneurysm clips: assessment of magnetic field interaction associated with a 0.2-T extremity MR system, *Radiology*, 208, 407, 1998.

24. Shellock, F. G., O'Neil, M., Ivans, V., Kelly, D., O'Connor, M., Toay, L., and Crues, J. V., Cardiac pacemakers and implantable cardioverter defibrillators are unaffected by operation of an extremity MR imaging system, *AJR*, 172, 165, 1999.

25. Kulkarin, M. V., Patton, J. A., and Price, R. P., Technical considerations for the use of surface coils in MRI, *AJR*, 147, 373, 1986.

26. Wall, B. E., Wolfman, N. T., Williams, R., and Moran, P. R., Dedicated MR receiver coils: a simple design and construction method, *Radiology*, 160, 273, 1986.

27. Carlson, J. W., Arakawa, M., Kaufman, L., McCarten, B. M., and George, C., Depth-focused radio frequency coils for MR imaging, *Radiology*, 165, 251, 1987.

28. Lufkin, R. B., Sharpless, T., Flannigan, B., and Hanafee, W., Dynamic-range compression in surface-coil MRI, *AJR*, 147, 379, 1986.

29. Axel, L., Constantini, J., and Listerud, J., Intensity correction in surface-coil MR imaging, *AJR*, 148, 418, 1987.

30. Kneeland, J. B., Jesmanowicz, A., Froncisz, W., Grist, T. M., and Hyde, J. S., High-resolution MR imaging using loop-gap resonators: work in progress, *Radiology*, 158, 247, 1986.

31. Hyde, J. S., Froncisz, J. W., Kneeland, J. B., and Grist, T. M., Parallel image acquisition from noninteracting local coils, *J. Magn. Reson.*, 70, 512, 1986.

32. Erickson, S. J., Prost, R. W., and Timins, M. E., The "magic angle" effect: background physics and clinical relevance, *Radiology*, 188, 23, 1993.

33. Zanetti, M., Ledermann, T., Zollinger, H., and Hodler, J., Efficacy of MR imaging in patients suspected of having Morton's neuroma, *AJR*, 168, 529, 1997.

34. Hricak, H. and Amparo, E. G., Body MRI: alleviation of claustrophobia by prone positioning, *Radiology*, 152, 819, 1984.

35. Erickson, S. J., Canale, P. B., Carrera, G. F., Johnson, J. E., Shereff, M. J., Gould, J. S., Hyde, J. S., and Jesmanowicz, A., Interdigital (Morton) neuroma: high-resolution MR imaging with a solenoid coil, *Radiology*, 181, 833, 1991.

36. Traughber, P., Correct terminology for foot CT (letter), *AJR*, 161, 1114, 1993.

37. Herring, C., Nomenclature for imaging planes of the feet (letter), *AJR*, 168, 277, 1997.

38. Rubin, D. A., Nomenclature for imaging planes of the feet (letter). Reply, *AJR*, 168, 278, 1997.

39. Rubin, D. A., Towers, J. D., and Britton, C. A., MR imaging of the foot: utility of complex oblique imaging planes, *AJR*, 166, 1079, 1996.

40. Edelman, R. R., Strak, D. D., Saini, S., Ferrucci, J. T., Jr., Dinsmore, R. E., Ladd, W., and Brady, T. J., Oblique planes of section in MR imaging, *Radiology*, 159, 807, 1986.

41. Schwaighofer, B. W., Yu, K. K., and Mattrey, R. F., Diagnostic significance of interslice gap and imaging volume in body MR imaging, *AJR*, 153, 629, 1989.
42. Winkler, M. L., Ortendahl, D. A., Mills, T. C., Crooks, L. E., Sheldon, P. E., Kaufman, L., and Kramer, D. M., Characteristics of partial flip angle and gradient reversal MR imaging, *Radiology*, 166, 17, 1988.
43. Mills, T. C., Ortendahl, D. A., Hylton, N. M., Crooks, L. E., Carlson, J. W., and Kaufman, L., Partial flip angle MR imaging, *Radiology*, 162, 531, 1987.
44. Klein, M. A., Reformatted three-dimensional Fourier transform gradient-recalled echo MR imaging of the ankle: spectrum of normal and abnormal findings, *AJR*, 161, 831, 1993.
45. Tsuruda, J. S., Norman, D., Dillon, W., Newton, T. H., and Mills, D. G., Three-dimensional gradient-recalled MR imaging as a screening tool for the diagnosis of cervical radiculopathy, *AJNR*, 10, 1263, 1989.
46. Yao, L., Sinha, S., and Seeger, L. L., MR imaging of joints: analytic optimization of GRE techniques at 1.5 T, *AJR*, 158, 339, 1992.
47. Elster, A. D., Gradient-echo MR imaging: techniques and acronyms, *Radiology*, 186, 1, 1993.
48. Petersein, J. and Saini, S., Fast MR imaging: technical strategies, *AJR*, 165, 1105, 1995.
49. Erlemann, R., Reiser, M. F., Peters, P. E., Vasallo, P., Nommensen, B., Kusnierz-Glaz, C. R., Ritter, J., and Roessner, A., Musculoskeletal neoplasms: static and dynamic Gd-DTPA-enhanced MR imaging, *Radiology*, 171, 767, 1989.
50. Reiser, M. F., Bongartz, G. P., Erlemann, R., Schneider, M., Pauly, T., Sittek, H., and Peters, P. E., Gadolinium-DTPA in rheumatoid arthritis and related disease: first results with dynamic magnetic resonance imaging, *Skeletal Radiol.*, 18, 591, 1989.
51. Gyngell, M. L., The application of steady-state free precession in rapid 2DFT NMR imaging: FAST and CE-FAST sequences, *Magn. Reson. Imaging*, 6, 415, 1988.
52. Sebag, G. H. and Moore, S. G., Effect of trabecular bone on the appearance of marrow in gradient-echo imaging of the appendicular skeleton, *Radiology*, 174, 855, 1990.
53. Rosenthal, H., Thulborn, K. R., Rosenthal, D. I., Kim, S. H., and Rosen, B. R., Magnetic susceptibility effects of trabecular bone on magnetic resonance imaging of bone marrow, *Invest. Radiol.*, 25, 173, 1990.
54. Melki, P. S., Mulkern, R. V., Panych, L. P., and Jolesz, F. A., Comparing the FAISE method with conventional dual-echo sequences, *J. Magn. Reson. Imaging*, 1, 319, 1991.
55. Listerud, J., Einstein, S., Outwater, E., and Kressel, H. Y., First principles of fast spin echo, *Magn. Reson. Q.*, 8, 199, 1992.
56. Jones, K. M., Mulkern, R. V., Schwartz, R. B., Oshio, K., Barnes, P. D., and Jolesz, F. A., Fast spin-echo MR imaging of the brain and spine: current concepts, *AJR*, 158, 1313, 1992.
57. Jaramillo, D., Laor, T., and Mulkern, R. V., Comparison between fast spin-echo and conventional spin-echo imaging of normal and abnormal musculoskeletal structures in children and young adults, *Invest. Radiol.*, 29, 803, 1994.
58. Rubin, D. A., Kneeland, J. B., Listerud, J., Underberg-Davis, S. J., and Dalinka, M. K., MR diagnosis of meniscal tears of the knee: value of fast spin-echo vs. conventional spin-echo pulse sequences, *AJR*, 162, 1131, 1994.
59. Constable, R. T., Smith, R. C., and Gore, J. C., Signal-to-noise and contrast in fast spin echo (FSE) and inversion recovery FSE imaging, *J. Comput. Assist. Tomogr.*, 16, 41, 1992.
60. Eustace, S., Jara, H., Goldberg, R., Fenlon, H., Mason, M., Melhem, E. R., and Yucel, E. K., A comparison of conventional spin-echo and turbo spin-echo imaging of soft tissues adjacent to orthopedic hardware, *AJR*, 170, 455, 1998.
61. Mirowitz, S. A., Fast scanning and fat-suppression MR imaging of musculoskeletal disorders, *AJR*, 161, 1147, 1993.
62. Beltran, J., Munchow, A. M., Khabiri, H., Magee, D. G., McGhee, R. B., and Grossman, S. B., Ligaments of the lateral aspect of the ankle and sinus tarsi: an MR imaging study, *Radiology*, 177, 455, 1990.
63. Kneeland, J. B., Shimakawa, A., and Wehrli, F. W., Effect of intersection spacing on MR image contrast and study time, *Radiology*, 158, 819, 1986.
64. Harned, E. M., Mitchell, D. G., Burk, D. L., Jr., Vinitski, S., and Rifkin, M. D., Bone marrow findings on magnetic resonance images of the knee: accentuation by fat suppression, *Magn. Reson. Imaging*, 8, 27, 1990.

65. Simon, J. H. and Szumowski, J., Chemical shift imaging with paramagnetic contrast material enhancement for improved lesion depiction, *Radiology*, 171, 539, 1989.

66. Simon, J. H. and Szumowski, J., Proton (fat/water) chemical shift imaging in medical magnetic resonance imaging: current status, *Invest. Radiol.*, 27, 865, 1992.

67. Wedeen, V. J., Chao, Y. S., and Ackerman, J. L., Dynamic range compression in MRI by means of a nonlinear gradient pulse, *Magn. Reson. Med.*, 6, 287, 1988.

68. Keller, P.J., Hunter, W. W., Jr., and Schmalbrock, P., Multisection fat-water imaging with chemical shift selective presaturation, *Radiology*, 164, 539, 1987.

69. Smith, D. K. and Wright, J., Water bags: an inexpensive method for improving fat suppression in MR imaging of the extremities (letter), *AJR*, 162, 1252, 1994.

70. Dixon, W. T., Simple proton spectroscopic imaging, *Radiology*, 153, 189, 1984.

71. Maas, M., Dijkstra, P. F., and Akkerman, E. M., Uniform fat suppression in hands and feet through the use of two-point Dixon chemical shift MR imaging, *Radiology*, 210, 189, 1999.

72. Szumowski, J. and Plewes, D. B., Separation of lipid and water MR imaging signals by Chopper averaging in the time domain, *Radiology*, 165, 247, 1987.

73. Szumowski, J., Coshow, W. R., Li, F., and Quinn, S. F., Phase unwrapping in the three-point Dixon method for fat suppression MR imaging, *Radiology*, 192, 255, 1994.

74. Bydder, G. M. and Young, I. R., MR imaging: clinical use of the inversion recovery sequence, *J. Comput. Assist. Tomogr.*, 9, 659, 1985.

75. Fleckenstein, J. L., Archer, B. T., Barker, B. A., Vaughan, J. T., Parkey, R. W., and Peshock, R. M., Fast short-tau inversion-recovery MR imaging, *Radiology*, 179, 499, 1991.

76. Weinberger, E., Shaw, D. W. W., White, K. S., Winters, W. D., Stark, J. E., Nazar-Stewart, V., and Hinks, R. S., Nontraumatic pediatric musculoskeletal MR imaging: comparison of conventional and fast-spin-echo short inversion time inversion-recovery technique, *Radiology*, 194, 721, 1995.

77. Greco, A., McNamara, M. T., Escher, M. B., Trifilio, G., and Parienti, J., Spin-echo and STIR imaging of sports-related muscle injuries at 1.5 T, *J. Comput. Assist. Tomogr.*, 15, 994, 1991.

78. Krinsky, G., Rofsky, N. M., and Weinreb, J. C., Nonspecificity of short inversion time inversion recovery (STIR) as a technique of fat suppression: pitfalls in image interpretation, *AJR*, 166, 523, 1996.

79. Van Hecke, P. E., Marchal, A. L., and Baert, A. L., Use of shielding to prevent folding in MR imaging, *Radiology*, 167, 557, 1988.

80. Wood, M. L. and Henkelman, R. M., MR image artifacts from periodic motion, *Med. Phys.*, 12, 143, 1985.

81. Edelman, R. R., Atkinson, D. J., Silver, M. S., Loaiza, F. L., and Warren, W. S., FRODO pulse sequences: a new means of eliminating motion, flow, and wraparound artifacts, *Radiology*, 166, 231, 1988.

82. Haacke, E. M. and Lenz, G. W., Improving MR image quality in the presence of motion by using rephasing gradients, *AJR*, 148, 1251, 1987.

83. Soila, K., Viamonte, M., Jr., and Starewicz, P., Chemical shift misregistration effect in magnetic resonance imaging, *Radiology*, 153, 819, 1984.

84. Dick, B. W., Mitchell, D. G., Burk, D. L., Levy, D. W., Vinitski, S., and Rifkin, M., The effect of chemical shift misregistration on cortical bone thickness on MR imaging, *AJR*, 151, 537, 1988.

85. Ebraheim, N. A., Savolaine, E. R., Zeiss, J., and Jackson, W. T., Titanium hip implants for improved magnetic resonance and computed tomography examinations, *Clin. Orthop.*, 275, 194, 1992.

86. Suh, J., Jeong, E., Shin, K., Cho, J. H., Na, J., Kim, D., and Han, C., Minimizing artifacts caused by metallic implants at MR imaging: experimental and clinical studies, *AJR*, 171, 1207, 1998.

87. Mueller, P. R., Stark, D. D., Simeone, J. F., Saini, S., Butch, R. J., Edelman, R. R., Wittenberg, J., and Ferrucci, J. T., Jr., MR guided aspiration biopsy: needle design and clinical trials, *Radiology*, 161, 605, 1986.

88. Petersilge, C. A., Lewin, J. S., Durek, J. L., Yoo, J. U., and Ghaneyem, A. J., Optimizing imaging parameters for MR evaluation of the spine with titanium pedicle screws, *AJR*, 166, 1213, 1996.

89. Helgason, J. W., Chandnani, V. P., and Yu, J. S., MR arthrography: a review of current technique and applications, *AJR*, 168, 1473, 1997.

90. Wolf, G. L., Joseph, P. M., and Goldstein, E. J., Optimal pulsing sequences for MR contrast agents, *AJR*, 147, 367, 1986.

91. Palmer, W. E., Brown, J. H., and Rosenthal, D. I., Rotator cuff: evaluation with fat-suppressed MR arthrography, *Radiology*, 188, 683, 1993.
92. Terk, M. R., Kwong, P. K., Suthar, M., Horvath, B. C., and Colletti, P. M., Morton neuroma: evaluation with MR imaging performed with contrast enhancement and fat suppression, *Radiology*, 189, 239, 1993.
93. Hugo, P. C., III, Newburg, A. H., Newman, J. S., and Wetzner, S. M., Complications of arthrography, *Semin. Musculoskeletal Rad.*, 2, 345, 1998.
94. Hajek, P. C., Baker, L. L., Sartoris, D. J., Neumann, C. H., and Resnick, D., MR arthrography: anatomic-pathologic investigation, *Radiology*, 163, 141, 1987.
95. Engel, A., Magnetic resonance knee arthrography: enhanced contrast by gadolinium complex in the rabbit and in humans, *Acta Orthop. Scand. (Suppl.)*, 240, 1, 1990.
96. Vahlensieck, M., Peterfy, C. G., Wischer, T., Sommer, T., Lang, P., Schlippert, U., Genant, H. K., and Schild, H. H., Indirect MR arthrography: optimization and clinical applications, *Radiology*, 200, 249, 1996.
97. Chandnani, V. P., Harper, M. T., Ficke, J. R., Gagliardi, J. A., Rolling, L., Christensen, K. P., and Hansen, M. F., Chronic ankle instability: evaluation with MR arthrography, MR imaging, and stress radiography, *Radiology*, 192, 189, 1994.
98. Kramer, J., Recht, M. P., Imhof, H., Stiglbaüer, R., and Engel, A., Postcontrast MR arthrography in assessment of cartilage lesions, *J. Comput. Assist. Tomogr.*, 18, 218, 1994.
99. Kramer, J., Stiglbaüer, R., Engel, A., Prayer, L., and Imhof, H., MR contrast arthrography (MRA) in osteochondrosis dissecans, *J. Comput. Assist. Tomogr.*, 16, 254, 1992.
100. Brossmann, J., Priedler, K. W., Daenen, B., Pedowitz, R. A., Andresen, R., Clopton, P., Trudell, D., Pathria, M., and Resnick, D., Imaging of osseous and cartilaginous intraarticular loose bodies in the knee: comparison of MR imaging and MR arthrography with CT and CT arthrography in cadavers, *Radiology*, 200, 509, 1996.
101. Applegate, G. R., Flannigan, B. D., Tolin, B. S., Fox, J. M., and Del Pizzo, W., MR diagnosis of recurrent tears in the knee: value of intraarticular contrast material, *AJR*, 161, 821, 1993.

2 Normal Anatomy of the Ankle and Foot

Monique Starok and Joel Rubenstein

CONTENTS

INTRODUCTION

Magnetic resonance (MR) imaging of the ankle and foot, when performed with high-field-strength magnets and dedicated extremity coils, provides the radiologist and the orthopedic surgeon with excellent demonstration of normal anatomic structures, as well as pathology. Interpretation of MR images demonstrating such detailed structure requires an in-depth knowledge of the anatomy. The anatomic structures have been well delineated by anatomic dissection and, more recently, have been correlated with MR images.[1-4]

This chapter is a summary of the important osseous, ligamentous, muscular, and neurovascular structures of the ankle and foot, with illustrations of their appearance on select axial, coronal, and sagittal images (Figures 2.1 through 2.17).

OSSEOUS STRUCTURES

MR is an excellent tool for evaluating osseous abnormalities that is complementary, and often superior, to plain radiographs and computed tomography (CT).

The ankle (or talocrural) joint is a "mortise" formed by the distal end of the tibia and its malleolus plus the lateral malleolus of the fibula, which articulates with its "tenon" formed by the articular surfaces of the talus.

The distal tibia extends along its medial side as the medial malleolus. The articular surface of the tibial plafond consists of two shallow depressions separated by a slight central elevation. A rough surface is present at the anterior articular margin of the tibia for attachment of the ankle joint capsule; similarly, the posterior surface is rough for capsular attachment, but also has shallow grooves for passage of the flexor hallucis longus, flexor digitorum longus, and tibialis posterior tendons. The lateral tibial surface contains a triangular rough depression for attachment of the interosseous ligament, below which it is smooth and articulates with the fibula.

The fibula expands at its distal extent to form the lateral malleolus, which articulates with a corresponding facet on the lateral aspect of the talus. The posterior border contains a shallow malleolar sulcus for the two peroneal tendons. Rough depressions are located anterior and posterior to the articular surface, which serve as the respective attachment sites for the anterior and posterior talofibular ligaments.

The talus is the second largest of the tarsal bones and is a structural member of both the ankle and foot. The talus has no muscular or tendinous attachments and approximately 60% of its surface area is covered by articular cartilage, resulting in a limited surface area for vascular perforation.[5] The trochlea (i.e., the superior convex surface of the talar body) articulates with the corresponding concave articular surface of the distal tibia. The trochlear articular surface is continuous with medial and lateral talar facets that articulate with the medial and lateral malleoli, respectively. The talar body extends anteriorly into a constricted neck and a convex head, which articulate with the anterior and middle subtalar facets of the calcaneus, as well as the navicular. Two processes extend from the body of the talus: (1) the posterior process, which is divided into medial and lateral tubercles and separated by the groove for flexor hallucis longus tendon and (2) the lateral process, which is the site of attachment of the lateral talocalcaneal ligament, forms the lateral third of the posterior subtalar articulation inferiorly, and articulates with the fibula superolaterally.

The foot is divided into three segments: (1) the hind foot, comprising the talus and calcaneus; (2) the mid-foot, comprising the remaining tarsal bones; and (3) the forefoot, comprising the metatarsals and phalanges.

The calcaneus is the largest of the tarsal bones and is divided into an anterior articular half and a posterior tuberosity. The Achilles tendon inserts into the posterior cortex of the tuberosity. The plantar surface of the tuberosity serves as a site of attachment for the plantar fascia and intrinsic muscles of the foot.[6] The anterior calcaneus contains three articular facets on its superior surface, posterior, middle, and anterior, corresponding to those of the talus. The middle articular facet is situated on the sustentaculum tali, a broad osseous process on the medial aspect of the calcaneus. The undersurface of the sustentaculum contains a groove for the flexor hallucis longus tendon. The anterior and middle subtalar facets are often confluent. The talocalcaneal joint is divided into two separate articulations, the posterior subtalar and the talocalcaneonavicular joints, which are separated by the tarsal canal and tarsal sinus.

The Lisfranc joint represents the articulation between the mid-foot and forefoot, and is collectively composed of all five tarsometatarsal joints. The medial and lateral margins of each of the wedge-shaped cuneiform bones (medial, intermediate, and lateral) articulate with the corresponding wedge-shaped proximal articular surface of the medial three metatarsals, whereas the cuboid has two facets for articulation with the fourth and fifth metatarsals, respectively. The wedge shape of these bones further serves to create a transverse arch across the Lisfranc joint.

LIGAMENTOUS STRUCTURES

The ligaments, composed of dense collagen, normally appear hypointense on all MR sequences (Figures 2.1 through 2.3). The demonstration of all the ankle ligaments is difficult on conventional MR imaging planes because of their size and orientation.

The tibia and fibula are bound together by numerous short, oblique fibrous bands known collectively as the interosseous membrane constituting the primary stabilizer between the tibia and fibula.[1] At the level of the ankle joint, the anterior and posterior tibiofibular ligaments and the transverse ligament provide additional stabilization.

Lateral supporting ligaments of the ankle include the anterior and posterior talofibular and calcaneofibular ligaments. The anterior talofibular ligament passes from the anterior fibula to the anterolateral surface of the talus. The posterior talofibular ligament extends from the posterior fibula to the lateral tubercle of the talus; the posterior intermalleolar ligament is a variant in 56% of individuals that extends from the posterior fibula to the posterior margin of the medial malleolus. The

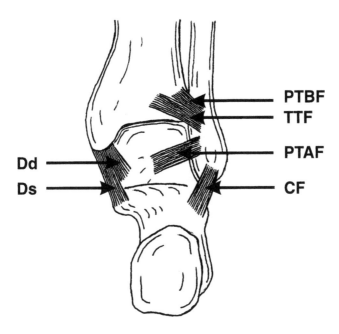

FIGURE 2.1 Diagram of the ligaments of the ankle as seen posteriorly.

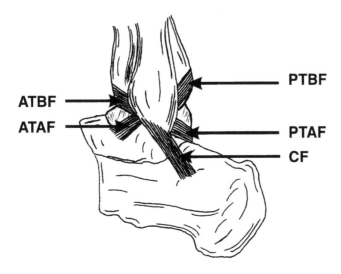

FIGURE 2.2 Diagram of the lateral ligaments of the ankle.

calcaneofibular ligament extends from the lateral malleolus deep to the peroneal tendons and attaches to the lateral calcaneus.

Medially, the deltoid ligament is composed of superficial and deep fibers. The superficial fibers extend from the medial malleolus to the navicular tuberosity, spring ligament, sustentaculum tali, and talus. The deep fibers pass from the medial malleolar tip to the adjacent medial talus.

Ligaments in the tarsal canal include the interosseous talocalcaneal ligament, the cervical ligament, as well as the medial, intermediate, and lateral roots of the inferior extensor retinaculum.[7] Additional talocalcaneal supporting ligaments include the anterior talocalcaneal ligament, which

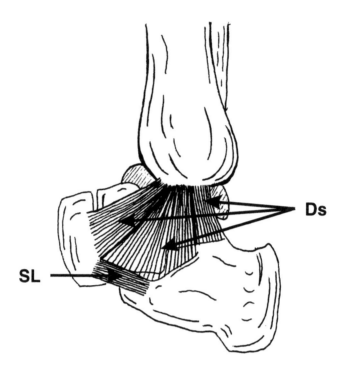

FIGURE 2.3 Diagram of the medial ligaments of the ankle.

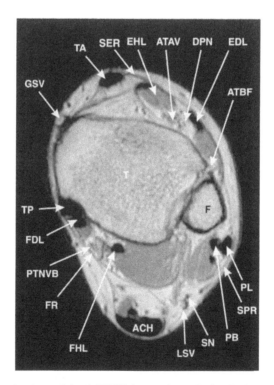

FIGURE 2.4 Axial proton-density-weighted (PDW) image above the level of the ankle joint. (Abbreviations are on pages 50 and 51.)

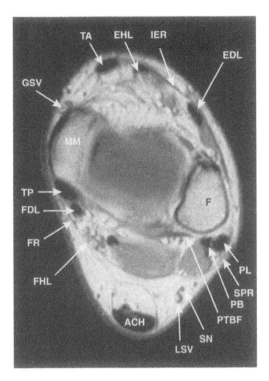

FIGURE 2.5 Axial PDW image at the level of the ankle joint. (Abreviations are on pages 50 and 51.)

extends from the lateral talar neck to the superior calcaneus, and the posterior talocalcaneal ligament, which extends from the lateral tubercle of the talus to the medial calcaneus. Laterally, the lateral talocalcaneal ligament passes from the lateral process of the talus beneath the fibular facet to the lateral surface of the calcaneus deep to, but parallel with, the calcaneofibular ligament. Medially, the medial talocalcaneal ligament connects the medial tubercle of the talus with the sustentaculum tali calcaneonavicular ligament.

Although the calcaneus and navicular do not articulate directly, the plantar calcaneonavicular or "spring" ligament passes from the sustentaculum tali to the plantar surface of the navicular. This ligament serves to support the head of the talus. Additional support of the talocalcaneonavicular joint includes the dorsal talonavicular ligament and the calcaneonavicular limb of the bifurcate ligament.

The calcaneus articulates with the cuboid bone laterally. Supporting ligaments include the long plantar ligament. This ligament passes from the plantar surface of the calcaneus just anterior to the tuberosity to the cuboid and the third, fourth, and fifth metatarsal bases. The deeper, short plantar ligament passes from the plantar aspect of the calcaneus to the cuboid. Dorsally, the calcaneocuboid ligament and the cuboid limb of the bifurcate ligament support the calcaneocuboid joint.

Multiple plantar, dorsal, and interosseous ligaments support the mid-foot. The five metatarsals articulate with the cuneiforms and cuboid bones and each has three phalanges except for the first, which only has two. Dorsal, plantar, and interosseous ligaments strengthen and limit the motion of the tarsometatarsal and intermetatarsal joints. Distally, the transverse metatarsal ligament connects the heads of all five metatarsals. Deep in the transverse ligament are dense fibrous bands crossing each metatarsophalangeal joint known as the plantar ligaments. Collateral ligaments are present medially and laterally at the metatarsophalangeal joints and interphalangeal joints. Tendons and tendon sheaths provide additional stability to the interphalangeal joints.

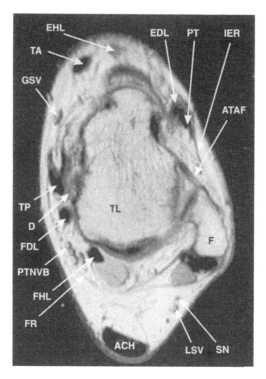

FIGURE 2.6 Axial PDW image at the level of the upper body of the talus. (Abbreviations are on pages 50 and 51.)

RETINACULA

Five fibrous bands or retinacula are present about the ankle to bind the tendons close to the underlying osseous structures. The superior extensor retinaculum extends between the distal tibia and fibula above the level of the ankle joint. The inferior extensor retinaculum is a Y-shaped band extending with its stem from the lateral calcaneus to the medial malleolus and plantar aponeurosis. The extensor retinacula secure the tendons of tibialis anterior, extensor hallucis longus, extensor digitorum longus, and peroneus tertius at and below the ankle joint.

The flexor retinaculum extends from the medial malleolus to the medial calcaneus. Fibrous septae divide the tarsal tunnel into separate canals for each of the flexor tendons and neurovascular bundle. From medial to lateral, the compartments formed transmit the tibialis posterior tendon, flexor digitorum longus tendon, posterior tibial vessels and tibial nerve, and the flexor hallucis longus tendon.

The superior peroneal retinaculum attaches to the lateral malleolus and lateral surface of the calcaneus. The inferior peroneal retinaculum is continuous with the fibers of the inferior extensor retinaculum and is attached to the lateral calcaneus. Together, the peroneal retinacula secure the peroneal tendons. Slips from the inferior retinaculum form a septum between the peroneus longus and brevis tendons.

TENDONS AND MUSCLES

There are three distinct groups or compartments of lower leg musculature: posterior, lateral, and anterior.[8]

The posterior muscles are divided into superficial and deep groups. The origins and insertions of these muscles are summarized in Table 2.1. The superficial group consists of gastrocnemius, soleus, and plantaris. The gastrocnemius and soleus unite to form the Achilles tendon that inserts into the tuberosity of the calcaneus. The Achilles tendon is not surrounded by a tendon sheath as are other ankle tendons, but does have a peritenon covering.[4] The fibers of the Achilles tendon are

TABLE 2.1
Muscles of the Superficial and Deep Posterior Compartments

Muscle	Origin	Insertion
Gastrocnemius	Medial and lateral femoral condyles	Posterior tuberosity calcaneus (Achilles tendon)
Soleus	Posterior and medial tibia and posterior fibula	Posterior tuberosity calcaneus (Achilles tendon)
Plantaris	Lateral femoral condyle	Posterior tuberosity calcaneus ± Achilles
Flexor hallucis longus	Lower 2/3 posterior fibula and interosseous membrane	Base of first distal phalanx
Flexor digitorum longus	Posterior tibia	Base of distal phalanges of digits 2 to 5
Tibialis posterior	Interosseous membrane, posterior tibia, and proximal 2/3 medial fibula	Navicular tuberosity, cuneiforms, calcaneus, 2nd to 4th metatarsals

homogeneous and low signal on all MR pulse sequences. On axial images the tendon has a flat or concave anterior surface. Anterior to the tendon is a fat-containing space known as Kager's fat pad. Between the distal Achilles tendon and the posterior calcaneal tuberosity lies the retrocalcaneal bursa. The plantaris is a small muscle between the gastrocnemius and soleus; this muscle is rudimentary and may be absent in 10% of the population.[4] Its long tendon runs along the medial border of the Achilles and inserts into the calcaneus, the Achilles tendon itself, or the flexor retinaculum.

The deep group of posterior muscles consists of the flexor hallucis longus, flexor digitorum longus, and tibialis posterior. All three muscles arise from the posterior tibia, fibula, and/or interosseous membrane. The tendons begin above the level of the ankle and all three pass beneath the flexor retinaculum. The larger posterior tibial tendon is most medial and inserts onto the navicular tuberosity as well as multiple smaller slips to the sustentaculum tali, cuneiforms, and the second through fourth metatarsal bases. The flexor digitorum tendon passes behind the medial malleolus posterior and lateral to the tibialis posterior tendon. It passes into the sole of the foot, crosses superficial to the flexor hallucis tendon, then divides into four tendons to insert into the bases of the second through fifth distal phalanges. The flexor hallucis, the most posterior tendon, passes through grooves in the posterior tibia, talus, and sustentaculum tali to the plantar aspect of the foot between the two heads of the flexor hallucis brevis to its insertion on the base of the first distal phalanx.

The anterior compartment contains the tibialis anterior, extensor hallucis longus, extensor digitorum longus, and peroneus tertius muscles. The origins and insertions of these muscles are summarized in Table 2.2. All the anterior compartment muscles arise from the anterior tibia, fibula, and/or interosseous membrane. The tibialis anterior tendon begins above the ankle and passes

TABLE 2.2
Muscles of the Anterior and Lateral Compartments

Muscle	Origin	Insertion
Tibialis anterior	Upper 1/2 lateral tibia and interosseous membrane	Medial cuneiform and base of first metatarsal
Extensor hallucis longus	Medial fibula and interosseous membrane	Base of first distal phalanx
Extensor digitorum longus	Lateral tibial condyle, upper 3/4 fibula and interosseous membrane	Middle and distal phalanges of digits 2 to 5
Peroneus tertius	Distal 1/3 of fibula and interosseous membrane	Base of the fifth metatarsal
Peroneus longus	Upper 2/3 fibula	Base of first metatarsal and medial cuneiform
Peroneus brevis	Distal 2/3 fibula	Tuberosity base of fifth metatarsal

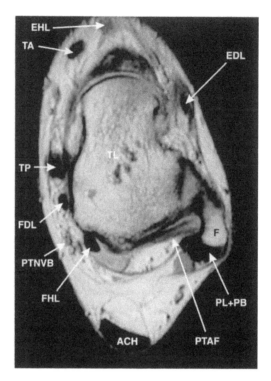

FIGURE 2.7 Axial PDW image at the level of the mid-body of the talus. (Abbreviations are on pages 50 and 51.)

beneath the extensor retinacula in the most medial position to insert onto the medial and plantar surfaces of the medial cuneiform and the base of the first metatarsal. The extensor hallucis tendon is situated between tibialis anterior and extensor digitorum longus as the tendon passes beneath the retinacula to its insertion on the base of the distal phalanx of the first toe. The extensor digitorum tendon passes beneath the retinacula with the peroneus tertius tendon before dividing into four slips that insert into the middle and distal phalanges of the second through fifth digits. Tendinous slips from the extensor digitorum brevis join the extensor digitorum longus tendons of the second to fourth digits, in addition to contributions from the lumbricals and interossei to form the dorsal extensor hood. The peroneus tertius tendon passes with the accompanying extensor digitorum longus tendon to its insertion into the base of the fifth metatarsal.

The lateral compartment muscles include the peroneus longus and brevis, and their origins and insertions are summarized in Table 2.2. Peroneus longus is the more superficial of the two muscles and ends in a long tendon, which passes behind the lateral malleolus with the peroneus brevis in a common sheath. The tendon then passes more posterior to the brevis tendon and crosses into the sole of the foot to its insertion into the lateral aspect of the base of the first metatarsal and medial cuneiform. The peroneus brevis has a shorter tendon and inserts into the lateral aspect of the fifth metatarsal base.

The muscles of the foot are grouped into four layers. The first layer includes the abductor hallucis, flexor digitorum brevis, and abductor digiti minimi. The abductor hallucis arises from the medial process of the tuberosity of the calcaneus, flexor retinaculum, and plantar aponeurosis and inserts into the medial aspect of the base of the proximal first phalanx. The flexor digitorum brevis arises as a narrow tendon from the medial process of the calcaneal tuberosity and plantar aponeurosis, and it divides into four tendons distally. Each tendon divides into two slips at the bases of the proximal phalanges and allows the flexor digitorum longus to pass through. The slips reunite and then divide again to insert on either side of the base of the middle phalanx of digits two through five. The abductor digiti minimi originates from the lateral process of the calcaneal tuberosity and plantar aponeurosis and inserts into the lateral aspect of the base of the fifth proximal phalanx.

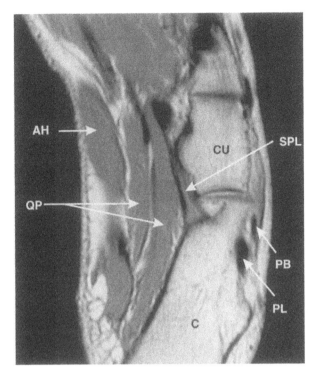

FIGURE 2.8 Axial PDW image at the level of the calcaneocuboid joint. (Abbreviations are on pages 50 and 51.)

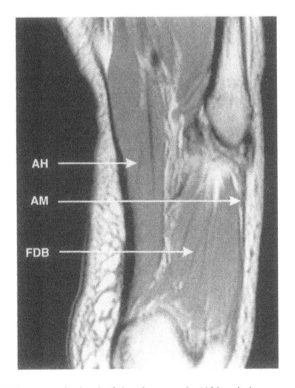

FIGURE 2.9 Axial PDW image at the level of the plantar arch. (Abbreviations are on pages 50 and 51.)

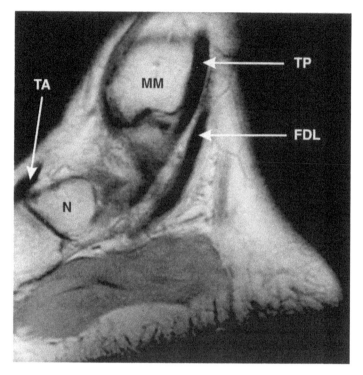

FIGURE 2.10 Sagittal PDW image of the medial aspect of the ankle. (Abbreviations are on pages 50 and 51.)

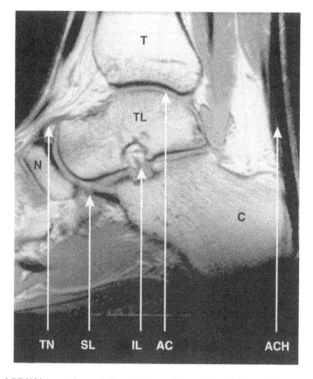

FIGURE 2.11 Sagittal PDW image through the midline of the ankle. (Abbreviations are on pages 50 and 51.)

The second layer consists of the quadratus plantae and the lumbrical muscles. The quadratus plantae arises by two heads from the medial plantar surface and lateral border of the calcaneus and separated by the long plantar ligament. Distally, its tendons blend with the tendons of the flexor digitorum longus. The four lumbricals arise from the tendons of the flexor digitorum longus and insert into the medial aspect of the metatarso-phalangeal joints of digits two to five.

The third layer consists of the flexor hallucis brevis, adductor hallucis, and flexor digiti minimi brevis muscles. Flexor hallucis brevis arises from the medial aspect of the plantar surface of the cuboid and adjacent cuneiform bone. Distally, its tendon divides allowing the flexor digitorum longus to pass between the two tendons and inserts into the medial and lateral aspect of the base of the proximal phalanx of the first digit. The adductor hallucis consists of an oblique head arising from the bases of the second through fourth metatarsals and a transverse head arising from the plantar metatarsophalangeal and transverse metatarsal ligaments of the third to fifth digits. The two heads insert with the lateral head of the flexor hallucis brevis on the lateral aspect of the base of the first proximal phalanx. The flexor digiti minimi brevis arises from the base of the fifth metatarsal bone and inserts into the lateral aspect of the base of the proximal fifth phalanx.

The fourth layer consists of the three plantar and four dorsal interossei muscles. The plantar interossei arise from the bases and medial sides of the third, fourth, and fifth metatarsals and insert into the medial aspects of the bases of the proximal phalanges of the same toes. The dorsal interossei arise via two heads from adjacent metatarsals. The tendons insert into the bases of the proximal phalanges. The first inserts into the medial side of the second digit, whereas the other three are inserted into the lateral aspect of the second, third, and fourth digits.

VESSELS AND NERVES

At the level of the ankle, the posterior tibial nerve lies between the flexor hallucis longus and the flexor digitorum longus tendons. Distal to the flexor retinaculum it divides into the medial and

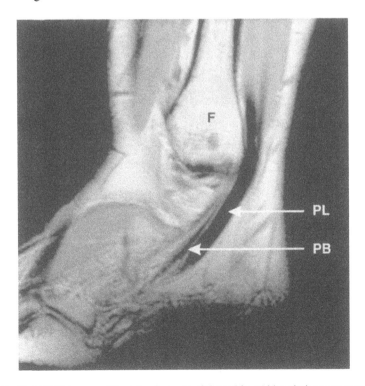

FIGURE 2.12 Sagittal PDW image of the lateral aspect of the ankle. (Abbreviations are on pages 50 and 51.)

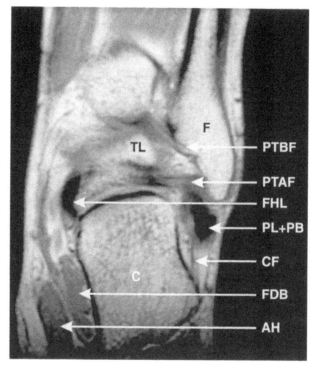

FIGURE 2.13 Coronal PDW image posterior to the tibiotalar joint. (Abbreviations are on pages 50 and 51.)

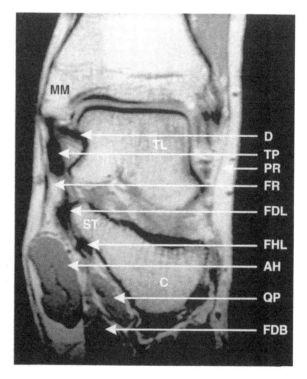

FIGURE 2.14 Coronal PDW image through the tibiotalar joint. (Abbreviations are on pages 50 and 51.)

lateral plantar and the calcaneal nerves. The posterior tibial artery, a branch of the popliteal artery, travels with the tibial nerve and also divides into medial and lateral branches.

At the ankle, the anterior tibial artery passes beneath the extensor retinacula between the extensor hallucis longus tendon and the extensor digitorum longus and then becomes the more superficial dorsalis pedis artery. The deep peroneal nerve accompanies the anterior tibial artery and terminates in medial and lateral branches.

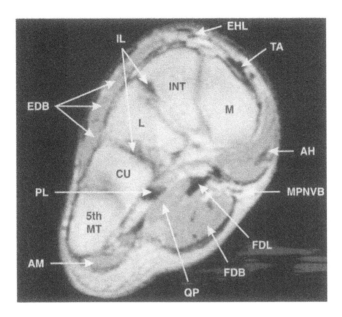

FIGURE 2.15 Coronal PDW image through the mid-foot at the level of the cuneiforms. (Abbreviations are on pages 50 and 51.)

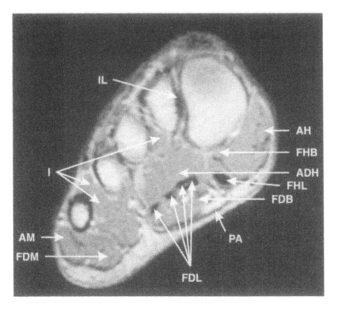

FIGURE 2.16 Coronal PDW image through the mid-foot at the level of the metatarsal bases. (Abbreviations are on pages 50 and 51.)

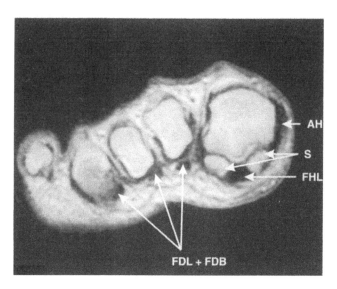

FIGURE 2.17 Coronal PDW image through the distal metatarsals. (Abbreviations are on pages 50 and 51.)

The peroneal artery, a branch of the posterior tibial artery high in the calf, runs behind the tibiofibular syndesmosis inferior to the lateral malleolus and ends on the calcaneal surface as the lateral calcaneal artery.

The great saphenous vein begins superficially on the medial aspect of the foot and continues proximally, anterior to the medial malleolus into the medial calf. The short saphenous vein begins on the lateral surface of the foot and passes behind the lateral malleolus into the calf. The sural nerve travels with the short saphenous vein.

SUMMARY

In summary, the ankle and foot are complex anatomic regions. MR imaging, because of its ability to depict soft-tissue detail, can demonstrate the major components of these areas. It is a very useful modality in the evaluation of patients with symptoms or signs referable to these areas.

ABBREVIATIONS

AC	articular cartilage
ACH	Achilles tendon
ADH	adductor hallucis
AH	abductor hallucis
AM	abductor digiti minimi
ATAV	anterior tibial artery and vein
ATAF	anterior talofibular ligament
ATBF	anterior tibiofibular ligament
C	calcaneus
CF	calcaneofibular ligament
CU	cuboid
D	deltoid ligament
Ds	superficial deltoid ligament
Dd	deep deltoid ligament
DPN	deep peroneal nerve

EDL	extensor digitorum longus
EDB	extensor digitorum brevis
EHL	extensor hallucis longus
F	fibula
FDB	flexor digitorum brevis
FDL	flexor digitorum longus
FDM	flexor digiti minimi brevis
FHL	flexor hallucis longus
FR	flexor retinaculum
GSV	greater saphenous vein
I	interossei muscles
IER	interior extensor retinaculum
IL	interosseous ligament
INT	intermediate cuneiform
L	lateral cuneiform
LSV	lesser saphenous vein
M	medial cuneiform
MM	medial malleolus
MPNVB	medial plantar neurovascular bundle
MT	metatarsal
N	navicular
PA	plantar aponeurosis
PB	peroneus brevis
PIML	posterior intermalleolar ligament
PL	peroneous longus
PT	peroneus tertius
PTAF	posterior talofibular ligament
PTBF	posterior tibiofibular ligament
PTNVB	posterior tibial neurovascular bundle
QP	quadratus plantae
S	sesamoids
SL	spring ligament
SN	sural nerve
SPL	short plantar ligament
SPR	superior peroneal retinaculum
ST	sustentaculum tali
T	tibia
TA	tibialis anterior
TL	talus
TN	talonavicular ligament
TP	tibialis posterior
TTF	transverse tibiofibular ligament

REFERENCES

1. *Gray's Anatomy*, 38th ed. Churchill Livingston, London, 1995, 710–895.
2. Schweitzer, M. E. and Resnick, D., Normal anatomy of the foot and ankle, in A. L. Deutsch, J. H. Mink, and R. Kerr, Eds., *MRI of the Foot and Ankle*, Raven Press, New York, 1992, 33–37.
3. Kneeland, B. J., Macrandar, S., Middleton, M. D., Cates, J. D., Jesmanowicz, A., and Hyde, J. S., MR imaging of the normal ankle: correlation with anatomic sections, *AJR*, 151, 117–123, 1988.
4. Lucas, P., Kaplan, P., Dussault, R., and Hurwitz, S., MRI of the foot and ankle, *Curr. Probl. Diagn. Radiol.*, 26(5), 209–266, 1997.

5. Rockwood, C. A., Green, D. P., Buchotlz, R. W., and Heckman, J. D., *Rockwood and Green's Fractures in Adults*, Vol. 2, Lippincott-Raven, New York, 1996, 2291–2318.
6. Rosenberg, Z. S., Cheung, Y. Y., Beltran, J., Sheskier, S., Leong, M., and Jahss, M., Posterior intermalleolar ligament of the ankle: normal anatomy and MR imaging features, *AJR*, 165, 387–390, 1995.
7. Klein, M. A. and Spreitzer, A., MR imaging of the tarsal sinus and canal: normal anatomy, pathologic findings, and features of the sinus tarsi syndrome, *Radiology*, 186, 233–240, 1993.
8. Cheung, Y., Rosenberg, Z. S., and Magee, T. et al., Normal anatomy and pathologic conditions of ankle tendons: current imaging techniques, *Radiographics*, 12, 429, 1992.

3 Bone Injuries and Related Abnormalities

Joshua M. Farber and Thomas L. Pope

CONTENTS

INTRODUCTION

Foot and ankle fractures can present as acute post-traumatic fractures, stress fatigue fractures, or stress insufficiency fractures. Diagnostically, acute post-traumatic fractures rarely present a problem; radiographs are usually diagnostic, and, if need be, MRI (magnetic resonance imaging) examinations can be performed in difficult cases, such as radiographically occult osteochondral defects (OCD). Stress fatigue fractures and stress insufficiency fractures present a more difficult diagnostic problem since radiographs are often normal or nondiagnostic. In these cases, MRI should be considered early in a patient's evaluation.

Stress fatigue fractures (or simply fatigue fractures) of the foot and ankle result from abnormal stress on normal bone and are a relatively common injury in young, active people such as athletes, dancers, and soldiers.[1-3] Stress insufficiency fractures (or simply insufficiency fractures) result from normal stress on abnormal bone, and are a common problem in the increasingly active, aging population.[4,5] Insufficiency fractures also are seen in debilitated patients with diseases such as diabetes.[6]

In all patient groups, foot and ankle fractures (acute, fatigue, or insufficiency) can lead to significant morbidity, and early diagnosis and treatment are essential.[6-9] Radiological evaluation of suspected foot and ankle fractures should always begin with radiography. If the initial studies are normal and clinical concern persists, patients at the authors' institution routinely undergo MRI examination, which has essentially replaced nuclear medicine bone scanning for the evaluation of radiographically occult fractures. Computed tomography (CT) examination is reserved for questions of alignment and articular surface interfaces.

The incidence of foot and ankle fractures is high in a wide spectrum of patient groups. Broadly, in patients less than 50 years of age, the majority of foot and ankle fractures are seen in males and involve sports; in patients over 50, the majority of these fractures are seen in women and involve falls,[10] although insufficiency fractures are an increasing problem.[4,5] More specifically, foot and ankle injuries account for 10 to 20% of all sports-related injuries,[11,12] and fatigue fractures of the metatarsal are the most common cause of foot injury in the athlete.[3] In dancers, 25 to 42% of all injuries involve foot and ankle injuries, with chronic abnormalities being more prevalent than acute.[2]

Fatigue fractures, first described in Prussian soldiers by Breilhaupt in 1853, are a well-known hazard of long marching in the military.[13-15] Stress fractures are also seen in patients with diabetes and other forms of peripheral neuropathy,[7-16] and in women with menstrual problems.[17,18] In car accidents, 4.5% of all fractures involve the foot and ankle.[19] In the pediatric population, 13% of all fractures involve the foot, of which 50% involve the metatarsals and phalanges.[20]

PATHOPHYSIOLOGY

Normal bone remodeling is a continuous process and results from a proper coupling between osteoclastic and osteoblastic activity. In response to the stress of muscle tension and weight bearing, hormonal activity, and diet, osteoclasts resorb bone and osteoblasts lay osteoid, which, in the normal situation, is mineralized to form bone. The primary hormonal influences are calcitonin, which is secreted by parafollicular cells of the thyroid and whose major function is to decrease serum calcium by reducing osteoclast activity and number and by enhancing calcium phosphate deposition; and parathormone, which is secreted by the parathyroid glands and whose major function is to increase serum calcium levels by increasing osteoclast activity and number and by causing a phosphate diuresis. Vitamin D is required also for proper bone remodeling by its action on the gut for calcium absorption and by potentiating parathormone effects. Adequate dietary intake of calcium and phosphate is essential, as well, for proper bone maintenance. Osteoporosis occurs when the remodeling process produces an abnormally low amount of histologically normal bone, while osteomalacia occurs when the bone produced is architecturally abnormal and is characterized by nonmineralized osteoid.

According to Wolff's law, every change in the form and/or function of a bone results in a specific change in its external conformation. Thus, athletes, because of Wolff's law and the presence of normal bone remodeling, presumably should have very strong bone not susceptible to fatigue fractures. This situation, as noted above, often is not the case. A number of external factors, such as anatomic variation, poor training, poor footwear, and poor conditioning, can be blamed.[1] In addition, intrinsic factors contribute to bone fatigue. In response to stress, bone remodeling accelerates, and osteoclastic activity can outpace osteoblastic activity, which can leave bone structurally weakened; this weakened state can lead to microfractures. With continued training, the bone cannot fully heal and fatigue fractures result. In addition, fatigued muscles can lose some of their ability to contract, which in turn diminishes their ability to absorb loading forces (pounding) and to protect underlying bone. In general, the amount and frequency of loading and the number of repetitions determine when bone will fail.[1] Foot shape in the athlete is important also, with a high, rigid arch placing the athlete at greater risk than a flexible, flat foot.[21]

Older people and debilitated patients have alterations in the osteoclastic–osteoblastic coupling mechanism from hormonal, dietary, and external influences. This alteration results in weakened bone, which can fracture under normal loading.

IMAGING

In cases of suspected stress fracture, radiologic evaluation always should begin with radiography, which is often normal in the acute phase.[22-24] Not until the subacute or chronic phase of stress fracture do radiographs become positive.[23,25] Once apparent on radiographs, stress fractures can be classified according to their radiographic appearance: Type I fractures have a lucent line; Type II fractures have sclerosis of cancellous bone or endosteal callus; Type III fractures have external callus; and Type IV fractures are mixed.[26]

Bone scanning and MRI can detect the early stages of stress fracture, bone scanning by detecting early metabolic changes and MRI by detecting early inflammatory and edematous changes. MRI is preferred because of its superior spatial resolution. This superior spatial resolution allows a variety of diagnoses to be made that can explain a patient's pain, such as, in addition to stress fracture, tenosynovitis, ganglion cyst, neuroma, myositis, and others. Also, bone scanning can yield a false-positive result in cases of periostitis, which can be differentiated from stress fracture on MRI. In addition to the initial diagnosis of stress fractures, MRI can be utilized to monitor a patient's progress and response to therapy.[27]

MRI for stress fracture relies heavily on T2-weighted sequences. Such sequences include spin-echo (SE) and fast-spin-echo (FSE) sequences with long TR and long TE and inversion recovery (IR) sequences with long TR and TE; all of these sequences demonstrate edema and inflammation as increased signal. Although IR sequences demonstrate edema and inflammatory changes more readily than SE and FSE sequences, they often suffer from poor spatial resolution. To correct this problem, a modified IR technique is employed. Typically, the inversion time for fat is approximately 110 msec at 0.5 T and 150 to 160 msec at 1.5 T. By lowering the inversion times to 70 to 80 and 110, respectively, spatial resolution and anatomic detail are improved without significant loss of edema and inflammation sensitivity. This technique is more sensitive than SE and FSE techniques for edema and inflammation detection, and, in addition, suffers less from field inhomogeneities and subsequent poor fat saturation. A form of this sequence is included in all musculoskeletal exams in at least one plane.

As noted previously, MRI is useful in evaluating OCD. A number of techniques are used for this evaluation, such as SE or FSE with or without fat saturation. Gradient echo (GRE) sequences are preferred, either two or three dimensional (2D or 3D) with mixed imaging parameters for the evaluation of articular surfaces. In the foot and ankle, a 2D GRE with TR-500, TE-15, and a 20° flip angle with magnetization transfer constant (MTC) obtained in the coronal plane nicely evaluates the talar dome, a common place for OCD.

MR APPEARANCE OF STRESS FRACTURES BY ANATOMIC SITE

The appearance of stress fractures, whether fatigue or insufficiency, on MRI is uniform regardless of location; stress fractures, and the edema and inflammation they cause, have low signal intensity on T1-weighted images and have high signal on T2-weighted sequences. About the ankle, MRI can be used to evaluate stress fractures just proximal to the medial or lateral malleolus, the most common sites for stress fractures in the ankle.[1] Such injuries are seen in activities that include repetitive impact, such as running, dancing, or gymnastics. In addition, distal fibular fatigue fractures have been described in dancers.[28] In all these types of stress fractures, patients present with pain over the fracture site.

In the hind foot, stress fractures are seen most commonly in the calcaneus, although they also may occur in the talus (Figure 3.1).[29] Again, the patient population for fatigue fractures involves participants in multiple-load activities, and the patient population for insufficiency fracture involves the elderly or debilitated. So, too, in the mid-foot — those who participate in multiple-load activities suffer from fatigue fractures and the elderly and debilitated suffer from insufficiency fractures. In the mid-foot, stress fractures most commonly involve the tarsal navicular, although stress fractures involving virtually all mid-foot bones are documented (Figure 3.2).[29-31] Although patients with hind foot and mid-foot stress fractures may present with localized pain, often the pain is diffuse, ill-defined, medial, and lateral, and, in the mid-foot, may be described as cramping.

The most common locations for stress fractures in the forefoot involve the shaft or neck of the second or third metatarsal.[1] Patients with a short first metatarsal (a Morton's foot) may be predisposed to this injury because of altered mechanics.[32] Stress fractures may also be seen in the proximal fifth metatarsal, and, in dancers, in the base of the second metatarsal at the Lisfrac joint.[28] Patients with metatarsal stress fractures usually present with a gradual onset of pain. Other stress fractures in the forefoot involve those of the sesamoids[33-35] and the proximal phalanx of the great toe.[36]

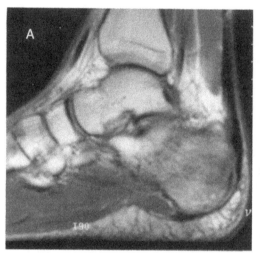
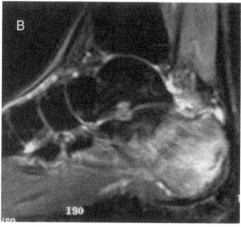

FIGURE 3.1 (A) Sagittal SE (500/15) and (B) IR (2000/40/150) images of a 21-year-old lacross player with heel pain. The SE images demonstrate abnormal low signal intensity and the IR images demonstrate abnormal increased signal intensity in the calcaneus. The MR imaging pattern reflects edema and is consistent with a stress fatigue injury. Radiographs were negative.

OCD injuries in the foot and ankle most commonly involve the talar dome and are post-traumatic. The common locations are posteromedial, which tend to be deep, and anterolateral, which tend to be shallow.[32,37] In either case, the patient presents with chronic pain. OCD injuries are staged as follows: Stage I, compression fracture; Stage II, partially avulsed osseous fragment; Stage III, nondisplaced avulsed osseous fragment; and Stage IV, displaced fragment.[38] These stages can be diagnosed with MRI, which has replaced conventional and CT arthrography in OCD evaluation (Figure 3.3).[39] The staging is clinically significant and impacts therapy directly. Stage I lesions are treated conservatively (no surgery), Stage II lesions are treated with drilling, and Stage III and Stage IV lesions usually are debrided, although large fragments sometimes are reattached surgically.[40]

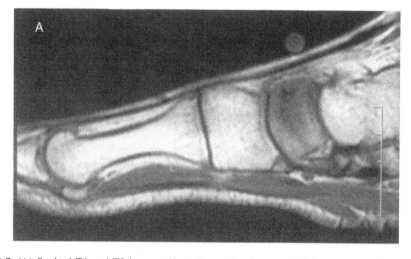

FIGURE 3.2 (A) Sagittal T1 and T2 images (the latter with fat saturation) demonstrate abnormal signal in the tarsal navicular bone of a 27-year-old female with multiple sclerosis and osteopenia. The abnormal signal is consistent with a stress insufficiency fracture. Note the dark area that extends from the dorsal surface of the tarsal navicular; this dark linear area indicates sclerosis.   (*continued*)

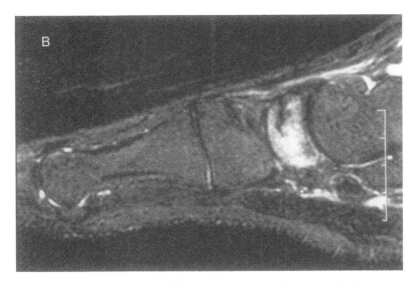

FIGURE 3.2 (continued) (B) Sagittal T1 and T2 images (the latter with fat saturation) demonstrate abnormal signal in the tarsal navicular bone of a 27-year-old female with multiple sclerosis and osteopenia. The abnormal signal is consistent with a stress insufficiency fracture. Note the dark area that extends from the dorsal surface of the tarsal navicular; this dark linear area indicates sclerosis.

CONCLUSION

Osseous injuries in the foot and ankle occur in a wide spectrum of patients from a variety of causes. Often foot and ankle bone abnormalities, such as fatigue and insufficiency fractures and OCD injuries, are radiographically occult. In these cases patients present with persistent and unexplained pain. MRI is the modality of choice in these circumstances, not only because of its ability to detect osseous injuries, but also because of its ability to diagnose soft tissue injuries that may mimic or accompany bone injuries.

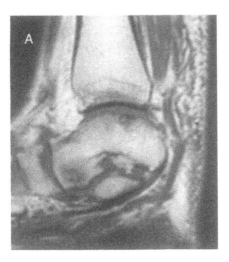
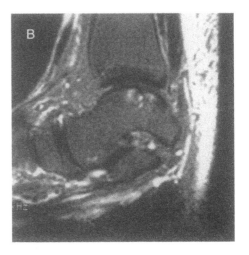

FIGURE 3.3 (A) Sagittal SE (650/14), (B) modified STIR (4300/104/120). The overlying cartilage appears to be intact, and the abnormality is consistent with a Stage II defect. MR arthrography allows definitive staging of these injuries.   (*continued*)

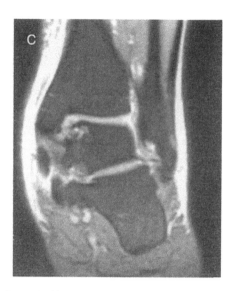

FIGURE 3.3 (continued) (C) Coronal FSE (3616/22) with fat saturation images demonstrate abnormal signal in the medial portion of the talar dome consistent with an osteochondral defect.

REFERENCES

1. Eisele, S. A. and Sammarco, G. J., Fatigue fractures of the foot and ankle in the athlete, *J. Bone Joint Surg.*, 75-A, 290–298, 1993.
2. Hardaker, W. T., Jr., Foot and ankle injuries in classical ballet dancers. *Orthop. Clin. North Am.*, 20, 621–627, 1989.
3. Fitch, K.D., Stress fractures of the lower limbs in runners, *Austr. Fam. Phys.*, 13, 511–515, 1984.
4. Court-Brown, C.M., McBirnie, J., and Wilson, G., Adult ankle fractures — an increasing problem? *Acta Orthop. Scand.*, 69(1), 43–47, 1998.
5. Carpintero, P., Berral, F. J., Baena, P., Garcia-Frasquet, A., and Lancho, J.L., Delayed diagnosis of fatigue fractures in the elderly, *Am. J. Sports Med.*, 25(5), 659–662, 1997.
6. Connolly, J.F. and Csencsitz, T.A., Limb threatening neuropathic complications from ankle fractures in patients with diabetes. *Clin. Orthop. Relat. Res.*, 348, 212–219, 1998.
7. McCormack, R. G. and Leith, J. M., Ankle fractures in diabetics. Complications of surgical management, *J. Bone Joint Surg.*, 80(4), 689–692, 1998.
8. Van der Sluis, C. K., Eisma, W. H., Groothoff, J. W., and ten Duis, H. J., Long-term physical, psychological and social consequences of a fracture of the ankle, *Injury*, 29(4), 277–280, 1998.
9. Kotter, A., Wieberneit, J., Braun, W., and Ruter, A., The Chopart dislocation. A frequently underestimated injury and its sequelae. A clinical study, *Unfallchirurg*, 100(9), 737–741, 1997.
10. Jensen, S. L., Andresen, B. K., Mencke, S., and Nielsen, P. T., Epidemiology of ankle fractures. A prospective population-based study of 212 cases in Aalborg, Denmark, *Acta Orthop. Scand.*, 69(1), 48–50, 1998.
11. MacAuley, D., Ankle injuries: same joint, different sports, *Med. Sci. Sports Exercise*, 31(7 Suppl.), S409–S411, 1999.
12. Fredericson, M., Bergman, A. G., and Matheson, G. O., Stress fractures in athletes, *Orthopade*, 26(11), 961–971, 1997.
13. Anderson, E. G., Fatigue fractures, of the foot, *Injury*, 21, 275–279, 1990.
14. Chillag, K. and Grana, W. A., Medial sesamoid stress fracture, *Orthopedics*, 8, 819–821, 1985.
15. Devas, M. B., *Stress Fractures*, Churchill Livingstone, Edinburgh, 1975.
16. Wolf, S. K., Diabetes mellitus and predisposition to athletic pedal fracture, *J. Foot Ankle Surg.*, 37(1), 16–22; Discussion 79, 1998.
17. Randt, T., Dahlen, C., Schikore, H., and Zwipp, H., Dislocation fractures in the area of the middle foot — injuries of the Chopart and Lisfranc joint, *Zentralbl. Chir.*, 123(11), 1257–1266, 1998.

18. Brukner, P. and Bennell, K., Stress fractures in female athletes. Diagnosis, management and rehabilitation, *Sports Med.*, 24(6), 419–429, 1997.

19. Richter, M., Thermann, H., von Rheinbaben, H., Schratt, E., Otte, D., Zwipp, H., and Tscherene, H., Fractures of the foot region of car drivers and passengers. Occurrence, causes and long-term results, *Unfallchirurg*, 102(6), 429–433, 1999.

20. Thermann, H., Schratt, H. E., Hufner, T., and Tscherne, H., Fractures of the pediatric foot, *Unfallchirurg*, 101(1), 2–11, 1998.

21. Nix, R. A., Stress fractures in the lower extremity, *J. Ark. Med. Soc.*, 80, 10–13, 1983.

22. Lazarus, M. L., Imaging of the foot and ankle in the injured athlete, *Med. Sci. Sports Exerc.*, 31(7 Suppl.), S412–S420, 1999.

23. Berquist, T. H., *Radiology of the Foot and Ankle*, Raven, New York, 1989.

24. Daffner, R. H., Stress fractures, *Skeletal Radiol.*, 2, 221–229, 1987.

25. Greaney, R. B., Gerber, F. H., and Laughlin, R. L., Distribution and natural history of stress fractures in U.S. Marine recruits, *Radiology*, 146, 339–346, 1983.

26. Wilson, E. S. and Katz, F. N., Stress fractures: an analysis of 250 consecutive cases, *Radiology*, 92, 481–486, 1969.

27. Ariyoshi, M., Nagata, K., Hiraoka, K., Sonoda, K., Hori, R., and Inoue, A., Stress fracture of the medial malleolus, *Kurume Med. J.*, 44(3), 233–236, 1997.

28. Sammarco, G. J. and Miller, E. H., Forefoot conditions in dancers, *Foot Ankle*, 3, 85–98, 1982.

29. Hardaker, W. T., Jr., Foot and ankle injuries in classical ballet dancers. *Orthop. Clin. North Am.*, 20, 621–627, 1989.

30. Orava, S., Puranen, J., and Ala-Ketola, L., Stress fractures caused by physical exercise. *Acta Orthop. Scand.*, 49, 19–27, 1978.

31. Shereff, M. J., Yang, Q. M., Kummer, F. J., Frey, C. C., and Greenidge, N., Vascular anatomy of the fifth metatarsal, *Foot Ankle*, 11, 350–353, 1991.

32. Drez, D., Jr., Young, J. C., Johnston, R. D., and Parker, W. D., Metatarsal stress fractures, *Am. J. Sports Med.*, 8, 123–125, 1980.

33. Dietzen, C. J., Great toe sesamoid injures in the athlete, *Orthop. Rev.*, 19, 966–972, 1990.

34. Pavlov, H., Torg, J. S., and Freiberger, R. H., Tarsal navicular stress fractures: radiographic evaluation, *Radiology*, 148, 641–645, 1983.

35. Van Hal, M. E., Keene, J. S., Lange, T. A., and Clancy, W. G., Jr., Stress fractures of the great toe sesamoids, *Am. J. Sports Med.*, 10, 122–128, 1982.

36. Yokoe, K. and Mannoji, T., Stress fracture of the proximal phalanx of the great toe. A report of three cases, *Am. J. Sports Med.*, 14, 240–242, 1986.

37. Flick, A. B. and Gould, N., Osteochondritis dissecans of the talus (transchondral fractures of the talus): review of the literature and new surgical approach for medial joint lesions, *Foot Ankle*, 5, 165–185, 1985.

38. Berndt, A. L. and Harty, M., Transchondral fractures (osteochondritis dissecans) of the talus, *J. Bone Joint Surg. (Am.)*, 41, 988, 1959.

39. Desmet, A. A., Fisher, D. R., and Burnstein, M. I., Value of MR imaging in staging osteochondral lesions of the talus (osteochondritis dissecans): results in 14 patients, *Am. J. Radiol.*, 254, 555, 1990.

40. Kneeland, B., *The Radiologic Clinics of North America, Update in Musculoskeletal Imaging*, W.B. Saunders, Philadelphia, 1997, 140–145.

4 Bone Tumors of the Foot and Ankle

Steven Shankman

CONTENTS

INTRODUCTION

Osseous tumors and tumor-like conditions of the ankle and foot are uncommon. Primary and secondary malignant neoplasms are especially rare. Benign lesions, particularly nonneoplastic tumor-like conditions such as simple and aneurysmal bone cysts, greatly outnumber true neoplasms, both benign and malignant.[1-3]

Most lesions present earlier in their course than lesions in other locations due to the inherent structure and function of the foot and ankle. The tight compartmental anatomy allows for small lesions to become symptomatic due to nerve and tendon encroachment during the constant mechanical demands of weight bearing. Scanty subcutaneous fat and muscle enable ready palpation of lesions.[4]

The evaluation of bone tumors of the foot and ankle begins with conventional radiographs. Radiographic characteristics of any bone tumor yields the most specific information regarding tumor histology. The aggressive or nonaggressive nature of the lesion may be ascertained and cartilaginous and osseous mineralization may be identified.[3]

Radiographs, may on the other hand, underestimate the extent of a bone lesion. This is particularly true for lesions involving the tarsal bones because of the many overlapping surfaces and undulating contours. MR (magnetic resonance) imaging is sensitive to the extent of soft-tissue involvement by bone tumors but is somewhat nonspecific. Its major role, therefore, is in anatomic localization and surgical staging.[3,5]

The most accepted staging system of bone and soft-tissue neoplasms is that devised by Enneking.[6] Staging of benign tumors is a function of the behavioral characteristics of the lesion. Stage I lesions are static or heal spontaneously. Stage II lesions appear more aggressive radiographically, are less mature histologically, and show continued growth. Stage III lesions are locally aggressive and histologically immature. They grow progressively, unrestricted by natural barriers. Anatomic location and size are not factors in the staging of benign lesions but are central to staging malignant ones.

Malignant tumors are first staged histologically as low grade (I) or high grade (II). Radiographic appearance is taken into account and anatomic location is determined as intracompartmental (A) or extracompartmental (B). A compartment is defined as an anatomic structure or space with natural barriers to tumor extension such as a bone, a joint, or a functional muscle group bounded by a major fascial septum. Interfascial planes containing neurovascular structures are not compartments because they have no proximal or distal borders. Other true compartments include subcutaneous fat and skin, rays of the feet, and periosseous potential spaces. The rays of the feet, but not the digits in isolation, are limited by natural barriers. Lesions with distant or regional metastasis are classified as Stage III regardless of any other features.[6]

This staging system excludes bone marrow malignancies and primary epithelial tumors of the feet. The lack of anatomic barriers in the foot often allows for extracompartmental extension at the patient's initial presentation. The close proximity to vital structures often makes limited excision incompatible with a functional foot. Even though the staging of malignant lesions appears straightforward, its utility in the foot is somewhat limited because of the lack of anatomic boundaries in the hind and mid-foot. A lesion confined to a ray is considered intracompartmental, whereas lesions in the hind and mid-foot are considered extracompartmental. For example, a malignant tumor at the toe distal to the metatarsal–phalangeal (MTP) joint requires ray resection, one in the mid-foot requires amputation in the ankle, and one in the hind foot necessitates below-knee amputation.[4,6]

MR imaging features of tumors and tumor-like conditions are often nonspecific. The majority of lesions show low to intermediate signal intensity on T1-weighted images and high signal intensity on T2-weighted images. Lesions of high signal intensity on T1-weighted images contain fat, proteinaceous fluid, or subacute hemorrhage. Lesions of low signal intensity on T2-weighted images contain dense fibrous tissue, abundant calcification, or hemosiderin. Most masses, however, are heterogeneous, indicative of a varied histologic composition, intralesion hemorrhage, necrosis, or cyst formation.

Despite the overall low specificity of MR imaging, there are certain benign lesions that have distinct morphology, signal characteristics, and location. For example, intraosseous lipomas show a pattern of signal intensity that parallels adjacent yellow marrow or subcutaneous fat.

MR imaging is also unreliable in estimating the extent and biological behavior of malignant lesions that appear well contained. In general, if the specific histologic diagnosis of the lesion cannot be made, then the aggressiveness of the lesion, especially in tumors that appear smooth, well-defined, and homogeneous, cannot be determined.[3]

MR imaging does, however, have a role in evaluating patients for local tumor recurrence following surgical resection and/or adjuvant therapy. Assessment of patients who have undergone recent radiation therapy can be difficult because of superimposed radiation-induced inflammation that can mimic local tumor recurrence. In this situation, dynamic gadolinium-enhanced MR imaging may be useful in distinguishing recurrent tumors from radiation-induced inflammation and necrosis.[1,7,8]

Although bone tumors and tumor-like conditions of the foot and ankle are rare, the differential diagnosis in some lesions is often predictable. Certain tumors have a predilection for anatomic bones of the foot and ankle. For example, simple bone cysts and lipomas favor the calcaneus, while osteoid osteoma, osteoblastoma, and chondroblastoma favor the talus. Intraosseous ganglions are commonly located about the ankle.[3]

UNICAMERAL BONE CYST

Nearly 90% of unicameral bone cysts (UBCs) occur in the proximal humerus and femur in children.[9] In the skeletally mature individual, simple bone cysts are usually seen in the iliac wing and calcaneus. UBCs are among the most common lesions of the calcaneus, although they are rare in the other bones of the foot and ankle. These lesions are not considered true neoplasms but are thought to represent a developmental or reactive process. On conventional radiographs, they appear as well-defined lytic lesions without central mineralization. MR imaging can confirm the diagnosis and better define the relation of the tumor to the subtalar and calcaneal–cuboid joints (Figure 4.1). Usually located in the anterior process of the calcaneus, UBCs contain serous or serosanguinous fluid, and the MR imaging examination shows homogeneous low to intermediate signal intensity on T1-weighted images and high signal intensity on T2-weighted images. Low-signal septa may be present. Hemorrhage may lead to a more heterogeneous appearance and fluid–fluid levels. A high protein content may result in increased signal intensity on T1-weighted images. Usually, however, signal characteristics on all sequences parallel that of simple fluid.[2,9,10]

ANEURYSMAL BONE CYST

The aneurysmal bone cyst (ABC) is typically a benign expansile lytic lesion named for its radiographic appearance. It is composed of distended, thin-walled, blood-filled spaces without an endothelial lining and is thought to be a reactive rather than a neoplastic process. ABC is almost always seen in children and young adults. In patients over 20 years old, ABC is usually associated with an underlying primary bone tumor such as giant cell tumor, fibrous dysplasia, chondroblastoma, or chondromyxoid fibroma. Although more commonly seen in the posterior elements of the spine

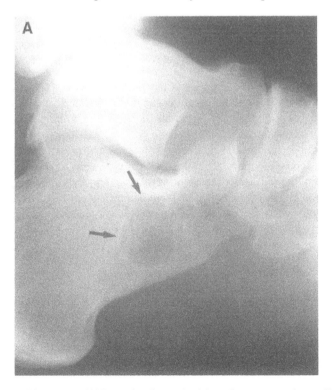

FIGURE 4.1 Unicameral bone cyst. (A) Lateral radiograph of the calcaneus reveals a well-defined lytic lesion with sclerotic borders (arrows) and no apparent mineralization in the anterior aspect of the calcaneus, typical of a UBC. (Courtesy of A. R. Spouge, M.D., London, Ontario, Canada.) (*continued*)

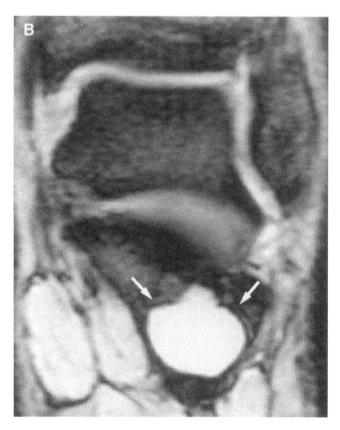

FIGURE 4.1 (continued) (B) Coronal gradient-echo image through the calcaneus shows homogeneous increased signal intensity (arrows) typical of a UBC. (Courtesy of A. R. Spouge, M.D., London, Ontario, Canada.)

and the long tubular bones, ABC can occur in any of the bones of the ankle and foot. ABC is usually an intramedullary lesion, although cortical and subperiosteal locations have been described.[12] Conventional radiographs demonstrate an expansile, nonmineralized lytic lesion marginated by a thin rim of periosteal new bone. The periosteal new bone may be so thin that it can only be appreciated on a computed tomography (CT) examination. The MR imaging findings of ABC consist of an expansile, lobulated, multiseptated mass with varying signal intensity within numerous cavities. Fluid–fluid levels representing hemoglobin byproducts may be seen and are typical of ABC. Although many tumors that undergo hemorrhage or cystic degeneration may cause fluid–fluid levels, these MR imagings or CT findings, in the correct clinical setting, are highly suggestive of ABC (Figures 4.2 through 4.4).[11-13]

INTRAOSSEOUS GANGLION

The intraosseous ganglion (IOG) is a subchondral lesion, reactive in nature, usually seen in young and middle-aged adults. It is most common in the ankle in the distal tibial plafond near the medial malleolus. Pathologically, the inner lining of an IOG is identical to that of a soft-tissue ganglion. The radiographic findings of an IOG consist of a nonexpansile, lytic subchondral lesion with a thin, well-defined sclerotic rim and no matrix mineralization. MR imaging shows a uni- or multilocular lesion with fluid characteristics, revealing low signal intensity on T1-weighted images and high signal intensity on T2-weighted images (Figure 4.5).[14] The differential diagnosis of an IOG includes an arthritic cyst or geode. The MR imaging characteristics of geodes may be identical to an IOG. However, the lack of an associated arthritis suggests the diagnosis of IOG (Figure 4.6).

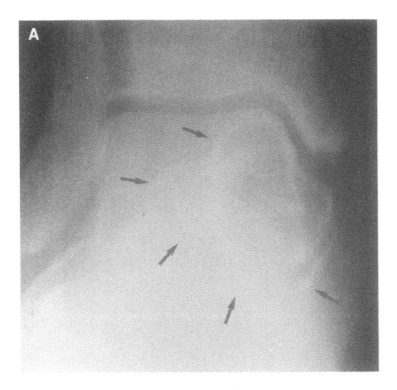

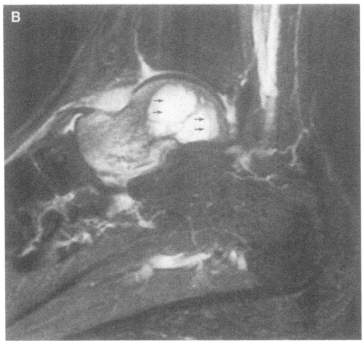

FIGURE 4.2 Aneurysmal bone cyst. (A) AP radiograph of the ankle shows a slightly expansile lytic lesion involving the medial talus with thin sclerotic borders (arrows). (B) Sagittal inversion recovery image of the hind foot reveals a lobulated, multiseptated lesion in the talus with varying signal intensities and multiple fluid–fluid levels (arrows) typical of an ABC. (Courtesy of A. R. Spouge, M.D., London, Ontario, Canada.)

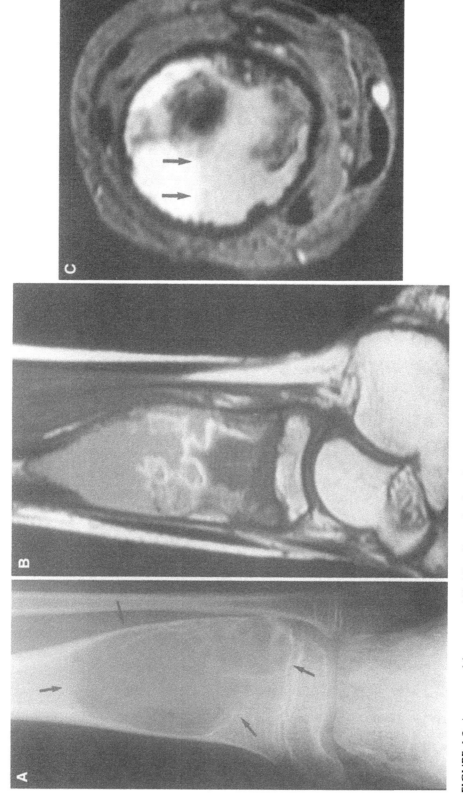

FIGURE 4.3 Aneurysmal bone cyst. (A) AP radiograph of an 8-year-old girl demonstrates an expansile, slightly lobulated lytic lesion in the distal tibial metastasis (arrows) associated with remodeling of the adjacent fibula. (B) Sagittal spin-echo T1 demonstrates the pronounced heterogeneous signal intensity of the lesion. (C) Axial T2* gradient-echo image demonstrates the concentric expansion and fluid–fluid levels (arrows). (Courtesy of A. R. Spouge, M.D., London, Ontario, Canada.

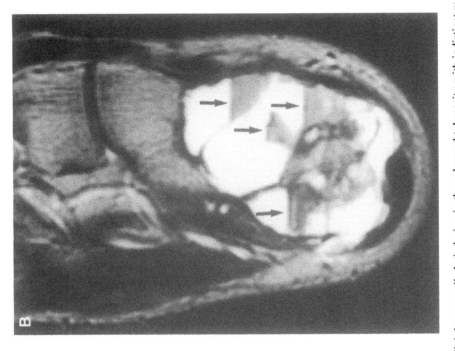

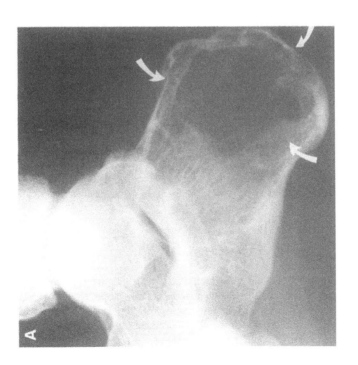

FIGURE 4.4 Aneurysmal bone cyst. (A) Lateral radiograph of the calcaneus shows a slightly expansile lytic lesion in the calcaneal tuberosity with indistinct margins anteriorly (arrows). (B) Axial convention spin-echo T2 confirms the presence of multiple fluid–fluid lesions (arrows). (Courtesy of A. R. Spouge, M.D., London, Ontario, Canada.)

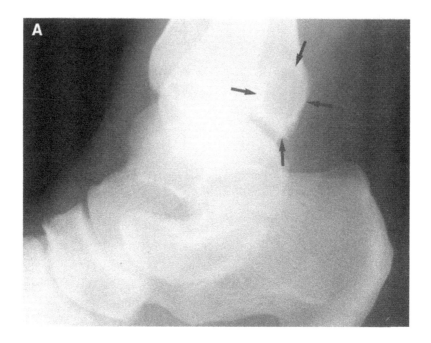

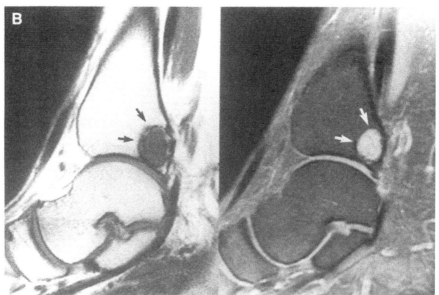

FIGURE 4.5 Intraosseous ganglion. (A) Lateral radiograph of the ankle and hind foot reveal a well-defined lytic lesion (arrows) with sclerotic borders and no apparent mineralization adjacent to the tibial plafond, typical of an IOG. (B) Sagittal T1-weighted spin-echo (left) and fast-spin-echo proton-density-weighted fat-suppressed (right) MR images show the subchondral lesion with signal characteristics typical of fluid (arrows). (Courtesy of A. R. Spouge, M.D., London, Ontario, Canada.)

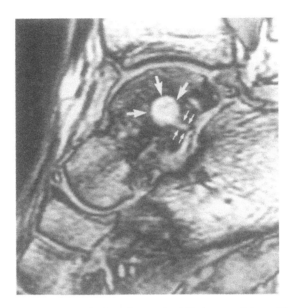

FIGURE 4.6 Arthritic cyst (Geode). Sagittal gradient-echo MR image of the ankle and hind foot shows a well-defined subchondral cyst in the talus extending from the posterior facet of the subtalar joint (arrows). The subchondral extension and arthritic change in the joint confirm the diagnosis of an arthritic cyst. (Courtesy of A. R. Spouge, M.D., London, Ontario, Canada.)

INTRAOSSEOUS LIPOMA

The intraosseous lipoma (IOL) is uncommon and considered by some to represent a degenerative phenomenon rather than a true neoplasm. Typically located in the tibia, fibula, femur, and especially in the anterior process of the calcaneus, the IOL may appear identical to UBC on conventional radiographs. Unlike UBC, however, the IOL may be expansile and show central calcification. MR imaging of an IOL shows signal intensity typical of fat, identical to the signal characteristics of subcutaneous fat. Low-signal-intensity areas may be caused by central calcification. Focal areas of cyst formation may be present and show fluid signal, manifested by low signal intensity on T1-weighted images and high signal intensity on T2-weighted images (Figure 4.7). This type of heterogeneity should not be confusing if the predominantly fatty nature of the lesion is appreciated. CT may also show the fat content of these tumors.[15]

GIANT CELL TUMOR

The giant cell tumor (GCT) occurs in skeletally mature individuals, usually 20 to 45 years of age. These lesions are typically in a subarticular location or in an apophysis, most commonly occurring in the distal femur, proximal tibia, distal radius, proximal humerus, and sacrum. The foot and ankle are rarely involved but the sites of predilection for GCT in this region are the distal tibia, talus, and calcaneus. Approximately 95% of GCTs are benign.[16] Radiographs show a lytic expansile lesion at the end of the bone without apparent matrix mineralization and no periosteal reaction unless there is callus formation from a pathologic fracture. MR imaging shows a varied signal pattern due to hemorrhage and cyst formation, typically demonstrating low to intermediate signal intensity on T1-weighted images and high signal intensity on T2-weighted images (Figures 4.8 and 4.9). Fluid–fluid levels may be seen. When present, cortical destruction and soft-tissue extension are easily appreciated on MR imaging (Figure 4.9).[16,17]

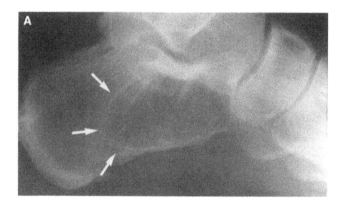

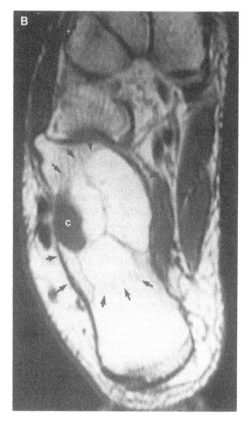

FIGURE 4.7 Intraosseous lipoma. (A) Coned-down lateral radiograph of the calcaneus reveals a nonexpansile lytic lesion with thin septations. There is a suggestion of a thin sclerotic border posteriorly (arrows). (Reprinted with permission from A. R. Spouge, *Postgraduate Radiology,* 19, No. 75, 2, 1999.) (B) Axial T1-weighted spin-echo MR image of the calcaneus shows a multilobulated lesion with signal characteristics typical of fat (arrows), consistent with an IOL. The low-signal-intensity region laterally represents an area of cyst formation. (Courtesy of A. R. Spouge, M.D., London, Ontario, Canada.)

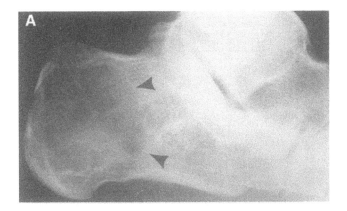

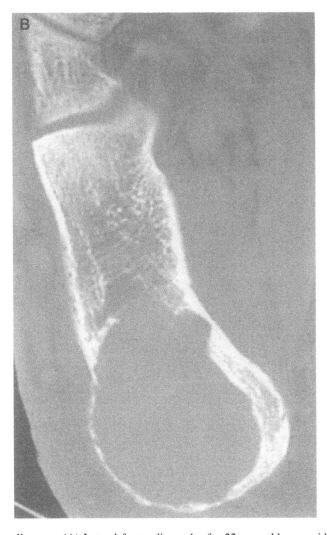

FIGURE 4.8 Giant cell tumor. (A) Lateral foot radiograph of a 22-year-old man with foot pain shows a lytic calcaneal lesion (arrowheads). (B) Axial CT scan shows lytic lesion in calcaneus with some bony expansion. (Courtesy of Mark Kransdorf, M.D., Mayo Clinic, Jacksonville, FL.)   (*continued*)

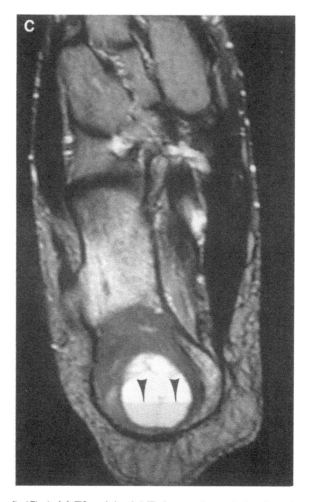

FIGURE 4.8 (continued) (C) Axial T2-weighted MR image shows lesion in calcaneus with high signal intensity and fluid–fluid levels (arrowheads). Biopsy showed GCT. (Courtesy of Mark Kransdorf, M.D., Mayo Clinic, Jacksonville, FL.)

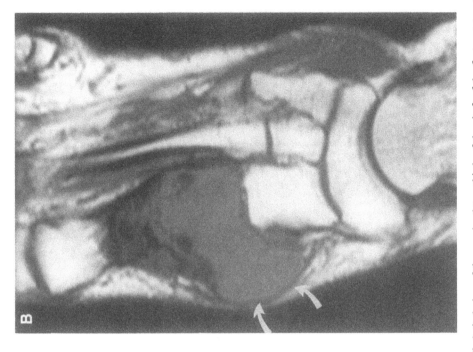

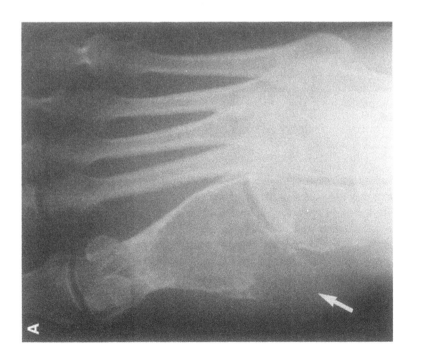

FIGURE 4.9 Giant cell tumor. (A) AP radiograph of the foot shows a markedly expansile lytic lesion of the proximal two thirds of the shaft of the first metatarsal with an intermediate zone of transition. There is cortical breakthrough medially at the base of the metatarsal (arrow). (B) Axial spin-echo T1 shows the relative sharp margination of the lesion and optimally demonstrates the soft-tissue extension medially (arrows). (Courtesy of A. R. Spouge, M.D., London, Ontario, Canada.) *(continued)*

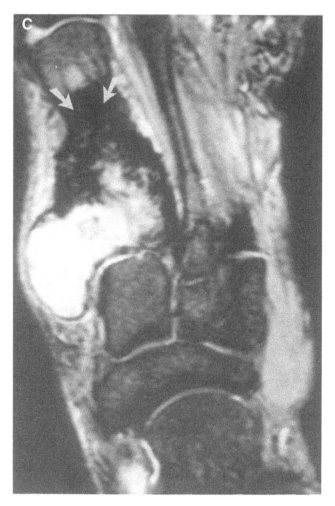

FIGURE 4.9 (continued) (C) Axial T2* gradient in the same location shows signal loss in the distal aspect of the lesion with magnetic susceptibility, consistent with prominent hemosiderin deposition (arrows). Hemosiderin deposition can be present in GCTs due to intralesion hemorrhage. (Courtesy of A. R. Spouge, M.D., London, Ontario, Canada.)

ENCHONDROMA

The majority of enchondromas occur in the metacarpals and phalanges of the hand. However, these benign cartilage tumors may also occur in the metacarpals and phalanges of the foot. Conventional radiographs show a lytic lesion with well-defined and frequently lobulated margins. Typically, central cartilaginous calcification and endosteal scalloping are present. MR imaging shows a homogeneous pattern of high signal intensity consistent with cartilage matrix on T2-weighted and short-tau inversion recovery (STIR) images. Focal low-signal-intensity areas usually represent cartilaginous calcification (Figures 4.10 and 4.11).[8]

OSTEOCHONDROMA

The osteochondroma is the most common benign bone tumor. These lesions rarely involve the foot but when they occur in the ankle, the distal tibia and fibula are the usual sites of involvement. The radiographic finding of continuity of the medullary and cortical bone of the lesion with that of the

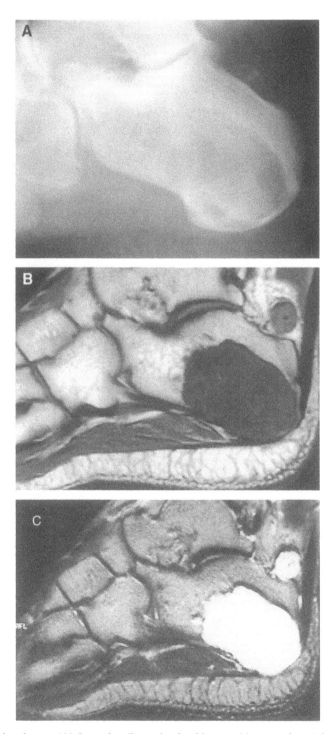

FIGURE 4.10 Enchondroma. (A) Lateral radiograph of a 39-year-old man referred for a "calcaneal cyst" shows a lytic expansile septated lesion in the calcaneus. (B) Sagittal T1-weighted MR image shows well-demarcated region of marrow replacement in posterior aspect of the calcaneus. (C) Sagittal fat-suppressed T2-weighted image shows well-demarcated region of mixed high and low signal intensity characteristic of cartilage. The man had a history of cysts removed as a child and histology of these was hemangioma. This man had Maffucci's syndrome (enchondromatosis and soft-tissue cavernous hemangiomas). (Courtesy of Mark Kransdorf, M.D., Mayo Clinic, Jacksonville, FL.)

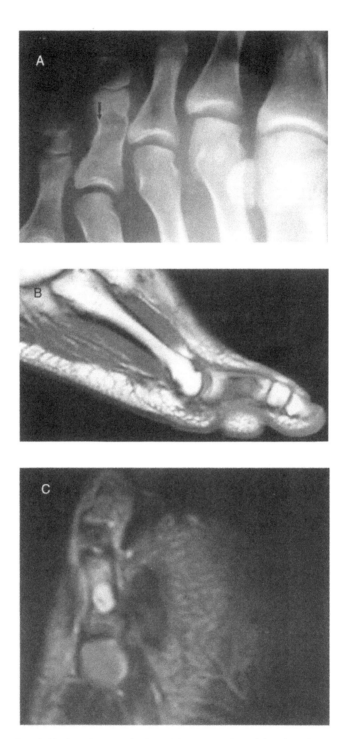

FIGURE 4.11 (continued) Enchrondroma. (A) Coned down AP view of foot in a 34-year-old man with pain shows a lytic lesion scalloping the cortex in the proximal phalanx of the fourth toe with a pathologic fracture (arrow). (B) Sagittal T1-weighted MR image draws intermediate-signal-intensity marrow replacement in proximal phalanx of the fourth toe. (C) Axial T2-weighted MR image shows the high signal intensity of the intraosseous lesion and in the adjacent soft tissues representing the sequelae of the fracture. (Courtesy of Mark Kransdorf, M.D., Mayo Clinic, Jacksonville, FL.)

parent bone are diagnostic. MR imaging is helpful in evaluating encroachment of the lesion on adjacent neurovascular structures, the thickness of the cartilage cap, and demonstrating associated bursal formation (Figures 4.12 and 4.13). The cartilage cap demonstrates low to intermediate signal intensity on T1-weighted and proton-density-weighted images and very high signal intensity on T2-weighted images. The relationship of the thickness of the cartilage cap and malignant transformation remains controversial, but growth of the cap in a skeletally mature individual should be considered a finding requiring further evaluation.

An osteochondroma should not be confused with a subungual exostosis, which is a common entity arising from the dorsal surface of the distal phalanx of the first toe. A subungual exostosis is regarded to be a post-traumatic lesion rather than a true neoplasm, although it may cause pain, swelling, ulceration, and infection (Figure 4.14).[18]

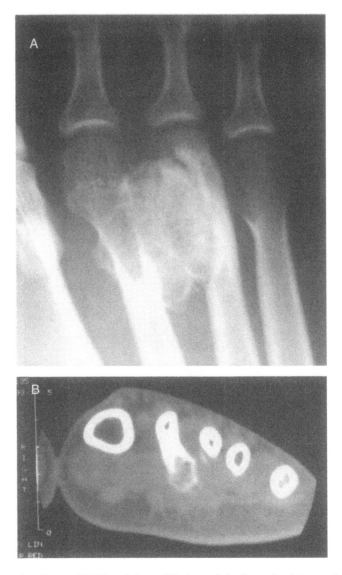

FIGURE 4.12 Osteochondroma. (A) Coned-down AP view of the foot of a 21-year-old runner with pain shows a bony mass extending from the lateral aspect of the shaft of the second metatarsal. (B) Coronal CT image shows the continuity of the cortex of the cartilaginous lesion with the native metatarsal. (Courtesy of Mark Kransdorf, M.D., Mayo Clinic, Jacksonville, FL.) *(continued)*

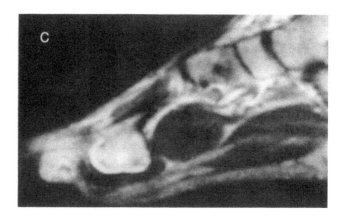

FIGURE 4.12 (continued) (C) Sagittal T2-weighted MR image shows bone marrow edema and high signal intensity of the osteochondroma. (Courtesy of Mark Kransdorf, M.D., Mayo Clinic, Jacksonville, FL.)

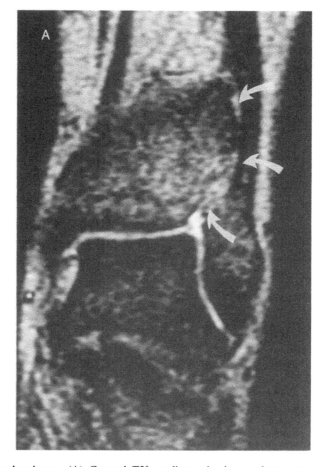

FIGURE 4.13 Osteochondroma. (A) Coronal T2* gradient-echo image demonstrates an osteochondroma protruding from the lateral tibial cortex (arrows) associated with remodeling of the distal fibula. (Courtesy of A. R. Spouge, M.D., London, Ontario, Canada.)   (continued)

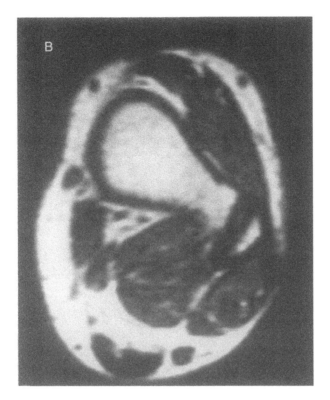

FIGURE 4.13 (continued) (B) Axial spin-echo T1 reveals continuity of the adjacent cortex and marrow into the tumor. The remodeled concave medial fibular cortex is well shown. No appreciable cartilage cap is evident in this mature osteochondroma. (Courtesy of A. R. Spouge, M.D., London, Ontario, Canada.)

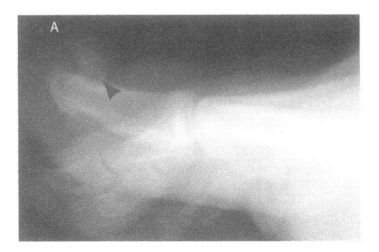

FIGURE 4.14 Subungual exostosis. A 15-year-old girl with toe pain. (A) Lateral radiograph of the foot shows an exostosis of the distal aspect of the distal phalanx of the first toe (black arrowhead). (Courtesy of Mark Kransdorf, M.D., Mayo Clinic, Jacksonville, FL.)   (*continued*)

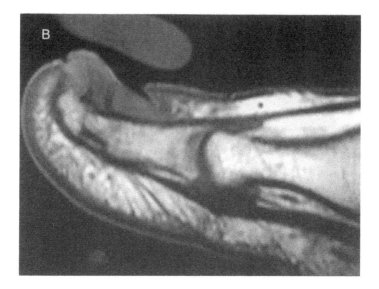

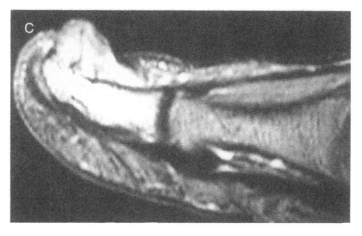

FIGURE 4.14 (continued) (B) Sagittal T1-weighted MR image shows exostosis extending off first distal phalanx. (C) Sagittal T2-weighted MR image shows bone marrow edema in distal phalanx and in the subungual exostosis. (Courtesy of Mark Kransdorf, M.D., Mayo Clinic, Jacksonville, FL.)

CHONDROBLASTOMA

Chondroblastoma is an uncommon benign cartilage neoplasm, although it is the most common benign tumor of the epiphysis or epiphysoid bones of children and adolescents. Chondroblastomas are most commonly located about the knee, shoulder, and hip, but they are one of the most common primary tumors of the talus, calcaneus, and navicular bones. Conventional radiographs typically show a small well-circumscribed lytic lesion with sclerotic borders. Central calcification may be present in one third of the cases. In the calcaneus, the lesion tends to rest beneath the posterior subtalar joint or at the calcaneal apophysis. MR imaging shows intermediate signal intensity on T1-weighted images and increased signal intensity on T2-weighted images. Cystic change or secondary aneurysmal bone cyst formation may produce fluid–fluid levels (Figures 4.15 and 4.16).[19]

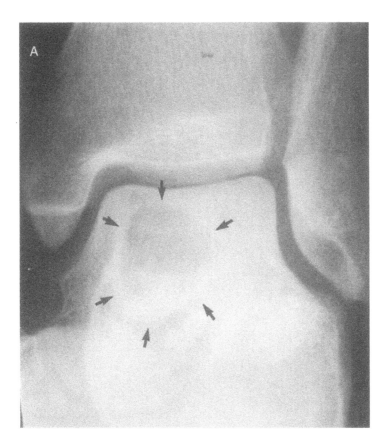

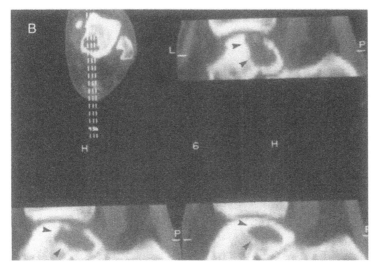

FIGURE 4.15 Chondroblastoma. (A) AP radiograph of the left ankle reveals a well-defined lytic lesion in the talus with sclerotic borders (arrows) typical of a chondroblastoma. (B) CT examination of the left ankle with sagittal reformats shows a well-defined lytic lesion in the talus extending to the articular surface (arrowheads).   (*continued*)

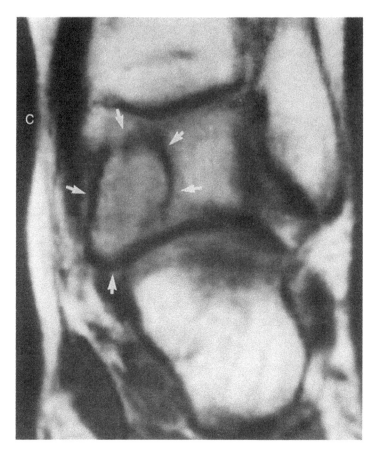

FIGURE 4.15 (continued) (C) Coronal proton-density spin-echo MR image shows a low-signal-intensity lesion (arrows).

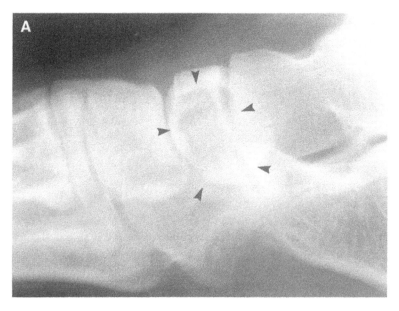

FIGURE 4.16 (A) Lateral radiograph of the mid-foot reveals a well-defined lytic lesion in the navicular bone with sclerotic borders and no matrix mineralization (arrowheads).   (*continued*)

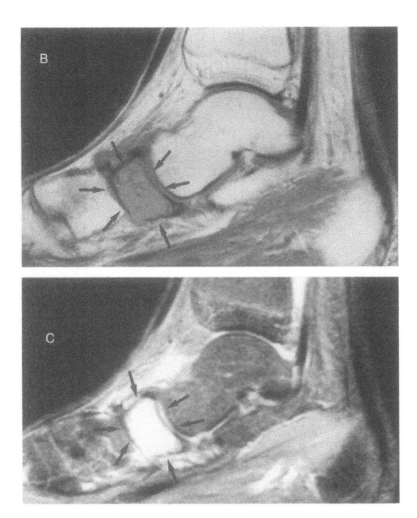

FIGURE 4.16 (continued) (B) Sagittal T1-weighted spin-echo and (C) inversion recovery images of the mid-foot show complete marrow replacement of the navicular (arrows). The lesion is nearly obscured by edematous change in the surrounding bone marrow. The importance of the conventional radiograph is again stressed.

OSTEOID OSTEOMA

Osteoid osteoma (OO), a benign bone-forming lesion seen in children and young adults, most commonly affects the femur, tibia, humerus, and spine. OO is rare in the foot and usually involves the distal tibia and talus when it occurs in the ankle. In the talus, OO typically involves the talar neck and is subperiosteal in location. In children, OO may cause premature fusion of the growth plate and overgrowth of the involved long bone secondary to hyperemia. About one half of the patients with OO present with pain, worse at night, relieved by aspirin and other nonsteroidal anti-inflammatory medication. The tumor is small, often measuring only a few millimeters in diameter. Cortical and extra-articular lesions provoke an exuberant periostitis that is a clue to the underlying lesion. Intra-articular lesions cause an intense synovitis and periarticular osteopenia while the nidus itself may not be radiographically evident. The radionuclide bone scan always identifies the location of the lesion and thin-section CT will usually demonstrate it. MR imaging may also show the nidus as an area of low to intermediate signal intensity on T1-weighted images and varied signal intensity on T2-weighted images depending on the extent of tumor mineralization (Figures 4.17 through 4.19). Because these tumors may provoke abundant adjacent bone marrow edema, the nidus itself may be less conspicuous on the MR examination.[20–26]

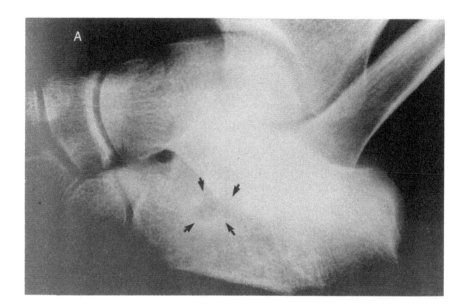

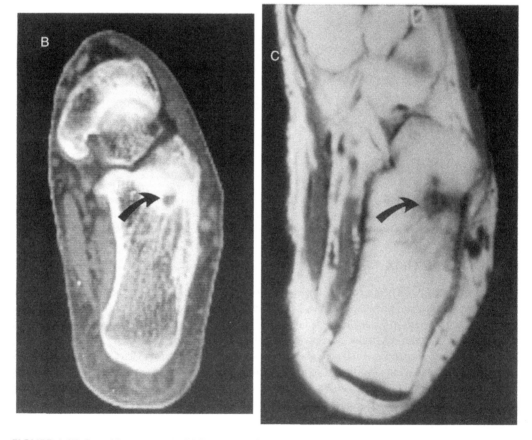

FIGURE 4.17 Osteoid osteoma. (A) Oblique view of the hind foot reveals a small lytic lesion in the calcaneus with fine sclerotic borders (arrows). (B) CT of the hind foot reveals a nidus with minimal surrounding sclerosis in the anterior portion of the calcaneus (arrow). (C) Axial MR T1-weighted spin-echo image of the hind foot shows a low-signal-intensity nidus (arrow) with central lower-signal-intensity calcification and lower-signal-intensity reactive bone at its periphery.

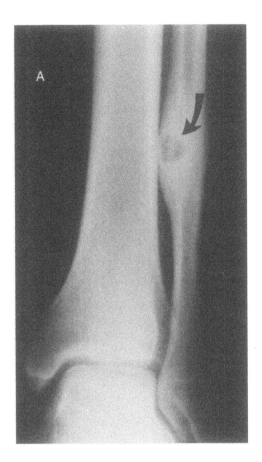

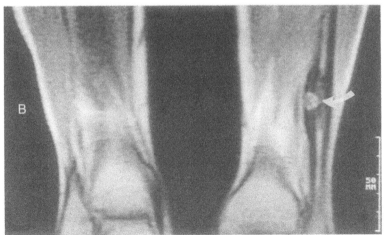

FIGURE 4.18 Osteoid osteoma. (A) AP radiograph of the left distal tibia and fibula reveal a well-defined round lytic lesion in the distal medial fibular cortex (arrow) associated with abundant reactive new bone formation and central calcification, consistent with a cortical OO. (B) Coronal T2-weighted spin-echo MR images show the high-signal-intensity nidus (arrow) with central low-signal-intensity calcification and reactive peripheral bone formation.   (*continued*)

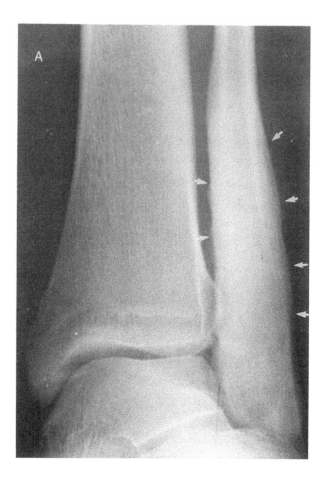

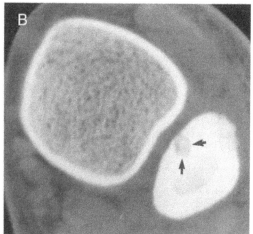

FIGURE 4.19 Osteoid osteoma. (A) Oblique radiograph of the ankle reveals abundant periosteal reaction in the distal fibula (arrows). (B) Axial CT shows a small nidus in the medial cortex of the distal fibula (arrows) with central calcification and adjacent periosteal new bone formation.   (*continued*)

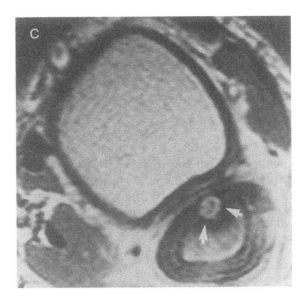

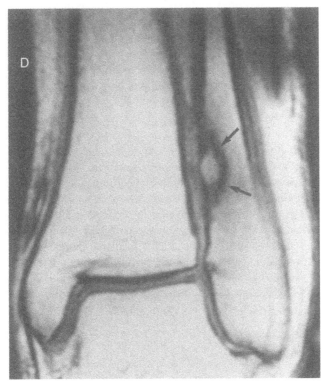

FIGURE 4.19 (continued) (C) Axial T2-weighted spin-echo MR images show the high-signal-intensity nidus (arrows) of a cortical OO. (D) Coronal T2-weighted spin-echo MR images reveal the high-signal-intensity nidus (arrows) of a cortical OO.

OSTEOBLASTOMA

Osteoblastomas most commonly occur in the posterior elements of the spine and are rare in the foot and ankle. These tumors are histologically similar to osteoid osteomas but are larger and may extend into the joint or adjacent soft tissues. The talus is the preferred site of involvement when osteoblastoma occurs in the ankle or foot regions. MR imaging readily demonstrates the local extent of this lesion. Low to intermediate signal intensity is seen on T1-weighted images and intermediate signal intensity is seen on T2-weighted images.[20,27,28]

CHONDROSARCOMA

Excluding myeloma, chondrosarcoma (CS) is the most common primary bone malignancy in middle-aged to older adults. Although it may occur at any age, CS is most common in patients aged 30 to 60 years. It may be central in location, arising in the medullary bone, usually *de novo*. Malignant transformation of an enchondroma into CS is rare except in patients with enchondromatosis or Ollier's disease. Peripheral chondrosarcoma always arises in a preexisting osteochondroma and usually occurs in patients with multiple hereditary exostosis (diaphyseal achlasia). CS typically affects the pelvis, femur, and shoulder girdle and involvement of the foot and ankle is extremely rare. When CS occurs in the foot and ankle, the sites of involvement in descending order are the calcaneus, the tarsal bones, and the phalanges (Figure 4.20). The radiographic appearance is determined by the grade of the tumor. Low-grade central lesions show a lobulated border, whereas higher-grade lesions destroy the cortex and produce a soft-tissue mass. Central cartilaginous calcification may be present. Peripheral chondrosarcoma arising from a preexisting osteochondroma shows scattered calcifications within the enlarging, malignantly transformed cartilaginous cap. The MR imaging features of low-grade CS are a homogeneous low-signal-intensity mass on T1-weighted images with high signal intensity on T2-weighted images. Intervening low-signal-intensity fibrous septa are usually present. Matrix calcification is best seen on CT.[29]

OSTEOSARCOMA

Osteosarcoma (OS) typically occurs in children and adolescents. Approximately 2% of all cases occur in the distal tibia and fibula and about 1% arise in the foot, primarily in the tarsal and metatarsal bones. OS has been classified according to location (i.e., central, cortical, or surface), histology (i.e., telangiectatic, fibrohistiocytic, small cell, or chondroblastic), and grade (i.e., I, II, or III). All of these categories overlap; for instance, a parosteal osteosarcoma can be a low-grade surface tumor or a periosteal osteosarcoma can be intermediate grade and predominantly chondroblastic. These histologic patterns are more accurately predicted by radiography. The major role of MR imaging is to delineate the anatomic extent of the lesion and to identify "skip" lesions. Most OS show low signal intensity on T1-weighted images and varied signal intensity on T2-weighted images corresponding to the degree of bone formation and necrosis. Fluid–fluid levels may be seen in both necrotic lesions and telangiectatic OS (Figure 4.21).[2,13,30,31]

EWING'S SARCOMA

Ewing's sarcoma primarily involves the pelvis and lower extremities, but is uncommon in the foot and ankle. Children and young adults are typically affected by Ewing's sarcoma, and, when this lesion is encountered in the foot and ankle, the calcaneal lesions have a poorer prognosis than metatarsal lesions. Radiographs show a permeative or moth-eaten pattern of bone destruction with cortical breakthrough, periostitis, and a soft-tissue mass. The soft-tissue mass is often quite large and indicative of the invasive properties of the tumor. Sclerosis may be present secondary to reactive new bone formation. The MR imaging appearance varies with the degree of sclerosis and hemorrhage (Figure 4.22).[30]

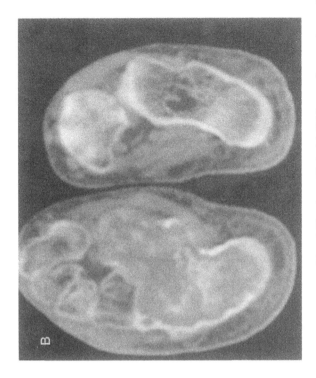

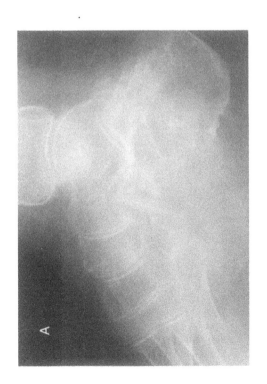

FIGURE 4.20 Chondrosarcoma. (A) Lateral foot radiograph shows destructive lytic lesion in calcaneus with calcification. (B) Axial CT image shows a destructive lesion of the calcaneus with extensive cartilaginous calcification characteristic of CS. (Courtesy of Mark Kransdorf, M.D., Mayo Clinic, Jacksonville, FL.)

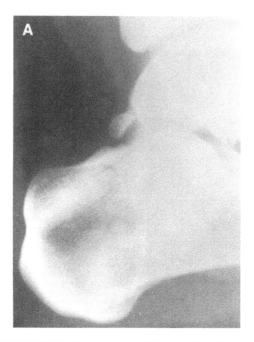 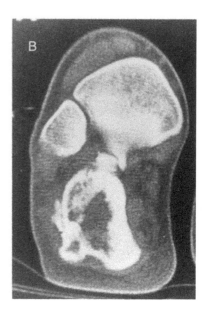

FIGURE 4.21 Osteosarcoma. (A) Lateral radiograph of calcaneus shows mixed lytic and sclerotic lesion involving the posterior facet. (B) Coronial CT image shows destructive lytic and sclerotic lesion of calcaneus with osseous matrix and cortical violation typical of OS.

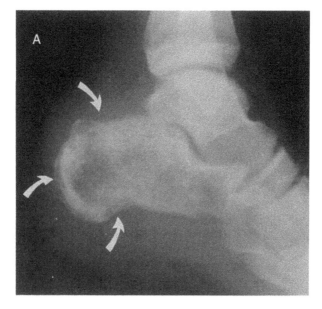

FIGURE 4.22 Ewing's sarcoma. (A) Lateral radiograph of the foot reveals a poorly defined lytic calcaneal lesion with patchy sclerosis (arrows) and possible breakthrough of the cortical tuberosity superiorly.

(*continued*)

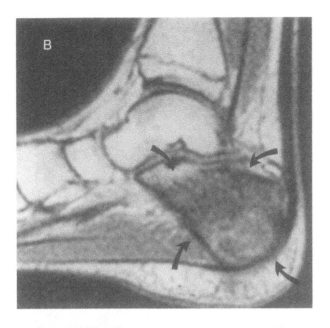

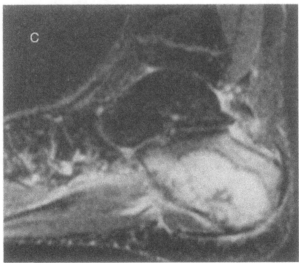

FIGURE 4.22 (continued) (B) Sagittal spin-echo T1-weighted and (C) inversion recovery MR images show complete marrow replacement of the calcaneus with low signal intensity on T1-weighted and high signal intensity on the inversion recovery images (arrows). It is unusual that the soft-tissue extension is limited in this Ewing's sarcoma.

METASTATIC DISEASE

Metastatic disease or myelomatous involvement of the foot and ankle is rare. When metastases occur in this anatomic region, the most common primary lesions are renal cell, colorectal, and lung carcinoma, and the calcaneus, metatarsals, and phalanges are most often affected. In this situation, metastatic disease is usually found in other skeletal sites. Radiographs generally show an aggressive lytic lesion and the MR imaging characteristics of myeloma and metastatic disease in this region are not specific (Figures 4.23 and 4.24).[10,32]

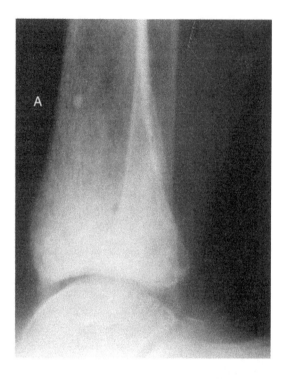

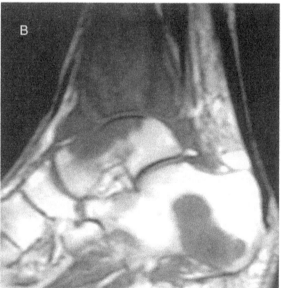

FIGURE 4.23 Metastatic disease. (A) Lateral radiograph of a 65-year-old female with symptoms of arthritis shows a mixed sclerotic/lytic pattern in the distal tibia and talus. (B) Sagittal T1-weighted MR image shows narrow replacement pattern in the distal tibia, talus, and calcaneus. (Courtesy of Don Fleming, National Naval Medical Center, Bethesda, MD.)   (*continued*)

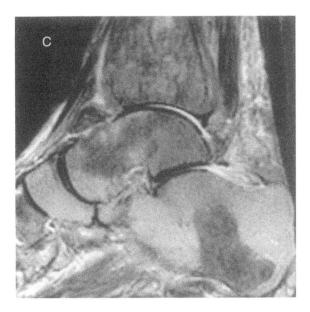

FIGURE 4.23 (continued) (C) Sagittal gradient-echo image shows mixed signal intensity. Chest radiograph on the woman later showed lung carcinoma. (Courtesy of Don Fleming, National Naval Medical Center, Bethesda, MD.)

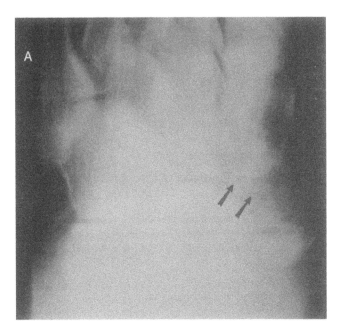

FIGURE 4.24 Plasmacytoma. A 57-year-old man with foot pain. (A) AP radiograph shows lytic lesion of right navicular (arrow). (Courtesy of Mark Kransdorf, M.D., Mayo Clinic, Jacksonville, FL.) *(continued)*

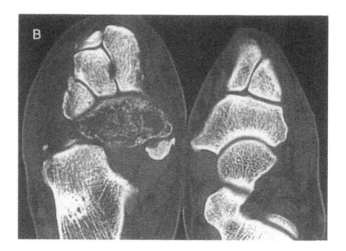

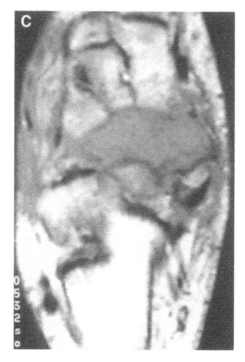

FIGURE 4.24 (continued) (B) Axial CT scan shows permeative expansile lesion of navicular bone. (C) Axial T1-weighted MR image shows marrow replacement of navicular, which is high signal intensity on T2-weighted image. (D) The findings of myeloma and metastatic disease are nonspecific. (Courtesy of Mark Kransdorf, M.D., Mayo Clinic, Jacksonville, FL.)   (*continued*)

SUMMARY

Bone tumors and tumor-like conditions of the ankle and foot are uncommon, and malignant lesions are especially rare. Radiographic characteristics are the most reliable predictors of specific tumor histology, whereas MR imaging remains more sensitive to the anatomic extent of the tumor. A working knowledge of which lesions occur most commonly in the foot and ankle may be the best aid to the diagnosis of lesions in this anatomic region.

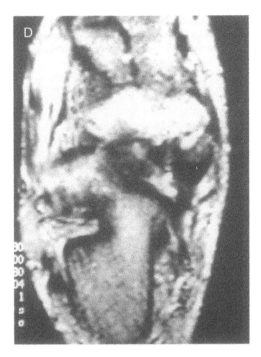

FIGURE 4.24 (continued) (D) The findings of myeloma and metastatic disease are nonspecific. (Courtesy of Mark Kransdorf, M.D., Mayo Clinic, Jacksonville, FL.)

REFERENCES

1. Berlin, S. J., A laboratory review of 67,000 foot tumors and lesions, *J. Am. Podiatr. Assoc.*, 74, 341–347, 1984.
2. Dahlin, D. C. and Unni, K. K., *Bone Tumors: General Aspects and Data on 8,542 Cases*, 4th ed. Charles C Thomas, Springfield, IL, 1986, 440–442.
3. Shankman, S., Cisa, J., and Present, D., Tumors of the ankle and foot, in *MRI of the Foot and Ankle*, Beltran, J., Ed., MRI Clinics of North America, W. B. Saunders, Philadephia, 1994, 139.
4. Harrelson, J. M., Tumors of the foot, in *Disorders of the Foot and Ankle*, Jahss, M.H., Ed., W. B. Saunders, Philadelphia, 1991, 1654–1677.
5. Bloem, J. L., Taminiau, A. H. M., Eulderink, F., et al., Radiographic staging of primary bone sarcoma: MR imaging, scintigraphy, angiography, and CT correlated with pathologic examination, *Radiology*, 169, 805–810, 1988.
6. Enneking, W. F., *Musculoskeletal Tumor Surgery*, Churchill Livingstone, New York, 1983, 719–741.
7. Deutsch, A. L., Mink, J. H., and Kerr, R., in *MRI of the Foot and Ankle*, Raven Press, New York, 1992, 348–354, 1992.
8. Erlemann, R., Reiser, M. F., Peters, P. E., et al., Musculoskeletal neoplasms; static and dynamic Gd-DTPA-enhanced MR imaging, *Radiology*, 171, 767–773, 1989.
9. Norman, A. and Schiffman, M., Simple bone cysts: factors of age dependency, *Radiology*, 124, 779–782, 1997.
10. Resnick, D. and Niwayama, G., *Diagnosis of Bone and Joint Disorders*, 2nd ed., W. B. Saunders, Philadelphia, 3854–3864.
11. Beltran, J., Simon, D. C., Levy, M., et al., Aneurysmal bone cysts: MR imaging at 1.5 T, *Radiology*, 158, 689–690, 1986.
12. Schoedel, K., Shankman, S., and Desai, P., Intra-cortical and subperiosteal aneurysmal bone cyst, *Skeletal Radiol.*, 25, 455–459, 1996.

13. Tsai, J. C., Dalinka, M. K., Fallon, M.D., et al., Fluid–fluid level: a nonspecific finding in tumors of bone and soft tissue, *Radiology*, 175, 779–782, 1990.
14. Feldman, F. and Johnson, A., Intraosseous ganglion, *Am. J. Roentgenol.*, 118, 328–343, 1973.
15. Milgram, J. W., Intraosseous lipomas: radiologic and pathologic manifestations, *Radiology*, 167, 155–160, 1988.
16. Herman, S. D., Mesgarzadeh, M., Bonakdarpour, A., et al., The role of magnetic resonance imaging in giant cell tumor of bone, *Skeletal Radiol.*, 16, 635–643, 1987.
17. Mechlin, M. B., Kricum, M. E., Stead, J., et al., Giant cell tumor of tarsal bones: report of three cases and review of the literature, *Skeletal Radiol.*, 11, 266–270, 1984.
18. Fuselier, C. O., Binning, T., Kushner, D., et al., Solitary osteochondroma of the foot: an in-depth study with case reports, *J. Foot Surg.*, 23, 3–24, 1984.
19. Dahlin, D. C. and Ivins, J. C., Benign chondroblastoma. A study of 125 cases, *Cancer*, 30, 401–413, 1972.
20. Capanna, R., Van Horn, J. R., Ayala, A., et al., Osteoid osteoma and osteoblastoma of the talus, *Skeletal Radiol.*, 15, 360–364, 1986.
21. Glass, R. G. J., Poznanski, A. K., Fisher, M. R., et al., Case report. MR imaging of osteoid osteoma. *J. Comput. Assist. Tomogr.*, 10, 1065–1067, 1986.
22. Jaffe, H. L., *Tumors and Tumorous Conditions of the Bones and Joints*, Lea & Febiger, Philadelphia, 92–105, 1950.
23. Klein, M. H. and Shankman, S., Osteoid osteoma: radiologic and pathologic correlation, *Skeletal Radiol.*, 21, 23–31, 1992.
24. Shankman, S., Desai, P., and Beltran, J., Sub-periosteal osteoid osteoma: radiology–pathology correlation, *Skeletal Radiol.*, 26, 457–462, 1997.
25. Shereff, M. J., Cullivan, W. T., and Johnson, K. A., Osteoid osteoma of the foot, *J. Bone Joint Surg.*, 65A, 638–641, 1983.
26. Yeager, B. A., Schiebler, M. L., Wertheim, S. B., et al., Case report. MR imaging of osteoid osteoma of the talus, *J. Comput. Assist. Tomogr.*, 11, 916–917, 1987.
27. Crim, J. R., Mirra, J. M., Eckardt, J. J., et al., Widespread inflammatory response to osteoblastoma: The flare phenomenon, *Radiology*, 177, 835–836, 1990.
28. Giannestras, N. J. and Diamond, J. R., Benign osteoblastoma of the talus. A review of the literature and report of a case, *J. Bone Joint Surg.*, 40A(2), 469–478, 1958.
29. Wu, K. K., Tumor review: Chondrosarcoma of the foot, *J. Foot Surg.*, 26, 269–271, 1987.
30. Boyko, O. B., Cory, D. A., Cohen, M.D., et al., MR imaging of osteogenic and Ewing's sarcoma. *Am. J. Roentgenol.*, 148, 317–322, 1987.
31. Wu, K. K., Tumor review: Osteogenic sarcoma of the foot, *J. Foot Surg.*, 26, 449–455, 1987.
32. Zindrick, M. R., Young, M. P., Daley, R. J., et al., Metastatic tumors of the foot. Case report and literature review, *Clin. Orthop. Relat. Res.*, 170, 219–225, 1982.

5 Tendons and Ligaments

Nancy M. Major and Clyde A. Helms

CONTENTS

TENDON AND LIGAMENT PATHOLOGY

Magnetic resonance (MR) imaging is playing an increasingly important role in examination of the foot and ankle. One of the more common reasons to perform an MR exam of the foot and ankle is to visualize the tendons and ligaments. Critical diagnostic information can be obtained, which the referring clinicians rely on to guide therapy. In many cases the result of the MR study determines the decision whether to operate or treat conservatively.[1]

PROTOCOL

Ideally, imaging of the ankle and foot should be done with the foot at right angles to the lower leg with the patient supine. Only the abnormal extremity should be imaged. A standard extremity coil is employed. Placing both feet in a head or torso coil leads to decreased spatial resolution from the increase in the field of view required. A field of view as small as possible is generally employed

(8 to 12 cm). A support may be required for the sole of the foot to maintain the alignment. Keeping the patient's foot immobile is necessary to avoid degrading the images due to motion. This may require additional padding. It is important to orient the plane of imaging perpendicular to the tendons to avoid the appearance of abnormal thickening of a tendon by the oblique orientation.

The imaging protocol should consist of T1-weighted or proton-density-weighted and some type of T2-weighted sequences such as conventional or fast-spin-echo (FSE) with fat suppression, (fast) short tau inversion recovery (STIR), or gradient-echo. Imaging should be performed in all three orthogonal planes. In general, the T1-weighted images define the anatomy while the T2-weighted images demonstrate pathology. Intravenous contrast is not necessary for evaluating ligament or tendon pathology.

TENDONS

The tendons of the ankle are conveniently divided into four groups based on their location in the ankle: anterior, posterior, medial, and lateral.

Tendons can be injured directly or by overuse. Abnormalities of the tendons on MR imaging consist of fluid completely surrounding a normal-appearing tendon (tenosynovitis), abnormal shape or size with increased signal intensity (tendinopathy), absence of a tendon segment (complete tear), or abnormal position (dislocation). Tendinopathy can be seen as focal or fusiform swelling of the tendon with increased intrasubstance signal intensity on the T2-weighted images (Type I tendon injury). Thinning or attenuation of the tendon reflects a more severe tendinopathy and is often a precursor to tendon rupture (Type II tendon injury). Complete tendon disruption (Type III tendon injury) is best visualized on axial imaging. The obliquity of the course of tendons in the ankle and foot can falsely demonstrate absence on the sagittal or coronal images.

POSTERIOR TENDONS

Achilles Tendon

The Achilles tendon comprises the conjoined tendons of the gastrocnemius and soleus muscles in the midline of the posterior ankle. The normal tendon is low signal intensity on all imaging sequences and shaped like a kidney bean. The Achilles does not have a tendon sheath and, therefore, a diagnosis of tenosynovitis is not applicable. Inflammatory change surrounding the Achilles tendon is referred to as paratenonitis. Anterior to the Achilles is a triangular fat pad called Kager's fat pad, which may show secondary features of tendon pathology.

If the Achilles loses its normal kidney bean shape and becomes more rounded anteriorly, the tendon is abnormally thickened. Complete disruption is commonly seen in athletes and often occurs spontaneously in males around 40 years of age. Rupture is also associated with other systemic disorders that cause tendon weakening such as rheumatoid arthritis, collagen vascular disease, crystal deposition disease, and hyperparathyroidism.[2] Tears may occur at the musculotendinous junction, but usually occur about 4 cm above the calcaneal insertion.[3] Therefore, the field of view on the sagittal MR images must be large enough to include this area.

Some surgeons use MR imaging to evaluate the size of the gap in complete disruption of the tendon (Figure 5.1). A large gap (retracted ends of the torn tendon) may indicate a need for surgical repair. If the ends of the tendon are not retracted, nonsurgical treatment is preferred. To date, however, no studies have been published to show this is in fact valid.

Xanthomas occur in the Achilles tendon in patients with familial hyperlipidemia types II and III.[4] The tendinous involvement is characterisitic of but not pathognomonic for xanthoma (Figure 5.2). The xanthomas are usually bilateral and cause fusiform focal or diffuse swelling with heterogeneous low and intermediate signal intensity on T1- and T2-weighted images. In some instances it may be difficult to distinguish between xanthomatous involvement and a partial tear of the Achilles tendon. The former diagnosis can be confirmed with laboratory studies.

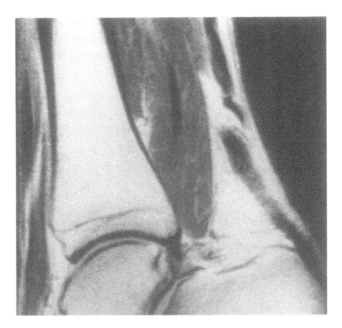

FIGURE 5.1 Achilles tendon rupture. T1-weighted sagittal image shows a torn Achilles tendon about 4 cm proximal to the calcaneal insertion without retraction. This patient elected for nonoperative treatment.

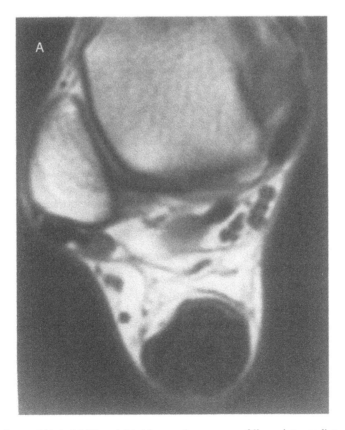

FIGURE 5.2 Xanthoma. (A) Axial T1-weighted image shows areas of linear intermediate signal faintly seen within a markedly enlarged Achilles tendon. *(continued)*

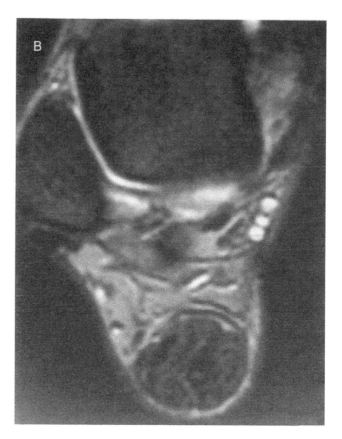

FIGURE 5.2 (continued) (B) Fast-spin-echo T2-weighted image with fat suppression shows heterogeneous signal in the markedly enlarged tendon.

Plantaris Tendon

As many as 90% of individuals have a small plantaris tendon, which lies anteromedial to the Achilles tendon and inserts onto the Achilles tendon, the posterior calcaneus, or the flexor retinaculum. The importance of identifying a plantaris tendon is to avoid mistakenly diagnosing a partial tear of the Achilles tendon because of the high-signal-intensity plane between the two tendons. Similarly, a completely torn Achilles tendon should not be misinterpreted as having some medial fibers intact, which are the fibers of the intact plantaris tendon. Evaluation of adjacent images will further clarify this situation (Figure 5.3).

MEDIAL ANKLE TENDONS (FLEXOR TENDONS)

The medial ankle tendons can easily be remembered by using the mnemonic "Tom, Dick, and Harry." "Tom" represents the posterior *t*ibial tendon and is the most medial tendon. "Dick" is the flexor *d*igitorum longus. "And" indicates the *n*eurovascular bundle, posterior tibial artery, vein, and nerve. "Harry" represents the flexor *h*allucis longus and is the most lateral tendon. The tendons are surrounded by individual tendon sheaths and they pass through the tarsal tunnel.

Posterior Tibial Tendon

The posterior tibial tendon (PTT) is the most common medial tendon to be abnormal at MR imaging. It is the largest of the three flexor tendons, roughly twice as large as the flexor digitorum longus, and demonstrates an oval shape. It passes beneath the medial malleolus and inserts onto the medial

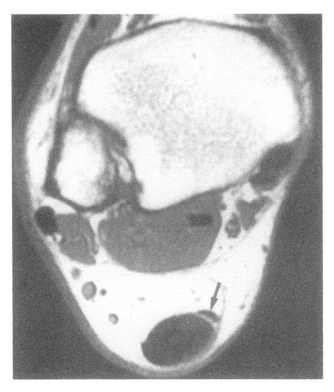

FIGURE 5.3 Normal plantaris tendon. Axial T1-weighted image demonstrates the low-signal-intensity curvilinear plantaris tendon (arrow) as it approaches the Achilles tendon. The high signal between the plantaris and Achilles tendon should not be mistaken for pathology.

navicular, cuneiforms, and the bases of the first through fourth metatarsals. As it sweeps under the foot, it supports the longitudinal arch. Tears of the tendon may result in loss of the longitudinal arch and a flat-foot deformity and are commonly encountered in patients with rheumatoid arthritis and middle-aged or older women. Additionally, there is a higher incidence of PTT tears in people with accessory navicular bones or those with large medial tubercles of the navicular (cornuate process). These bony anomalies result in altered stress and premature tendon degeneration.[5]

Most PTT tears occur more commonly at the level of the medial malleolus than they do distally. High signal intensity and thickening of the PTT can normally be seen as it inserts onto the medial aspect of the navicular and this appearance must not be confused with a tear. Abnormal signal intensity on the T2-weighted images in the tendon other than at the insertion is considered pathologic. It is not uncommon to see a longitudinal split tear of the posterior tibial tendon. In this situation the axial images will show "two" posterior tibial tendons (Figure 5.4) and has the same clinical significance as a complete rupture requiring surgery.[6] The secondary signs of PTT tears include loss of the longitudinal arch, a small spur or periosteal reaction along the posterior aspect of the medial malleolus.[7]

Thinning or attenuation of the PTT occasionally occurs as a prelude to complete rupture. It may be a chronic process, and, therefore, high signal intensity associated with inflammation or tenosynovitis may not be present. This abnormality is best identified on the axial T2-weighted images by noting that the PTT is smaller than the adjacent flexor digitorum longus[7] (Figure 5.5).

The PTT rarely subluxes or dislocates. When it dislocates the tendon is usually displaced in a medial and anterior direction relative to the medial malleolus.

The magic angle phenomenon can affect the PTT, and can mimic a tear. High signal intensity is seen in the tendon distal to the medial malleolus on a T1-weighted image. In fact, any short TE

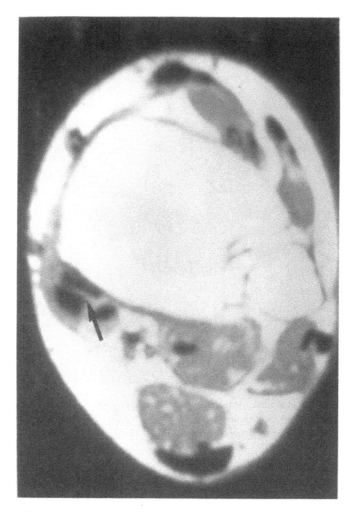

FIGURE 5.4 Longitudinal tear of posterior tibial tendon. Axial T1-weighted image demonstrates a longitudinal split tear of the posterior tibial tendon (arrow). Note the appearance of "two posterior tibial tendons."

sequence can result in the magic angle effect because of the anisotropic property of the PTT as it courses 55° to the bore of the magnet.[8,9] Note should be made of the appearance of the tendon on the T2-weighted images. If the high signal intensity disappears on the T2-weighted images, the conclusion can be drawn that magic angle effect was the cause of abnormal signal on the T1-weighted images.[8]

Flexor Digitorum Longus

The flexor digitorum longus (FDL) is rarely involved with pathology. It passes lateral to the PTT and divides to insert on the plantar aspect of the distal phalanges of the second through fifth toes.[10]

Flexor Hallucis Longus

The flexor hallucis longus (FHL) tendon is easily identified near the tibiotalar joint because it is typically the only tendon in the medial aspect of the ankle that still has muscle present at this level. It passes in a groove on the medial aspect of the posterior process of the talus, then beneath the sustentacululm tali, which serves as a pulley. It then continues between the hallux sesamoids and attaches to the base of the distal phalanx. The tendon sheath of the FHL communicates with the

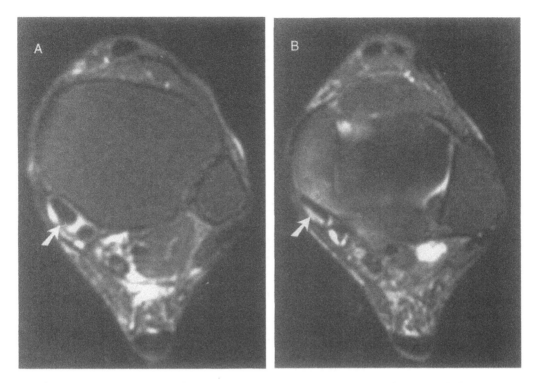

FIGURE 5.5 Attenuated posterior tibial tendon. (A) Fast-spin-echo T2-weighted image with fat suppression obtained above the level of the ankle joint shows fluid in the tendon sheath around the posterior tibial tendon. The tendon is normal in size and signal (arrow), but fluid is noted in the tendon sheath. (B) Axial image at the level of the talar dome. The posterior tibial tendon, in addition to fluid in the tendon sheath, shows marked attenuation. This appearance can be seen in a prerupture state. Note the bone edema adjacent to the posterior tibial tendon.

joint in about 20% of people. Therefore, fluid surrounding the FHL in the presence of a joint effusion is not considered pathologic.

The FHL is known as the "Achilles tendon of the foot" in ballet dancers because of the extreme flexion they use for prolonged periods.[11] Ballet dancers often have tenosynovitis of the FHL, manifested as fluid in the tendon sheath out of proportion with the quantity of tibiotalar joint fluid on T2-weighted images.

Focal asymmetric fluid within the tendon sheath is indicative of stenosing tenosynovitis, which is a result of focal areas of synovitis or fibrosis within the tendon sheath. This is often associated with os trigonum syndrome, which results from extreme plantar flexion causing the FHL to get trapped between the posterior malleolus and the calcaneus. This is one cause of posterior impingement syndrome, and has characteristic findings on MR imaging consisting of high signal intensity in the posterior soft tissues and/or talus on T2-weighted images, abnormal signal in the os trigonum, and FHL tenosynovitis (Figure 5.6).[12]

The distal end of the FHL tendon may be partially torn or develop tenosynovitis where it passes through the hallux sesamoid. These injuries are common in runners and ballet dancers.[13] FHL rupture is rare.

LATERAL TENDONS

Peroneal Tendons

The peroneus longus and brevis tendons are located posterior to the distal fibula and serve as the major everters of the foot. They are bound by a thin fibrous structure, the superior retinaculum. Proximally,

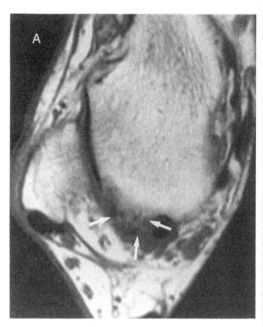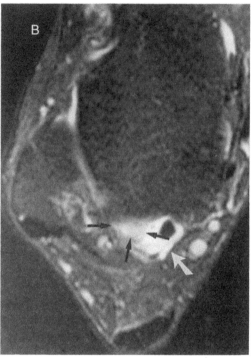

FIGURE 5.6 Os trigonum syndrome. (A) Axial T1-weighted image below the ankle joint shows low signal in the region of the os trigonum (arrows). (B) Fast-spin-echo T2-weighted axial image with fat suppression at the same level as (A) showing high signal in the os trigonum (arrows) as well as fluid in flexor hallucis longus tendon sheath (large arrow).

these tendons share a common sheath, then divide to form their own sheath distally. The tendons are located in close proximity to each other, using the fibula as a pulley and course adjacent to the calcaneus. The peroneus brevis runs anterior and slightly medial to the peroneus longus. Its muscle belly is also identified more distal than that of peroneus longus. The tendons can be separated by a small tubercle on the calcaneus with the peroneus brevis passing anterior to the tubercle; however, both tendons are usually located anterior to the tubercle. This information is useful to the surgeon to aid in planning the operative approach to the lateral ankle. The peroneus brevis inserts onto the base of the fifth metatarsal. The peroneus longus crosses the base of the foot to insert on the base of the first metatarsal.[10]

Entrapment of the peroneal tendons in a fractured calcaneus or fibula can occur and is easily recognized on MR imaging. This diagnosis can be overlooked clinically. Surgical intervention is required for treatment.[14–16]

A longitudinal split tear of the peroneus brevis is not uncommon, and can be a source of chronic lateral ankle pain. Patients usually have sustained an inversion injury accompanied by marked dorsiflexion. This mechanism forces the peroneus longus against the fibula, traps the peroneus brevis, and produces a longitudinal tear. The peroneus longus continues to invaginate into the peroneus brevis, resulting in delayed healing. The split tear usually originates at the level of the lateral malleolus and propagates proximally and distally. Surgical treatment is usually required. A few predisposing factors can lead to longitudinal split tears of the peroneus brevis. These include a thickened or torn superior retinaculum, a peroneus quartus muscle (an accessory muscle located adjacent to the peroneus brevis), a flattened peroneal groove on the posterolateral aspect of the fibula, a low-lying peroneus brevis muscle belly, and a bone spur.[17] It can be difficult to distinguish a low-lying peroneus brevis muscle from a peroneus quartus. A search for the small tendon of the peroneus quartus within the muscle can sometimes aid in the evaluation.

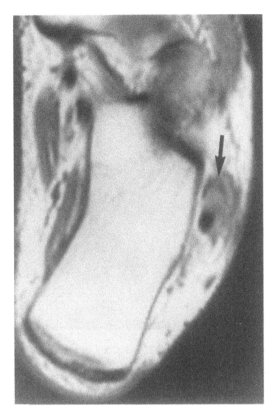

FIGURE 5.7 Longitudinal split tear of peroneus brevis. Axial proton-density-weighted image through the calcaneus shows a chevron-shaped peroneus brevis (arrow). This is characteristic of a longitudinal split tear of the peroneus brevis.

The axial images are important in evaluating longitudinal split tears of the peroneus brevis. A round or flattened low-signal tendon is considered normal. A chevron-shaped tendon is abnormal (Figure 5.7). Occasionally, high signal can be seen within the tendon, but is not essential for the diagnosis. The diagnosis should be made using the T2-weighted images because the "magic angle" phenomenon can show increased signal intensity within the tendon with short TE images.

The bifurcate or trifurcate peroneus brevis tendon is a normal variant, which may mimic a longitudinal split tear. In this instance, however, muscle bellies will be seen with each of the tendon slips, whereas a longitudinal split tear demonstrates a single muscle belly.[17]

Subluxation or dislocation of the peroneal tendons can occur. These tendons more commonly dislocate lateral to the fibula and are best seen on axial MR imaging (Figure 5.8). A predisposing factor for dislocation is a flattened peroneal groove. Usually the superior retinaculum is torn or has been injured producing laxity. Disruption of the superior retinaculum often occurs in skiing accidents and may result in displacement of the tendons (Figure 5.9).[18] This injury is often associated with a small avulsion fracture at the attachment of the superior retinaculum on the fibula. Retinacular tears usually require surgical correction.[19] Medial dislocation of the peroneal tendons is rare.

ANTERIOR ANKLE TENDONS (DORSIFLEXORS)

The four tendons found anterior to the ankle are the tibialis anterior (most medial), extensor hallucis longus, extensor digitorum longus, and peroneus tertius (most lateral). These structures dorsiflex

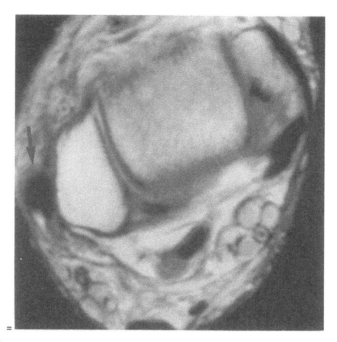

FIGURE 5.8 Dislocated peroneal tendons. Axial T2-weighted image at the level of the talar dome shows lateral dislocation of the peroneal tendons (arrow).

the foot and ankle and are infrequently involved by pathology. Of the anterior tendons, the tibialis anterior is most frequently subjected to injury.[20]

Tibialis Anterior

The tibialis anterior is the largest of the anterior tendons. Tears of this tendon are uncommon but have been reported in downhill runners and hikers. Patients may present with a mass rather than symptoms referable to a tendon abnormality.[21,22]

LIGAMENTS

ANKLE LIGAMENTS

Acute ankle ligament abnormaltites can be diagnosed clinically. In clinically equivocal cases or in patients with chronic lateral ankle pain, MR imaging is useful for evaluating the ligaments because many ligamentous abnormalities present with chronic lateral ankle pain. The anatomy of the ligaments around the ankle is straightforward and easily learned.

MEDIAL ANKLE LIGAMENTS

The deltoid ligament (medial collateral ligamentous complex) is a broad band and lies deep to the flexor tendons. It is composed of several structures: tibiotalar, tibiocalcaneal, talonavicular, and plantar calcaneonavicular (spring) ligaments. Because of its variable anatomic positions, only the tibiotalar and tibiocalcaneal ligaments are routinely identified on coronal images. The tibiotalar ligament courses between the medial malleolus and talus and is seen best on coronal MR images. It is inconsistently visualized on axial imaging as a striated structure. The tibiocalcaneal component of the deltoid has a vertical orientation and lies deep to the flexor retinaculum, but superficial to the tibiotalar component of the deltoid.[23]

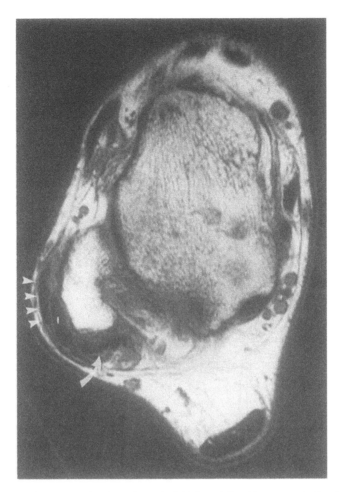

FIGURE 5.9 Torn superior peroneal retinaculum. Axial T1-weighted image at the level of the ankle demonstrates a thickened torn peroneal retinaculum (arrowheads) adjacent to a dislocated peroneus longus tendon (l). The peroneus brevis tendon (arrow) is split longitudinally. (Courtesy of A. R. Spouge, M.D., London, Ontario, Canada.)

The spring ligament is a thick triangular sheet that arises from the undersurface of the sustentaculum tali and attaches to the inferior and medial surfaces of the navicular. The spring ligament is a vital stabilizer of the longitudinal arch of the foot. It fills the gap between the anterior aspect of the calcaneus and the navicular. The plantar expansion of the posterior tibial tendon provides some support to the inferior aspect of the spring ligament. Laterally, the spring ligament is contiguous with the medial band of the bifurcate ligament, a Y-shaped structure joining the antero-superomedial aspect of the calcaneus with navicular and cuboid. Because of the complex orientation of the spring ligament, it cannot be imaged in a single plane. From an imaging perspective, the spring ligament has two parts: a medial, vertical portion that is continuous with the deltoid ligament (best seen axially) and a plantar, horizontal portion that is contiguous with the bifurcate and short plantar ligament (best imaged coronally). The spring ligament should not be confused with adjacent related structures such as the expansion of the posterior tibial tendon.[24]

The MR imaging appearance of an injury to the deltoid ligament depends on which components are injured. The T2-weighted coronal images may show a discontinuous ligament with or without hemorrhage and edema. A thickened ligament may indicate a chronic tear. The deltoid ligament is less frequently injured than the lateral collateral ligament complex.

LATERAL ANKLE LIGAMENTS

The lateral collateral ligamentous complex is responsible for over 90% of all ankle ligament injuries. It is composed of two parts: a superior (more proximal) group, the anterior and posterior tibiofibular ligaments, which make up part of the syndesmosis; and an inferior (more distal) group, the anterior and posterior talofibular ligaments and the calcaneofibular ligament (Figure 5.10). These ligaments are best evaluated on T2-weighted axial images with the exception of the calcaneofibular ligament, which is optimally identified on T2-weighted coronal images. The anterior and posterior tibiofibular ligaments are identified at, or slightly above, the tibiotalar joint. These two ligaments along with the interosseous membrane make up the syndesmosis. On

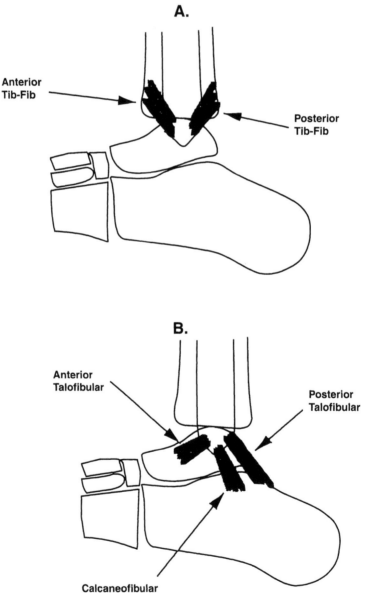

FIGURE 5.10 Proximal and distal lateral ankle ligaments. Schematic drawing demonstrating the proximal (A) and distal (B) lateral ankle ligaments.

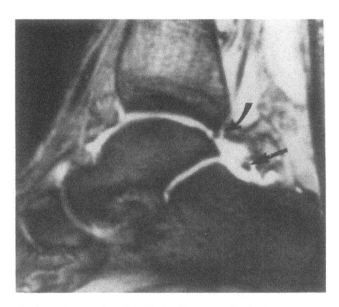

FIGURE 5.11 Loose body and posterior tibiofibular ligament. Sagittal gradient-echo image shows the posterior tibiofibular ligament as a round, low-signal structure mimicking a loose body (curved arrow). An additional round low-signal-intensity structure (straight arrow) represents a loose body identified on radiographs.

axial images, these ligaments are short, taut, low-signal structures on all sequences. The posterior tibiofibular ligament resembles an intra-articular loose body on sagittal images because it is surrounded by joint fluid. Knowledge of this appearance will eliminate an incorrect diagnosis of a loose body. Following the structure on adjacent images will identify this structure as the posterior tibiofibular ligament (Figure 5.11).

The anterior and posterior talofibular ligaments are seen on axial images below the tibiotalar joint emanating from a concavity in the distal fibula called the malleolar fossa. The calcaneofibular ligament is located just deep to the peroneal tendons best seen on the coronal images.

The most commonly torn ankle ligament is the anterior talofibular ligament. It is a thickening of the joint capsule, and is easily identified when joint fluid is present (Figure 5.12). It may be absent, attenuated, or disrupted when it is acutely torn (Figure 5.13) and joint fluid may be seen leaking out beyond the capsule. A chronic tear appears as a thickened, fibrotic ligament that may or may not be disrupted.[25,26] The anterior talofibular ligament is usually torn in isolation; however, with more severe trauma, ligament injury occurs in a predictable order. The calcaneofibular ligament is the next to tear and is rarely followed by a tear of the posterior talofibular ligament. The calcaneofibular ligament and posterior talofibular ligaments will not be torn without a tear of the anterior talofibular ligament.

The posterior intermalleolar ligament is a normal ligamentous variant of the posterior portion of the ankle. It is felt that this ligament plays a role in the development of posterior impingement syndrome. It is present in approximately 50% of the population and is variable in size, measuring from 1 to 8 mm wide and 5 to 8 mm in diameter. However, it is identified on MR examinations in only about 20% of patients.[27] The ligament has an appearance that resembles a meniscus. It is visualized on both coronal and axial images as a distinct low-signal band traversing between the posterior tibiofibular ligament and the posterior talofibular ligament (Figure 5.14). It originates from the posterior tibial margin and the lateral fibers may blend with the posterior tibiofibular ligament. A few fibers may reach as far as the medial malleolus. The ligament courses downward and laterally and inserts onto the fibula slightly superior to the attachment of the posterior

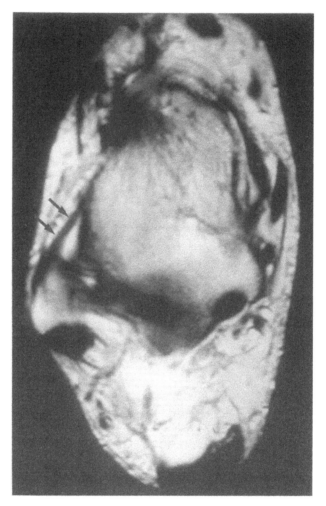

FIGURE 5.12 Normal anterior talofibular ligament. Axial T1-weighted image at the level of the malleolar fossa shows an intact anterior talofibular ligament as a linear low-signal structure (arrows).

talofibular ligament. Because it is located between the two malleoli, it has been termed the posterior intermalleolar ligament. Its meniscus-like shape and occasional extension into the ankle joint may account for the development of posterior impingement syndrome.[27]

Posterior Impingement Syndrome

Posterior impingement syndrome is a painful entity that is present in patients who assume extreme plantar flexion such as baseball catchers or ballet dancers. In this foot position, the intermalleolar ligament may herniate into the joint space. Patients complain of a locking sensation and pain in the posterior ankle joint. These lesions are treated surgically by removal of the ligament with relief of symptoms.[28] Other causes of posterior impingement, such as os trigonum syndrome, avulsion of the posterior tibiofibular ligament and loose bodies need to be excluded.

Several entities have an association with lateral ankle ligament tears. These include sinus tarsi syndrome, anterolateral impingement, and longitudinal split tears of the peroneus brevis tendon. Additional abnormalities such as osteochondral injuries and bone contusions can also be associated with inversion injuries and ankle ligament pathology, but are discussed in Chapter 3.

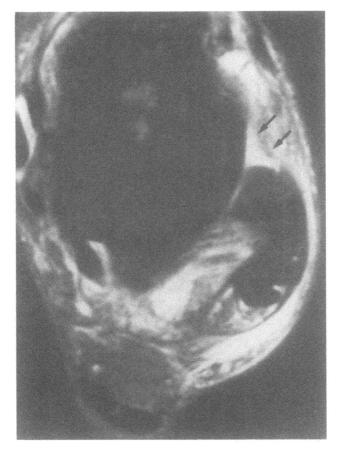

FIGURE 5.13 Torn anterior talofibular ligament. Axial fast-spin-echo T2-weighted image with fat suppression at the level of the malleolar fossa shows high-signal joint fluid (arrows) and absence of the anterior talofibular ligament.

Sinus Tarsi Syndrome

Sinus tarsi syndrome is frequently associated with lateral collateral ligament injuries. Torn lateral collateral ligaments are seen in up to 80% of patients with sinus tarsi syndrome, and up to one third of patients who tear the lateral collateral ligaments have been reported to have sinus tarsi syndrome.[29] Patients complain of lateral ankle pain and a feeling of hind foot instability.

The sinus tarsi is a fat-filled cone-shaped space that lies between the talus and calcaneus (Figure 5.15). The narrow portion of the cone is located medially. The large end opens beneath the lateral malleolus. Several ligaments are present within the fat-filled space. The most lateral of these ligaments are slips from the extensor retinaculum. Medial to these slips are the cervical ligament, and the interosseous ligament (most medial).[30]

The ligaments are not always well visualized in normal patients; therefore, inability to identify them does not necessarily correlate with pathology.[30]

MR imaging of the sinus tarsi syndrome shows obliteration of the fat in the sinus tarsi with low signal on T1-weighted images and high signal (inflammation) or low signal (fibrosis) on T2-weighted images (Figure 5.16). An acutely injured ankle may show replacement of the fat in the sinus tarsi because an effusion in a sprained ankle can obliterate the fat. Therefore, a diagnosis of "sinus tarsi syndrome" should not be made in the setting of an acute injury. Conditions associated with sinus tarsi syndrome include disrupted lateral collateral ligaments, posterior tibial tendon tears, and inflammatory arthritides.

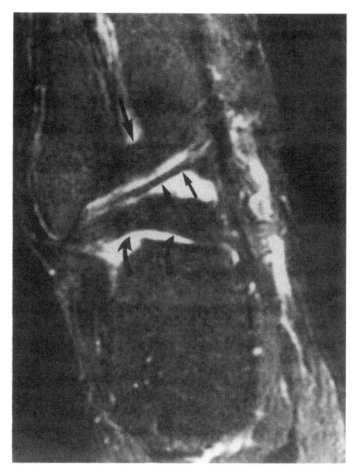

FIGURE 5.14 Posterior intermalleolar ligament. Coronal fast-spin-echo T2-weighted image with fat suppression at the posterior aspect of the ankle joint shows the posterior intermalleolar ligament (short arrows) bounded by the posterior tibiofibular ligament superiorly (long, straight arrow) and posterior talofibular ligament inferiorly (curved arrows).

In the past, the diagnosis has relied on clinical suspicion and therapy has included injection of xylocaine into the sinus tarsi to help resolve the pain. MR imaging now allows direct visualization of the sinus tarsi, and the treatment can vary depending on the findings, but includes steroid injections, tarsal sinus ligament reconstruction, surgical debridement, or joint fusion.

Anterolateral Impingement Syndrome

Anterolateral impingement syndrome is another cause of chronic lateral ankle pain. It results from entrapment of abnormal soft tissue in the lateral gutter of the ankle. The gutter is a space bounded anteriorly by the anterior tibiofibular and talofibular ligaments, medially by the talus, posteriorly by the posterior talofibular and tibiofibular ligaments, and laterally by the fibula. Superiorly, the space extends to the tibial plafond and inferiorly to the calcaneofibular ligament.[31] This space is an area where loose bodies can lodge.

Patients with anterolateral impingement syndrome usually complain of anterolateral ankle pain and swelling with limited dorsiflexion. They may experience a click or pop with dorsiflexion. Soft-tissue lesions causing this syndrome include hypertrophic synovium, fibrotic scar, or an accessory fascicle from the anterior tibiofibular ligament.

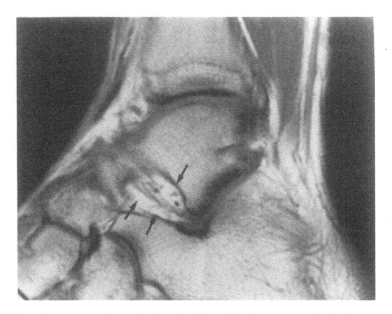

FIGURE 5.15 Normal sinus tarsi. Sagittal spin-echo T1-weighted image through the sinus tarsi demonstrates normal high signal intensity of fat (arrows) surrounding the linear low-signal subtalar ligaments.

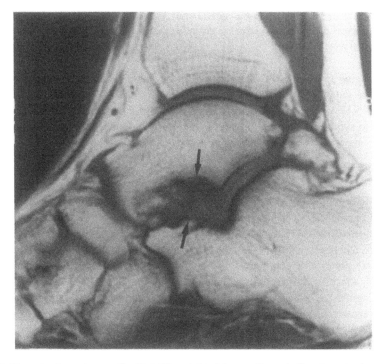

FIGURE 5.16 Sinus tarsi syndrome. Sagittal T1-weighted image through the sinus tarsi reveals abnormal low signal intensity filling the sinus tarsi (arrows) compatible with sinus tarsi syndrome.

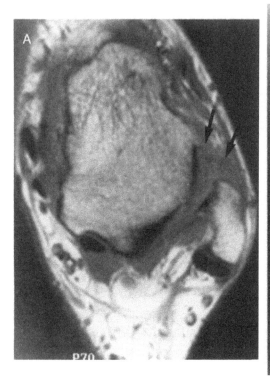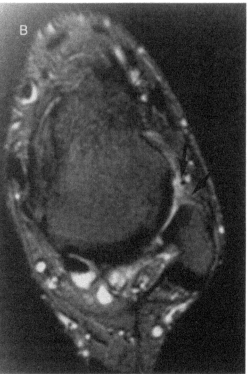

FIGURE 5.17 Anterolateral impingement syndrome. (A) Axial T1-weighted image at the level of the malleolar fossa shows low signal intensity in the anterolateral gutter (arrows). (B) Fast-spin-echo T2-weighted image with fat suppression shows low signal intensity in the anterolateral gutter (arrows) compatible with anterolateral impingement syndrome.

The MR imaging appearance of anterolateral impingement syndrome is manifested by abnormal soft tissue in the gutter with low to intermediate signal intensity on both T1- and T2-weighted images (Figure 5.17). It is postulated that injuries to the anterior tibiofibular and/or talofibular ligaments lead to synovitis resulting in anterolateral joint line tenderness and the subjective feeling of the ankle giving way. These lesions can be removed arthroscopically.[31]

PLANTAR PLATE OF THE FOOT

The plantar plate of the foot is formed by the plantar aponeurosis and plantar capsule, which arises from the distal plantar aspect of the metatarsal neck and inserts on the plantar aspect of the base of the proximal phalanges. The function of the plantar plate is to support the undersurface of the metatarsal heads and to resist hyperextension of the metatarsophalangeal joint. T1-weighted images show the plantar plate as a continuous low-signal structure abutting the plantar aspect of the metatarsal head, attaching at the proximal phalangeal base adjacent to the joint surface.[32] It can be difficult to distinguish the plate from the overlying flexor tendons. Because gradient-echo sequences show slight increased signal of the plantar plate, this sequence is recommended, as the plate can be more readily distinguished from the overlying flexor tendons, which remain lower in signal intensity. Three-dimensional (volume) acquisitions are also recommended to evaluate the plantar plate because of the higher resolution and ability to reformat in the appropriate oblique plane.[32] Poorly defined areas of high signal intensity may be seen in the plantar plate, but a diagnosis of rupture is made when the high signal intensity is more widespread and extends beyond the area of the plate attachment to the base of the proximal phalanx. Plantar plate disruption typically occurs

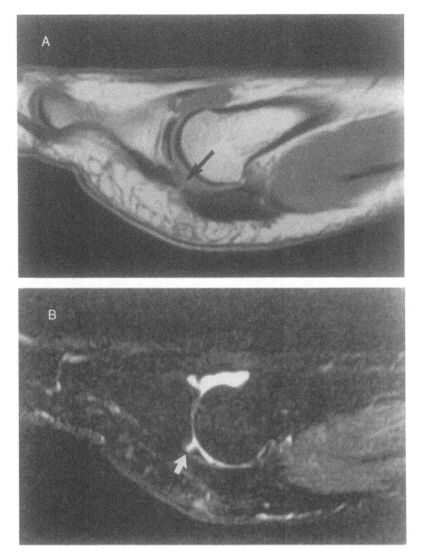

FIGURE 5.18 Plantar plate rupture. (A) Sagittal T1-weighted image through the metatarsal–phalangeal joint reveals abnormal high signal intensity in the plantar plate (arrow). (B) Sagittal fast-spin-echo T2-weighted image with fat suppression shows high signal intensity of joint fluid in the disrupted plantar plate (arrow).

below the metatarsal head, near the distal attachment of the plantar plate (Figure 5.18). Associated findings include synovitis of the metatarsal–phalangeal joint and hyperextension of the proximal phalanx. Additionaly, synovitis or effusion in the flexor tendon sheath may be a helpful secondary finding supporting the diagnosis of rupture.[32]

SUMMARY

In conclusion, MR imaging has improved the ability to identify pathologic processes involving the tendons and ligaments of the foot and ankle in a noninvasive fashion. Impingement syndromes and other associated pathologic processes of chronic ankle pain can accurately be assessed. Referring clinicians also find MR imaging extremely useful in guiding the clinical management of the patient with foot and ankle injury or pain.

REFERENCES

1. Anzilotti, K., Schweitzer, M. E., Hecht, P., Wapner, K., Kahn, M., and Ross, M., Effect of foot and ankle MR imaging on clinical decision making, *Radiology*, 201(2), 515–517, 1996.
2. Panageas, E., Greenberg, S., Franklin, P. D., Carter, A. P., and Bloom, D., Magnetic resonance imaging of pathologic conditions of the Achilles tendon, *Orthop. Rev.*, 19(11), 975–980, 1990.
3. Myerson, M. S. and McGarvey, W., Disorders of the insertion of the Achilles tendon and Achilles tendinitis, *J. Bone Joint Surg. (Am.)*, 80A, 1814–1824, 1998.
4. Dussault, R., Kaplan, P., and Roederer, G., MR imaging of Achilles tendon in patients with familial hyperlipidemia, *AJR*, 164, 403–407, 1995.
5. Miller, T. T., Staron, R. B., Feldman, F., Parisien, M., Glucksman, W. J., and Gandolfo, L. H., The symptomatic accessory tarsal navicular bone: assessment with MR imaging, *Radiology*, 195(3), 849–853, 1995.
6. Gazdag, A. R. and Cracchiolo, A. R., Rupture of the posterior tibial tendon. Evaluation of injury of the spring ligament and clinical assessment of tendon transfer and ligament repair, *J. Bone Joint Surg. (Am.)*, 79A (5), 675–681, 1997.
7. Khoury, N. K., Elkhoury, G. Y., Saltzman, C. L., and Brandser, E. A., MR imaging of posterior tibial tendon dysfunction, *AJR*, 167(3), 675–682, 1996.
8. Erickson, S., Cox, I., Hyde, J., Carrera, G., Strandt, J., and Estowski, L., Effect of tendon orientation on MR imaging signal intensity: a manifestation of the "magic angle" phenomenon, *Radiology*, 181, 389–392, 1991.
9. Erickson, S., Prost, R., and Timins, M., The "magic angle" effect: background physics and clinical relevance, *Radiology*, 188, 23–26, 1993.
10. Cheung, Y., Rosenberg, Z. S., Magee, T., and Chinitz, L., Normal anatomy and pathologic conditions of ankle tendons: current imaging techniques, *Radiographics*, 12(3), 429–444, 1992.
11. Kolettis, G. J., Micheli, L. J., and Klein, J. D., Release of the flexor hallucis longus tendon in ballet dancers, *J. Bone Joint Surg. (Am.)*, 78(9), 1386–1390, 1996.
12. Karasick, D. and Schweitzer, M. E., The os trigonum syndrome: imaging features, *AJR*, 166(1), 125–129, 1996.
13. Wakeley, C. J., Johnson, D. P., and Watt, I., The value of MR imaging in the diagnosis of the os trigonum syndrome, *Skeletal Radiol.*, 25(2), 133–136, 1996.
14. Rosenberg, Z. S., Feldman, F., Singson, R. D., and Price, G. J., Peroneal tendon injury associated with calcaneal fractures: CT findings, *AJR*, 149(1), 125–129, 1987.
15. Tjin, A., Ton, E., Schweitzer, M., and Karasick, D., MR imaging of peroneal tendon disorders, *AJR*, 168, 135–140, 1997.
16. Khoury, N. J., Elkhoury, G. Y., Saltzman, C. L., and Kathol, M. H., Peroneus longus and brevis tendon tears — MR imaging evaluation, *Radiology*, 200(3), 833–841, 1996.
17. Rosenberg, Z., Beltran, J., Cheung, Y. Y., Colon, E., and Herraiz, F., MR features of longitudinal tears of the peroneus brevis tendon, *AJR*, 168, 141–147, 1997.
18. Oden, R., Tendon injuries about the ankle resulting from skiing, *Clin. Orthop.*, 216, 63–69, 1987.
19. Sobel, M., Geppert, M., Olson, E., Bohne, W., and Arnoczky, S., The dynamics of peroneus brevis tendon splits: a proposed mechanism, technique of diagnosis, and classification of injury, *Foot Ankle*, 13, 413–422, 1992.
20. Deutsch, A., Mink, J., and Kerr, R., *MRI of the Foot and Ankle*, Raven Press, New York, 1992.
21. Khoury, N. J., Elkhoury, G. Y., Saltzman, C. L., and Brandser, E. A., Rupture of the anterior tibial tendon — diagnosis by MR imaging, *AJR*, 167(2), 351–354, 1996.
22. Dooley, B. J., Kudelka, P., and Menelaus, M. B., Subcutaneous rupture of the tendon of tibialis anterior, *J. Bone Joint Surg. [Br.]*, 471–472, 1980.
23. Klein, M., MR imaging of the ankle: normal and abnormal findings in the medial collateral ligament. Pictorial essay, *AJR*, 162, 377–384, 1994.
24. Rule, J., Yao, L., and Seeger, L., Spring ligament of the ankle: normal MR anatomy, *AJR*, 161, 1241–1244, 1993.
25. Schneck, C., Mesgarzadeh, M., Bonakdarpour, A., and Ross, G., MR imaging of the most commonly injured ankle ligaments. Part 1. Ankle anatomy, *Radiology*, 184, 499–506, 1992.

26. Schneck, C., Mesgarzadeh, M., and Bonakdarpour, A., MR imaging of the most commonly injured ankle ligaments. Part II. Ligament injuries, *Radiology,* 184, 507–512, 1992.

27. Rosenberg, Z. S., Cheung, Y. Y., Beltran, J., Sheskier, S., Leong, M., and Jahss, M., Posterior intermalleolar ligament of the ankle: normal anatomy and MR imaging features, *AJR*, 165(2), 387–390, 1995.

28. Hamilton, W. G., Foot and ankle injuries in dancers, *Clin. Sports Med.,* 7(1), 143–173, 1988.

29. Klein, M. and Spreitzer, A., MR imaging of the tarsal sinus and canal: normal anatomy, pathologic findings, and features of the sinus tarsi syndrome, *Radiology,* 186, 233–240, 1993.

30. Beltran, J., Munchow, A., Khabiri, H., Magee, D., McGhee, R., and Grossman, S., Ligaments of the lateral aspect of the ankle and sinus tarsi: an MR imaging study, *Radiology,* 177, 455–458, 1990.

31. Rubin, D. A., Tishkoff, N. W., Britton, C. A., Conti, S. F., and Towers, J. D., Anterolateral soft-tissue impingement in the ankle: diagnosis using MR imaging, *AJR*, 169(3), 829–835, 1997.

32. Yao, L., Do, H. M., Cracchiolo, A., and Farahani, K., Plantar plate of the foot: findings on conventional arthrography and MR imaging, *AJR*, 163(3), 641–644, 1994.

6 Soft-Tissue Tumors and Tumor-Like Lesions

Mark J. Lee and Peter L. Munk

CONTENTS

INTRODUCTION

Magnetic resonance (MR) imaging is accepted as the most effective and accurate way of evaluating known or suspected soft-tissue tumors of the foot and ankle. Although soft-tissue masses are relatively infrequently encountered compared with other conditions requiring imaging in the foot and ankle, accurate and detailed evaluation is critical in their proper management. With modern surgical techniques, even malignant tumors can often be readily treated with excellent clinical outcome. A variety of different conditions can also mimic both benign and malignant soft-tissue tumors and recognition of these is helpful in expediting treatment while avoiding unnecessary investigations or interventions.

MR imaging has generally been accepted as the primary modality for the evaluation of soft-tissue tumors because of its ability to delineate and stage lesions accurately.[1,2] The soft-tissue contrast available with MR imaging greatly exceeds that of its nearest competing imaging modality, computed tomography (CT) (although in skilled hands CT is reputedly as accurate as MR imaging in evaluation of soft-tissue masses). With current local coils and pulse sequences, it is also possible to evaluate adjacent bony structures accurately for possible involvement. The multiplanar capability of MR imaging is also advantageous in that it allows the surgeon to evaluate masses in a manner that would be analogous to the planned surgical approach should this prove necessary.[1]

Benign tumors are far more common than their malignant counterparts.[3–5] Their true incidence may well be much higher than reported as many patients with asymptomatic or minimally symptomatic lesions go unrecognized. Virtually all types of soft-tissue tumors found at other sites in the musculoskeletal system can also be encountered in the foot and ankle. In the following sections the more common entities will be briefly discussed and illustrated and a selection of more rarely encountered lesions will also be shown.

ROLE OF MR IMAGING

The role of MR imaging in the evaluation of soft-tissue tumors can be broadly divided into four principle categories:[6]

1. Detection

In general, patients who are sent for MR imaging of the foot and ankle will already have an established diagnosis of a soft-tissue mass. However, in many instances clinical evaluation does not allow definite confirmation of the presence of a mass and imaging may be required for further assessment. In some instances patients will have previous imaging studies that are equivocal. Occasionally patients will have conditions that are known to predispose to development of masses (such as neurofibromatosis) and monitoring of the lesion is required to evaluate for possible malignant transformation or other complications. In this circumstance, availability of previous imaging studies is invaluable. In cases where a questionable mass is noted clinically, detailed information is helpful in allowing imaging studies to be tailored to focus on the area most in need of evaluation.[1]

2. Characterization

Most benign soft-tissue masses have nonspecific findings. The vast majority of masses tend to show relatively low signal intensity on T1-weighted images, similar to that of surrounding muscle and increased signal intensity as T2-weighting is augmented.[1] Most lesions, unless they are very fibrous or have high nuclear-to-cytoplasmic ratios, demonstrate high signal intensity if fat-suppressed sequences are used. For this reason, specific characterization is often impossible.

The presence of specific signal characteristics in a soft-tissue lesion may occasionally allow the differential diagnosis to be greatly narrowed. For instance, the presence of hemosiderin, which is of low signal intensity on all sequences and tends to "bloom" on gradient-echo sequences, is strongly suggestive of pigmented villonodular synovitis or other hemorrhagic lesions. The presence of fat in a lesion suggests a diagnosis of lipoma or liposarcoma, or very occasionally, some other fat-containing lesion such as a hemangioma. Signal flow voids in a lesion are consistent with a vascular etiology such as an arteriovenous malformation (AVM).[1,8,9]

The location of the lesion will often also be helpful since some tumors occur in specific areas. Morton's neuroma, for example, is typically situated in the intermetatarsal space, usually toward the lateral aspect of the foot.

In general, specific characterization is often not possible and requires biopsy for definitive evaluation.[10]

3. Staging

It is in the role of staging soft-tissue tumors that MR imaging truly excels. This modality can more accurately evaluate the extent of a lesion and its relationship to surrounding structures than any other imaging technique,[1] permitting accurate surgical planning while minimizing unnecessary surgery or traumatization of normal tissues. Every effort should be made to determine which normal structures are involved, impinged on, or displaced by the soft-tissue mass.[11,12] Of particular importance is evaluation of any possible invasion or contact with surrounding bones, as well as encasement or impingement on neurovascular structures. The issue of accurate staging becomes critically important, particularly for malignant lesions, as it is vital that all involved structures be completely excised during the first surgery if the best long-term clinical outcome is to be achieved. In the case of malignant lesions, it may also be necessary to do other systemic staging examinations such as bone scintigraphy or chest CT to detect possible metastatic spread.

4. Post-Therapeutic Follow-Up

Subsequent to treatment, follow-up examination may prove necessary, particularly in the case of excision of malignant tumors. Occasionally, however, follow-up may be required following excision of some benign tumors that are prone to recur, particularly if a marginal excision has been performed.[1]

Follow-up examination is often difficult, especially in the acute setting as the anatomy has been distorted by surgery and/or radiation therapy. It is common to have abnormal high signal intensity in the treated region 3 to 6 months after therapy.[13] The abnormal signal may be focal or have a more diffuse feathery pattern. High-signal-intensity changes may persist on MR imaging for over a year.[14]

Postsurgical fluid collections (seromas) may also be encountered and, at times, can mimic a mass. In this situation, use of intravenous gadolinium is often helpful in proving a fluid collection is present. Blood tracks along fascial planes and septa result in apparent thickening and high signal intensity of these structures on T2-weighted and fat-suppressed sequences. With time, post-therapeutic edematous changes gradually regress, and comparison with baseline examinations 3 to 6 months after surgery often proves to be invaluable, often showing the development of low-signal-intensity scar formation. Use of intravenous contrast may occasionally be helpful in demonstrating nodules of a recurrent tumor. However, it should be noted that both immature scar and, to a lesser degree, edematous tissue can also enhance.

The Biopsy

Whenever possible, MR imaging should precede biopsy.[15] Performing a biopsy prior to MR imaging often introduces an undesirable artifact which may make interpretation of the examination difficult. Even fine-needle aspiration biopsies often produce a remarkable amount of hemorrhage, which may track along fascial planes and which, at times, can obscure the mass. Biopsy artifact may also potentially lead to overstaging.[15-17]

It is important to emphasize that prior to performing a biopsy, consultation with the surgeon who will provide definitive treatment of the lesion should be undertaken, as the biopsy track should follow the course of the anticipated surgical approach. Violation of this rule can significantly compromise patient prognosis as more extensive surgery and/or radiotherapy may be required occasionally, necessitating amputation.[11,16,17]

SPECIAL IMAGING CONSIDERATIONS

As a general rule, at least two imaging planes are desirable in the evaluation of the vast majority of soft-tissue tumors to appreciate fully the anatomic orientation of the lesion. The authors perform both T1- and T2-weighted sequences at a minimum for the evaluation of most tumors and usually also include a fat-suppressed sequence (either fat-suppressed fast-spin-echo T2-weighted or fat-suppressed inversion-recovery). These latter sequences are often helpful in demonstrating poorly defined or difficult to visualize tumors prior to planning subsequent sequences and are also helpful in confirming the presence of fat in a lesion.[18] In the situation where a soft-tissue mass abuts bone, fat-suppressed sequences can show subtle bone involvement by demonstrating bone marrow edema, even in the presence of minimal cortical change.

Gradient-echo sequences are useful in demonstrating the presence of degraded blood products such as hemosiderin. The presence of hemosiderin is frequently encountered in some hemorrhagic lesions, particularly pigmented villonodular synovitis or giant cell tumor of tendon sheath. Calcifications are also better demonstrated with gradient-echo sequences and may occasionally be encountered in lesions such as synovial sarcoma or soft-tissue chondrosarcoma.[1,9,19]

Most imaging can be performed with a standard extremity coil. However, in some instances it may be desirable to use other coils. In particular, examination of small lesions in the forefoot may be more optimally performed by positioning the patient prone in the bore of the magnet and placing a small surface coil adjacent to the area of interest. The authors have found this technique is particularly useful for superficial lesions or lesions in the intermetatarsal area, but some patients may find this position uncomfortable.

As a general rule, the field of view should be kept as small as possible while fully encompassing the lesion and demonstrating important adjacent structures. Use of the body coil results in a dramatic decrease in spatial resolution and should be avoided. Occasionally, imaging of the contralateral foot may be helpful if a variant of normal anatomy is suspected clinically; this is seldom necessary.

The use of routine intravenous gadolinium in the authors' experience is generally not warranted, as, in most instances, it does not typically add information useful in patient management except in selected situations. For instance, the use of intravenous gadolinium in evaluating large masses will occasionally help delineate the location of viable tissue, therefore permitting biopsy planning to avoid necrotic areas. In the postoperative setting, intravenous gadolinium is useful in delineating nodular tumor remnants or recurrent tumor. It should be remembered that immature scar is often highly vascular and may enhance significantly. Intravenous gadolinium can also be helpful both pre- and postoperatively in evaluation of suspected cystic lesions. The wall of a cyst shows enhancement, whereas the central fluid component does not.

DIFFERENTIATION OF BENIGN AND MALIGNANT TUMORS

It is often possible to differentiate between a benign and a malignant bone tumor on the basis of the radiographic appearance alone. The distinction between a benign and malignant soft-tissue mass is more difficult because the two cannot often be reliably separated.[10,20–25] Malignant tumors are frequently well-delineated lesions of uniform signal intensity just as benign lesions are. Certain features are suggestive of a more aggressive histology including bone invasion, aggressive destruction of tendons, and encasement of normal tissue structures. Bone invasion, however, is unusual even with malignant lesions, although when this finding is encountered, the histology will usually prove to be either malignant fibrous histiocytoma (MFH) or synovial sarcoma. Malignant lesions also frequently demonstrate inhomogeneous signal intensity.[20] However, this feature may be present in benign lesions as well, particularly in large traumatized (as not infrequently is the case in foot lesions) tumors. Assessment of the enhancement pattern of a mass following intravenous gadolinium administration is of very limited value as a significant fraction of benign and malignant tumors show overlapping enhancement patterns.[26–29]

For these reasons, in the absence of characteristic features of a benign lesion, most solid soft-tissue masses should be considered malignant until proved otherwise. This is particularly important in planning an imaging-guided biopsy since the biopsy route should be that which would be utilized if the lesion were known to be malignant (i.e., contamination of other muscle groups or tissue planes should always be avoided if at all possible).

SPECIFIC TUMOR TYPES

Several large series have demonstrated that the vast majority of tumors encountered in the foot are benign.[3,4] Kirby et al.[20] reported that 87% of foot tumors were benign, while the proportion reported by Berlin was even higher than this.[3,5] The proportion of benign tumors is likely even greater than that reported in the literature as many patients with benign lesions never present for evaluation. The following section briefly outlines the MR imaging features of a variety of benign and malignant tumors. This list is not comprehensive — the more common tumors have been included as well as a selection of less-often-encountered tumor types.[12,30,32]

BENIGN LESIONS

Morton's Neuroma (Interdigital Neuroma)

Morton's neuroma is one of the most common tumors of the foot. It arises from the intermetatarsal plantar digital nerves. It is characterized by neural degeneration and perineural fibrosis, and typically involves the nerves of the second or third intermetatarsal spaces. The diagnosis is usually made clinically by the typical history of pain radiating from the mid-foot into the toes which often can be elicited by lateral compression. Patients may also complain of numbness, typically worsened by walking and relieved with rest. Treatment requires surgical excision in most instances.[8,33,34]

Although the diagnosis may be simple if the classic findings are encountered on examination, at times, the clinical presentation can be atypical. In this situation it is desirable to have objective imaging findings of an abnormality in the suspected intermetatarsal space. Some success has been achieved in evaluation of patients using CT and ultrasound, but more recently numerous reports have suggested that MR imaging appears to be the most useful imaging technique in the diagnosis of these lesions.[8,33–35]

A variety of different MR imaging strategies have been proposed for visualization of Morton's neuromas. We position the patient prone with a surface coil and obtain images in the plane coronal to the forefoot through the region of the metatarsal–phalangeal joint, extending approximately as far as the proximal metaphysis of the metatarsals. Most authors have reported that T1- or proton-density-weighted images are most useful in visualizing these tumors (Figure 6.1). The tumors are seen as foci of diminished signal intensity and are generally well demarcated from adjacent fatty tissue. The use of fat suppression with concomitant intravenous gadolinium has been reported to be helpful in making these lesions even more conspicuous.[36] We have found the degree of enhancement is variable, making this strategy disappointing at times. On T2-weighted sequences, most Morton's neuromas do not brighten appreciably and the decreased signal-to-noise ratio and diminished signal intensity of the fat in this sequence actually may make these lesions more difficult to visualize.[37,38] The T2-weighted images, however, may be helpful in differentiating a suspected Morton's neuroma from fluid in an intermetatarsal bursa, a lesion that may resemble a

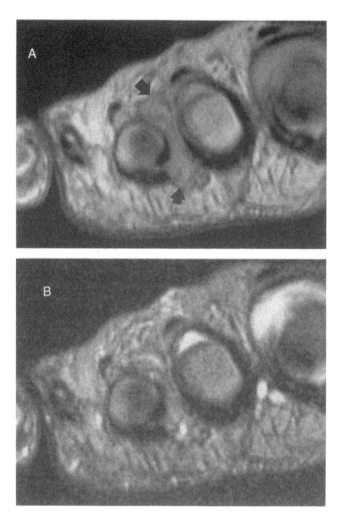

FIGURE 6.1 Morton's neuroma. (A) Coronal proton-density spin-echo image (TR2000/TE22) reveals a bulky dumbbell-shaped lesion (arrows) between the second and third metatarsals that shows low signal intensity relative to the surrounding higher-signal-intensity fat. (B) The coronal T2-weighted spin-echo image (TR2000/TE80) shows near complete obscuration of the neuroma. Note the small amount of high-signal-intensity fluid in the adjacent joints.

Morton's neuroma on T1-weighted images. The use of fat-suppressed inversion recovery (STIR) will occasionally show high signal intensity in a Morton's neuroma, but the acquisition time for this sequence is longer.[5,39]

One published report has suggested that the transverse diameter of symptomatic neuromas is generally 5 mm or greater. Occasionally smaller neuromas or multiple neuromas may be detected (Figure 6.2).

Pigmented Villonodular Synovitis and Related Lesions

Pigmented villonodular synovitis (PVNS) is an idiopathic proliferative lesion that can be either focal or diffuse and typically affects tendon sheaths and bursae, as well as the synovium of diarthrodial joints. Although this condition is most frequently encountered in the vicinity of the knee, virtually every joint has been reported to be affected. The lesion may be either villous or

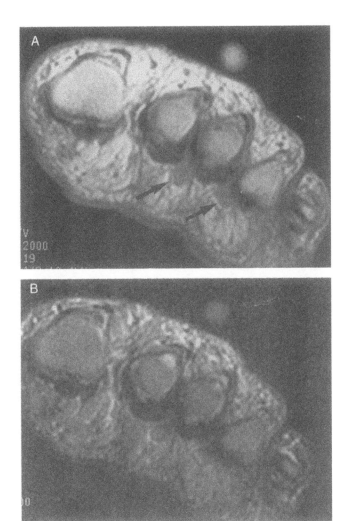

FIGURE 6.2 Multiple Morton's neuromas. (A) Coronal proton-density spin-echo image (TR2000/TE19) demonstrates two low-signal-intensity lesions (arrows) at the plantar aspect of the second and third interspaces, abutting the metatarsals. (B) The tumors are barely visible on the T2-weighted spin-echo image (TR2000/TE88).

frankly nodular. The nodular variety, which most commonly affects tendon sheaths, is sometimes referred to as giant cell tumor of tendon sheath[40,41] (Figure 6.3). Occasionally only a small focal area of a joint may be affected; however, it is not uncommon for the whole joint to demonstrate abnormal tissue and extension into the soft tissues surrounding the joint can occur in the foot and ankle.[3]

In most cases PVNS has a striking appearance on MR imaging because of the extensive hemosiderin deposition in the abnormal synovial tissue[42] (Figure 6.4). The lesion also contains fibrous tissue, which contributes to the low signal intensity typically seen on most sequences. Occasionally, fat in the lesion can also be identified due to the presence of abundant lipid-laden macrophages.[43]

Because of the large quantity of hemosiderin and extensive fibrous tissue, both T1- and T2-weighted sequences usually demonstrate generalized low signal intensity. In instances when a large amount of fat is present, areas of high signal intensity may occasionally be encountered on T1-weighted images.[44] Since these lesions are hemorrhagic, areas of inhomogeneity with high signal intensity on both T1- and T2-weighted sequences may be encountered, particularly in larger

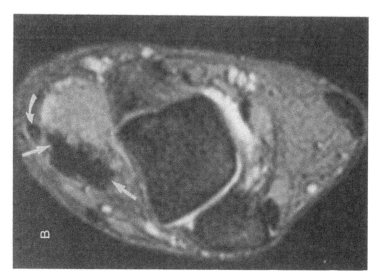

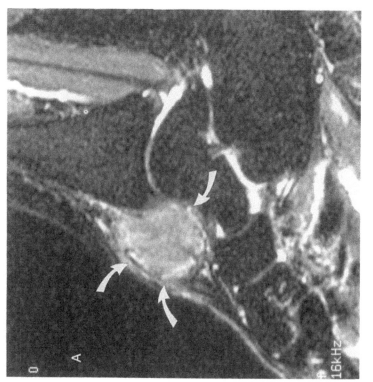

FIGURE 6.3 Giant cell tumor of tendon sheath. (A) Sagittal fast inversion recovery (TR3000/TI160/TEef34) demonstrates a globular mass at the anterior aspect of the ankle with slightly increased signal intensity (arrows), much less than that of the fluid in the surrounding joints. (B) Axial gradient-echo image (TR600/TE18 flip angle 40°) through the mass shows an irregular low-signal region (arrows) at the lateral aspect representing an area of hemosiderin deposition. Gradient-echo sequences make the presence of hemosiderin in tissues vividly apparent, as in this instance. The tendon of the tibialis anterior is separate from the mass (curved arrow).

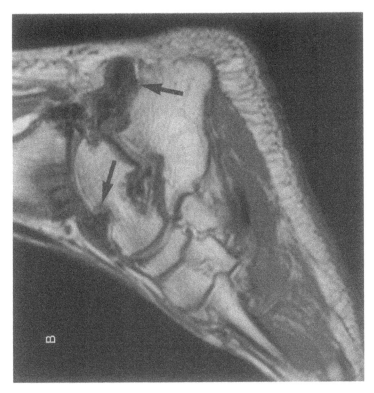

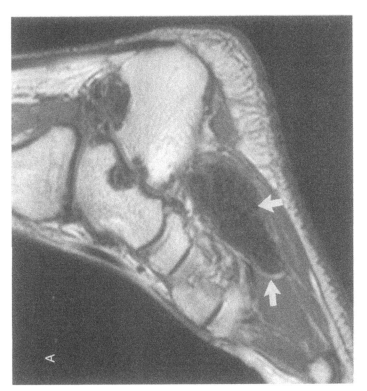

FIGURE 6.4 Multifocal pigmented villonodular synovitis. (A) Sagittal T1-weighted spin-echo image (TR 650/TE20) shows a bulky low-signal mass in the plantar musculature (arrows). (B) An adjacent image from the same sequence shows additional low-signal foci at the anterior and posterior aspects of the ankle joint (arrows). Degenerative changes in the anterior aspect of the tibiotalar joint are noted with narrowing of the joint and subarticular cysts. *(continued)*

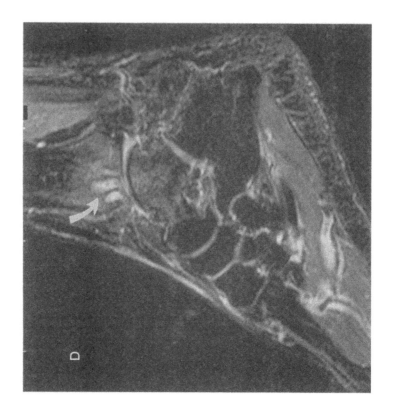

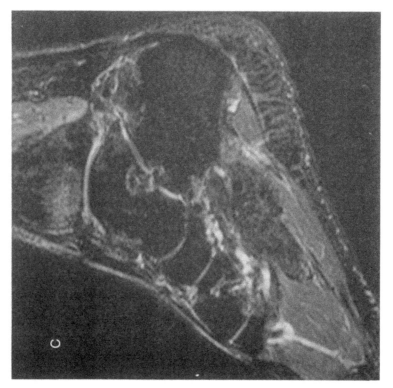

FIGURE 6.4 (continued) (C and D) Corresponding inversion recovery images (TR2000/TI160/TE30) demonstrate persistent low signal intensity of the lesions due to the extensive deposition of hemosiderin. Frequently, examples of PVNS with less hemosiderin show areas of increased signal intensity on this sequence. Note the high signal intensity in the subarticular cysts, which were found to contain only mucoid material and granulation tissue at surgery (arrow).

lesions.[41,43,45] The use of gradient-echo sequences accentuates the low-signal-intensity areas produced by hemosiderin deposition in the proliferative tissue due to magnetic susceptibility artifact inherent in this sequence. Demonstration of this "blooming" artifact on MR imaging should immediately suggest PVNS as one of the most likely diagnoses in the differential diagnosis. Administration of intravenous gadolinium typically demonstrates extensive enhancement, as these lesions are quite vascular.

In large lesions or those that have been present for a long period of time, adjacent bony erosion can be present, which may be detected on radiographs. Follow-up of patients who have been treated for PVNS is imperative because local tumor recurrence, even after extensive efforts such as complete synovectomy, is not uncommon.

Ganglia

A ganglion is a soft-tissue lesion that is commonly encountered and is usually associated with a joint or tendon sheath. On pathologic examination, a connection can often be demonstrated between the ganglion and the adjacent joint or tendon sheath, although frank communication is not usually present. Ganglion cysts may be either uni- or multiloculated and can insinuate between surrounding soft tissues. They are most frequently encountered on the dorsal aspect of the foot, but can occur at multiple sites and can produce significant symptoms, particularly if they occur in the tarsal tunnel or the sinus tarsi. Lesions that protrude dorsally may also interfere with footwear.[31,38]

Ganglia are often fluctuant and change in size, and may be associated with considerable inflammatory change should they rupture. At times, they may also present as a firm, hard mass. Sonographic examination often demonstrates the cystic nature of these lesions; however, sometimes ganglia can appear complex or solid on this modality because of the presence of a large amount of debris from hemorrhage or inflammation.

On MR imaging these lesions typically show low signal intensity on T1-weighted images unless they contain extensive proteinaceous debris or subacute hemorrhage.[46] Ganglia are often bright on T2-weighted images and, if they contain a considerable amount of debris, may appear very inhomogeneous (Figure 6.5). Intravenous administration of gadolinium will demonstrate peripheral enhancement unless the lesion is associated with considerable inflammation from previous traumatization and rupture, in which case the enhancement pattern may be more extensive and ill-defined. The cyst is usually located adjacent to a joint capsule or tendon sheath.

Plantar Fibromatosis

Plantar fibromatosis arises from the plantar aponeurosis where the fibrous tissue proliferates and eventually may involve adjacent skin or nearby deep structures. It typically occurs in young and middle-aged adults, and bilateral involvement may occur in up to 50% of patients. The usual presentation is that of one, and sometimes more, firm, fixed subcutaneous nodules on the plantar aspect of the foot, which frequently recur following excision. The mass may be painless, although involvement of an adjacent superficial plantar nerve can cause local paresthesia. Treatment is often conservative and typically involves the use of orthotics. Large or infiltrating lesions, or those that are particularly painful, may require excision.[38,47–49]

Plantar fibromatosis is most often found at the medial aspect of the plantar aponeurosis, which is not unexpected, as the aponeurosis is thickest in this location, and indeed it may be largely absent laterally. These lesions are usually well defined superficially due to the adjacent subcutaneous fat, but typically blend imperceptibly with the adjacent deep muscles and aponeurosis. On both T1- and T2-weighted sequences, the signal intensity is usually homogeneous but relatively low compared with that of adjacent skeletal muscle (Figures 6.6 and 6.7). Some brightening with fat-suppressed inversion recovery can occur and intravenous gadolinium demonstrates moderate enhancement in some cases.[48]

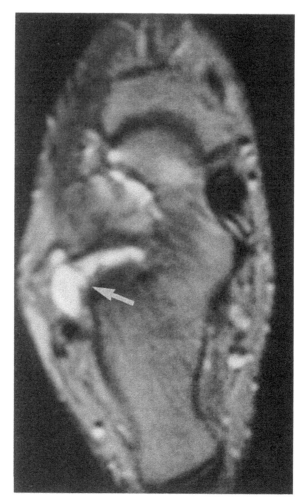

FIGURE 6.5 Ganglion of the tarsal tunnel. Axial T2-weighted spin-echo image (TR2000/TE80) demonstrates a high-signal-intensity lesion in the tarsal tunnel (arrow). The ganglion is elongated and slightly lobulated. The patient's pain resolved following excision.

Deep Fibromatosis

Deep fibromatosis is encountered less frequently than plantar fibromatosis and is seen most often in young adults. Usually solitary, these lesions may extend into the deep soft tissues and become applied to bone, which infrequently shows evidence of destruction.[50] The lesions are locally aggressive and are highly prone to recurrence after excision. For this reason, supplementary radiation therapy following surgery is frequently utilized.

Because of the significant fibrous content of these lesions, low signal intensity is often demonstrated on both T1- and T2-weighted sequences, although a modest increase in signal intensity on T2-weighted or fat-suppressed inversion recovery sequences may be encountered. Some enhancement is usually observed with infusion of intravenous gadolinium. Increased signal intensity on T2-weighted images and following intravenous gadolinium usually corresponds to the degree of cellularity, with more-fibrous lesions showing less signal intensity and enhancement.[50] The margination of the lesions is often fairly crisp, although recurrent lesions frequently show less well defined and more infiltrative margination as a result of adjacent scarring.

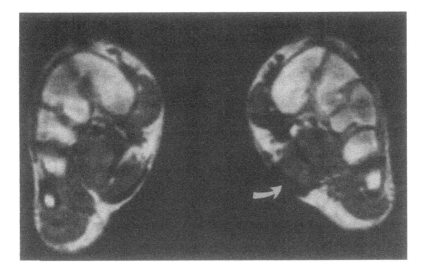

FIGURE 6.6 Plantar fibromatosis. Coronal T1-weighted spin-echo image (TR800/TE20) shows low-signal thickening of the plantar fascia of the left foot (curved arrow). The degree of thickening is well appreciated by comparison with the contralateral asymptomatic foot.

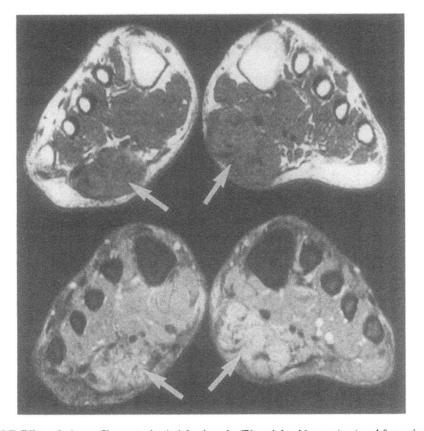

FIGURE 6.7 Bilateral plantar fibromatosis. Axial spin-echo T1-weighted image (top) and fast-spin-echo T2-weighted image with fat saturation (bottom) show a low- to intermediate-signal-intensity mass (arrows) extending deep from the plantar aponeurosis. The location and signal characteristics of the lesions are typical of plantar fibromatosis. (Courtesy of A. R. Spouge, M.D., London, Ontario, Canada.)

The neurovascular bundle is often ultimately involved by the lesion, at which time considerable symptomatology may be present, manifested by pain and numbness. Although histologically benign, the aggressive nature of these tumors is problematic and recurrent excisions and occasionally amputation is necessary.

Benign Neurogenic Tumors

The most common benign neurogenic tumors in the foot and ankle are neurofibromas, which may be part of the syndrome of neurofibromatosis (von Recklinghausen syndrome) and in this setting may be multiple (Figure 6.8). Neurofibromas often arise in small nerve branches and may therefore, at times, be very superficial.[38,51,52] These unencapsulated lesions are typically slow growing and may infiltrate the surrounding soft tissues, although this latter finding may not be appreciated on imaging.[53] Because of the infiltrative nature of these tumors, excision without sacrificing the affected nerve is usually not possible. A risk of malignant transformation of 10% is quoted and is more common in patients with neurofibromatosis.[54]

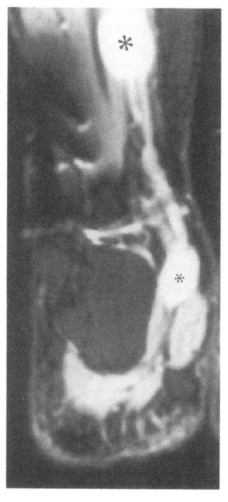

FIGURE 6.8 Multiple neurofibromas (von Recklinghausen syndrome). Coronal fat-suppressed inversion recovery image (TR2000/TI150/TE16) shows two medially situated lesions, at the level of the calcaneus (asterisk) and the second more proximally (asterisk). Both lesions show high signal intensity and are connected by the same nerve trunk. The patient had innumerable other neurogenic tumors throughout the body.

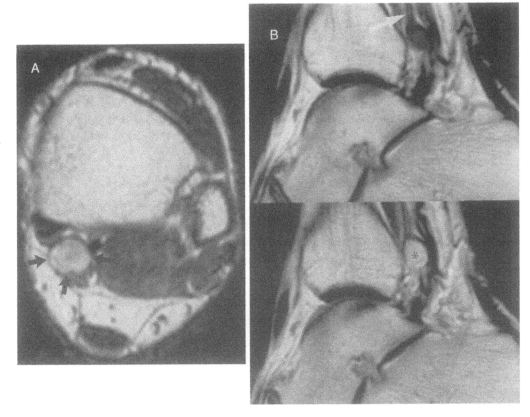

FIGURE 6.9 Schwannoma of the posterior tibial nerve. (A) Axial T2-weighted fast-spin-echo image (TR3000/TEef85) shows a well-defined lesion at the posteromedial aspect of the ankle immediately adjacent the tibia (arrows). The tumor is of mixed signal intensity. (B) Sagittal pre- (top) and post- (bottom) gadolinium-enhanced T1-weighted images (TR500/TE25). Precontrast the lesion is of low signal intensity, and brightens markedly after infusion (asterisk). Note that the nerve is thickened proximally (arrow).

On MR imaging, these tumors show low to intermediate signal intensity on T1-weighted images and increased signal intensity on T2-weighted images.[52–54] On T2-weighted images the lesions often appear inhomogeneous centrally, particularly with larger tumors, and cystic components may be present. The margins of the tumor are usually well defined and the adjacent nerve from which the tumor arises frequently demonstrates thickening over variable distance ("comet tail" sign) (Figure 6.9). Large chronic lesions may show remodeling of the adjacent bone.

Schwannomas are slightly less common than neurofibromas and demonstrate a true capsule on histologic examination. Surgical excision is more readily achieved than with neurofibromas as the nerve fascicles are not usually infiltrated. The MR imaging appearance of schwannomas is sufficiently similar to that of neurofibromas such that the two cannot be readily distinguished on this modality.

Lipoma

Lipomas are among the most common benign soft tissue tumors, but are not often seen in the foot. Lipomas are typically solitary lesions and usually present as an asymptomatic, poorly defined superficial mass. Less frequently, an intramuscular lipoma can present in the foot, although subcutaneous lesions are more common. Bulky tumors may require removal for cosmetic purposes, or, if particularly large, they can actually interfere with normal walking.[55]

The typical MR imaging appearance of a lipoma is manifested by a high-signal-intensity lesion on T1-weighted images with diminished signal intensity as T2 weighting is augmented (Figure 6.10). With fat suppression, the lesion will virtually disappear.[18] A thin capsule is not uncommon and tiny, thin septa can be present in the lesion. Nodularity within the septa or incomplete suppression on STIR sequences suggests that the lesion may be sarcomatous (i.e., liposarcoma) or may have undergone trauma with hemorrhagic foci. Small subcutaneous lesions may be difficult to detect on MR imaging and careful evaluation of surrounding subcutaneous septa is helpful, as the septa will be deformed or abnormal in the region of the tumor. If smaller lesions are palpable, the skin over the mass can be marked with a vitamin E capsule or similar means to help localize the tumor on the MR examination.

Synovial Osteochondromatosis

Synovial Osteochondromatosis (SOC) arises in joints but can occur in tendon sheaths and bursae. The process is characterized by synovial metaplasia, which results in the formation of multiple small cartilaginous or osteocartilaginous bodies usually associated with an effusion.[56,57] This SOC process typically involves a single joint and very rarely is associated with malignant

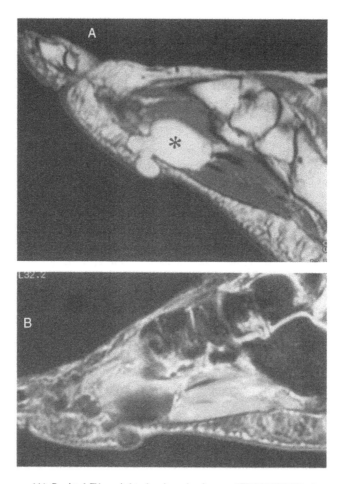

FIGURE 6.10 Lipoma. (A) Sagittal T1-weighted spin-echo image (TR800/TE17) shows a high-signal, lobulated homogeneous mass at the plantar aspect of the forefoot. The signal intensity is similar to that of the surrounding subcutaneous fat (asterisk). (B) Inversion recovery image shows near-complete signal drop-off in the lesion, consistent with a lipoma.

degeneration.[58–61] With time, the osteocartilaginous bodies gradually increase in size and number. The standard treatment involves complete excision of the metaplastic synovium and removal of the osteocartilaginous bodies. Large lesions may cause erosion of the adjacent bony structures.[57,62] Patients may present with a growing soft-tissue mass and/or painful joints or joint locking and grinding.

On T1-weighted images, the osteocartilaginous bodies are usually of low signal intensity unless they are sufficiently large to contain small areas of fatty marrow, which will be bright. The bodies may at times be difficult to differentiate from surrounding low-signal-intensity fluid. Rarely, these lesions may be hemorrhagic, in which case inhomogeneous areas of increased signal intensity can be seen. Calcified areas also show marked low signal intensity. On T2-weighted images, fluid in the joint becomes bright and often outlines the bodies (i.e., arthographic effect).[57,63] Gradient-echo sequences demonstrate the calcified foci to advantage with "blooming" in the areas of low signal intensity (Figure 6.11). If intravenous gadolinium is injected, pronounced enhancement of the metaplastic synovium at the margins of the fluid collection can be expected.

Hemangiomas and Other Vascular Malformations

This group of vascular lesions includes capillary and cavernous hemangiomata and arteriovenous malformations, all of which demonstrate abnormal-appearing blood vessels.[64,65]

Hemangiomas demonstrate abnormal small vessels, which are classified as capillary or cavernous depending on the vessel size. The vessels usually demonstrate stagnant blood flow and can be associated with phleboliths that may calcify. Not uncommonly, abnormally dispersed fat can be appreciated in the stroma of the lesion, although the relative proportion of fat in a given lesion varies considerably. These lesions can be located superficial or deep and involve muscle and other surrounding structures including bone.

On MR imaging, small vascular spaces with slowly flowing blood may be apparent, which, particularly on gradient-echo images, is of high signal intensity. T1-weighted images show the

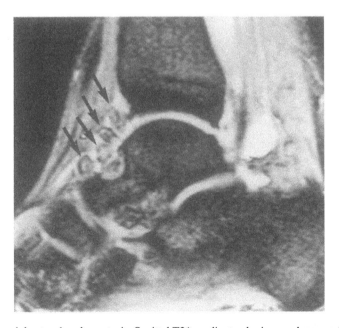

FIGURE 6.11 Synovial osteochondromatosis. Sagittal T2* gradient-echo image shows multiple intraarticular bodies (arrows) with rim and central punctate calcification in the anterior recess of the tibio–talar joint. Numerous bodies were found in the joint at arthroscopy, confirming the diagnosis. (Courtesy of A. R. Spouge, M.D., London, Ontario, Canada.)

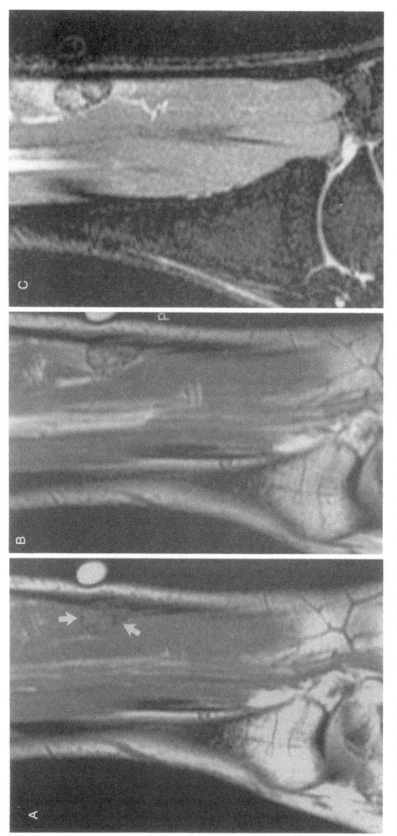

FIGURE 6.12 Epithelioid hemangioma. (A) Sagittal T1-weighted spin-echo image (TR650/TE15) reveals a small, mottled mass (arrows) applied to the anterior aspect of the Achilles tendon. Scattered low-signal-intensity areas are present within it. (B) Sagittal T1-weighted spin-echo image following intravenous administration of gadolinium better demonstrates the low-signal foci, which proved to be areas of hemosiderin. (C) Sagittal inversion recovery image (TR2000/TI150/TE16) shows high signal intensity in the lesion and a small amount of adjacent soft tissue edema.

vascular spaces as tubular areas of low signal intensity and also demonstrate any high-signal-intensity fat in the lesion to advantage. The lesion typically has a heterogeneous appearance with a globular configuration (Figure 6.12). On T2-weighted images, hemangiomas show increased signal intensity.[57,64] Phleboliths, if present, show low signal intensity on all sequences, and are seen to advantage on gradient-echo sequences.

Arteriovenous malformations usually demonstrate considerably larger vessels, which often have an irregular serpentine course. They may demonstrate enlarged feeding and draining vessels and/or aneurysms more proximally. If flow is sufficiently sluggish, fluid levels may even be seen within these vessels. Arteriovenous malformations may also involve adjacent structures including muscle and bone[64] (Figure 6.13).

MALIGNANT LESIONS

Synovial Sarcoma

Synovial sarcoma is one of the more common sarcomas of the lower extremity, although in terms of the total number of masses seen around the foot and ankle, it forms only a tiny subset. In spite of its name, synovial sarcomas rarely originate in an intra-articular location and are thought to arise from undifferentiated or mesenchymal cells. The only anatomic region more frequently afflicted by synovial sarcoma is the knee, and the vast majority are relatively deep. Typically, patients present

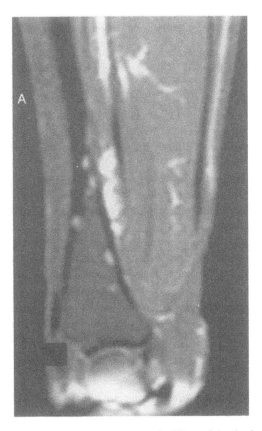

FIGURE 6.13 Arteriovenous malformation (AVM). (A) Sagittal T1-weighted spin-echo image (TR500/TR16) with fat saturation and gadolinium enhancement shows high-signal-intensity vessels immediately adjacent to the posterior cortex of the tibia. Punctate intramedullary high-signal foci can be seen.   (*continued*)

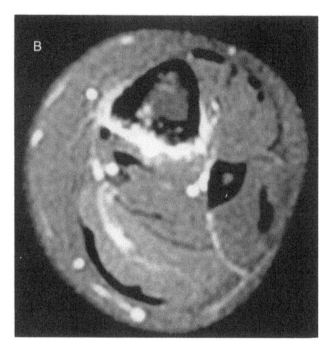

FIGURE 6.13 (continued) (B) Axial T1-weighted SE image (TR566/TR16) with fat saturation and gadolinium enhancement shows the irregularity of the posterior cortex and osseous involvement by the AVM.

with a long history of a slowly growing soft-tissue mass. Metastases are uncommon but they occur, generally involving the lungs and lymph nodes.

These tumors frequently have a fine sandlike or flourlike calcification, which may be visible on radiographs or CT. They are also quite vascular and generally show considerable enhancement with intravenous contrast on both CT and MR imaging.

On T1-weighted images these tumors typically show low signal intensity unless recent hemorrhage has occurred, in which case scattered areas of higher signal intensity are common. On T2-weighted images, synovial sarcoma shows increased signal intensity, although numerous foci of low signal intensity representing calcification or hemosiderin from previous hemorrhage may be visualized.[28,66,67] Due to the vascular and hemorrhagic nature of these lesions, fluid levels are not infrequently demonstrated.

The margination of these tumors is variable, but areas of invasion of surrounding structures should be sought.[68] Encasement of vascular structures and tendons may be encountered and synovial sarcoma, along with malignant fibrous histiocytoma, are the two sarcomas that demonstrate a propensity to invade surrounding bony structures. For this reason, close scrutiny of the osseous margins, as well as the intramedullary space of any contiguous bones, is important.

Intra-articular synovial sarcoma is rare and may present earlier as a result of hemorrhage into the joint. Subsynovial hemangiomas can also present in a similar fashion.

Leiomyosarcoma

Leiomyosarcomas are relatively rare tumors that are usually found in the retroperitoneum and gastrointestinal tract rather than in the soft tissues. The majority of these tumors probably arise from smooth muscle in small blood vessels and are much more common than soft-tissue chondrosarcoma or osteogenic sarcoma.[69,70] Peripheral leiomyosarcomas have a better prognosis than more central lesions as they tend to present when smaller and therefore at an earlier stage. They are also more amenable to complete excision. Leiomyosarcomas are often vascular and have a tendency to metastasize both to the lungs and liver.[71]

The MR imaging appearances of leiomyosarcoma tend to be relatively nonspecific and show low signal intensity on T1-weighted images and considerable brightening on T2-weighted images (Figure 6.14). Larger tumors may be quite inhomogeneous centrally on T2-weighted images if they are necrotic or have been traumatized. The borders of the lesions are relatively well defined.

Dermatofibrosarcoma Protuberans

This is a relatively well known clinical entity to oncologic surgeons, but is less familiar to radiologists. Patients typically present with slowly growing brownish nodules on the skin, which

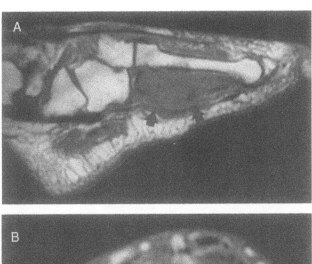

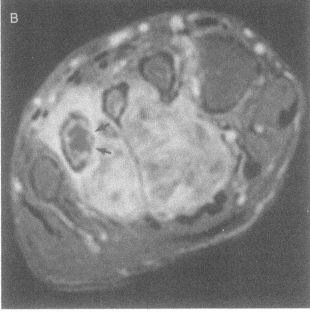

FIGURE 6.14 Leiomyosarcoma. (A) Sagittal T1-weighted spin-echo image (TR400/TE16) shows a mass of low signal intensity, similar to that of surrounding muscle at the plantar aspect of the foot (arrows). (B) Coronal T1-weighted spin-echo image (TR550/TE16) with fat suppression and gadolinium enhancement shows the bulky mass to better advantage. The tumor extends between the metatarsals. The medial cortex of the fourth metatarsal cannot be seen (arrows). At the time of surgery, partial destruction of the cortex was confirmed.

are frequently fixed to the underlying tissues. These lesions are often prone to trauma, particularly in the region of the foot and ankle, with ulceration and bleeding frequently occurring. Lesions that are neglected may demonstrate invasion of the adjacent soft tissues and bone. Treatment is by excision; however, local recurrence is extremely common. Distant metastases occur in a minority of cases, principally to the lungs and less commonly to lymph nodes although nodal metastases occur more frequently in association with dermatofibrosarcoma protuberans (DFSPs) than with many other types of soft-tissue sarcomas (with the possible exceptions of synovial sarcoma and embryonal rhabdomyosarcoma).[72]

The MR imaging characteristics of DFSP do not distinguish it from other soft-tissue lesions except for the superficial location of its epicenter. These lesions are often lobulated and frequently surrounded by subcutaneous fat. Deep penetration of the subcutaneous fat and extension to underlying fascia and muscle and, at times bone, may be seen on T1-weighted images. DFSP shows low signal intensity similar to that of adjacent muscle on T1-weighted images and moderate to marked increased signal intensity on T2-weighted images[72] (Figure 6.15). Enhancement of the lesion is to be expected with use of intravenous gadolinium.

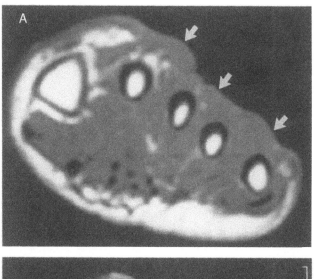

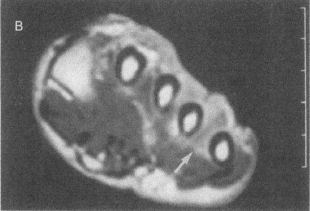

FIGURE 6.15 Dermatofibrosarcoma protuberans (DFSP). (A) Coronal T1-weighted spin-echo image (TR800/TE16) shows replacement of the high-signal-intensity fat at the dorsum of the foot by the tumor, which is isointense to the adjacent muscle (arrows). (B) Following intravenous infusion of gadolinium the tumor is more readily separated from the surrounding normal tissues. The lesion extends down to the dorsal surface of the metacarpals and into the intermetatarsal space at the lateral aspect of the foot (arrow).

Malignant Fibrous Histiocytoma

Malignant fibrous histiocytoma (MFH) is the most common soft tissue sarcoma encountered in adults. It frequently occurs in middle-aged to elderly individuals, but may be encountered at any age. MFH is notorious for its ability to recur following excision as well as its markedly infiltrating character, making confident surgical extirpation a challenge. Like synovial sarcoma, MFH may occasionally invade underlying bone and is the most common sarcoma to do so. The most common histologic varieties of MFH are storiform, myxoid, giant cell, and inflammatory, with storiform being the most frequently encountered.[73–75]

On T1-weighted sequences, MFH shows low to minimally increased signal intensity. With larger necrotic lesions, areas of inhomogeneity may be present and rarely tiny quantities of fat can be visualized. As T2 weighting is increased, inhomogeneity is frequently present, particularly with myxoid, cystic, or necrotic tumors.[74–76] At times, these tumors can show such pronounced increased signal on T2-weighted images that they may be mistaken for a cyst or abscess (Figure 6.16).

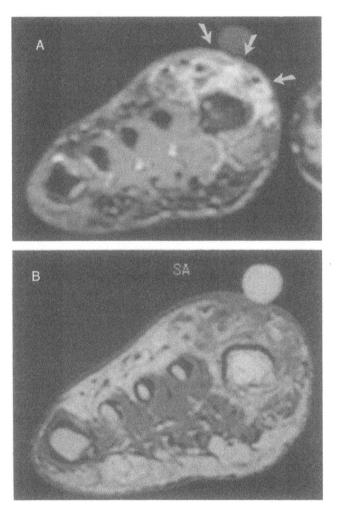

FIGURE 6.16 Malignant fibrous histiocytoma. (A) Coronal image through the great toe. Fat-suppressed fast inversion-recovery image (TR4000/TI150/TEef18) demonstrates a poorly marginated area of high signal intensity at the dorsal aspect of the digit, extending to the skin surface (arrows). (B) Precontrast spin-echo T1-weighted (TR800/TE15) contiguous images at the same level as (A) show the tumor is of low signal intensity and extends to the surface of the underlying bone. There is associated thickening of the overlying skin.   *(continued)*

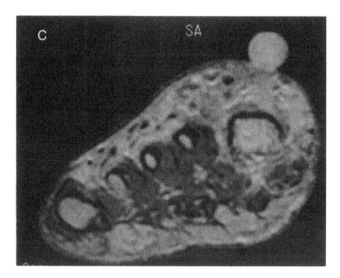

FIGURE 6.16 (continued) (C) Following infusion of gadolinium, the tumor enhances extensively. Without the use of fat suppression the tumor margins are less well appreciated than on the precontrast images. No cystic or necrotic foci were apparent.

Scattered areas of calcification are occasionally encountered and are seen as low-signal-intensity foci on all sequences that "bloom" if gradient-echo sequences are utilized.[73,77] Fat-suppressed sequences may demonstrate areas of bone marrow edema if the cortex has been violated.

MFH has a tendency to creep along fascial planes and inversion recovery sequences are sometimes helpful in demonstrating subtle changes in the fascia, which should alert the surgeon that a wide excision may be necessary. Use of intravenous gadolinium usually demonstrates extensive enhancement, which may be patchy as many of these tumors contain areas of necrosis, hemorrhage, or islands of myxoid material.

Melanoma

Melanoma is often also referred to as clear cell sarcoma of soft tissues if the lesion is intimately associated with a tendon, ligament, or an aponeurosis. Cutaneous melanomas are infrequently encountered in the foot and ankle and are usually demonstrated as small, intensely pigmented nodular lesions. Radiologists are frequently not called upon to image these superficial lesions.

The clear cell sarcoma variant of melanoma frequently occurs in a deeper location and often requires imaging.[78] Of these tumors, 75% occur in the lower extremity and are particularly common in the foot and ankle region. In spite of the fact that these tumors are not markedly pigmented on visual inspection, they usually contain melanin on microscopic examination. Treatment requires aggressive therapy, often involving amputation. Despite this, however, the prognosis is poor and metastases to lung and lymph nodes and, less frequently, to bone are commonly reported. Encasement of tendons and ligaments and, when present, invasion of adjacent bone can be visualized on MR imaging, the latter being optimally demonstrated on fat-suppressed T2-weighted sequences (Figure 6.17). The margins of the tumor may be indistinct because of the aggressive and invasive nature of these lesions. On T1-weighted images, these lesions are of low to intermediate signal intensity and may be of slightly higher signal intensity than adjacent muscle. On T2-weighted images, the lesions show greater inhomogeneity, but do not brighten significantly.[10] This latter feature may be attributed to the presence of melanin as well as the high nuclear-to-cytoplasmic ratio present in these tumors. A modest degree of enhancement with intravenous gadolinium can be expected. It should be noted that the involvement of tendons, muscles, and ligaments is usually best demonstrated in the short axis plane.

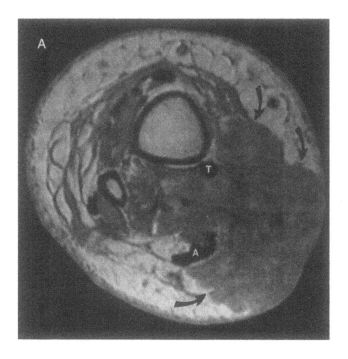

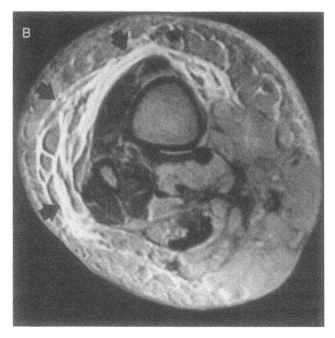

FIGURE 6.17 Clear cell variant of melanoma. (A) Axial proton-density spin-echo image (TR2000/TE16) shows a large, lobulated mass at the posteromedial aspect of the ankle and lower calf (arrows). The low-signal-intensity tumor is outlined by the surrounding fat. The mass partially encases both the Achilles (A) and the tibialis posterior (T) tendons. (B) The axial T2-weighted spin-echo image (TR2000/TE80) shows the tumor has increased only marginally in signal intensity and is now more poorly delineated from the surrounding fat. Note the high-signal-intensity edema anterolaterally extending along the fascia and sub-cutaneous septa (arrows).

Ewing's Sarcoma

This tumor usually arises from bone, but can also originate in the soft tissues. It is very closely related to primitive neuroectodermal tumor (PNET) and the radiologic manifestations are essentially congruent. The average age at presentation of soft-tissue Ewing's sarcoma is older than that of lesions arising in bone, although most cases are diagnosed before 30 years of age. Masses arising in the extremity are usually relatively painless. Lung metastases are not uncommon at the time of presentation.[79]

MR imaging demonstrates a low-signal-intensity mass on T1-weighted images, which brightens to a variable degree as T2 weighting is augmented. Foci of high signal intensity on both sequences are common as these tumors are frequently hemorrhagic (Figure 6.18). Changes in adjacent bone should raise the possibility of Ewing's sarcoma arising from bone rather than from soft tissue, but the treatment for both lesions is the same.

LESIONS THAT MAY MIMIC SOFT-TISSUE TUMORS

A variety of conditions can produce changes in the soft tissues of the foot, which can readily mimic a neoplastic mass.[23,80,81] At times, these conditions can be difficult to differentiate from a true soft-tissue tumor, but familiarity with some of the more common ones allows a correct diagnosis to be made.

Accessory Muscles

A variety of different accessory muscles are frequently encountered in the foot and ankle.[80] The accessory soleus is the best known of these; it presents as a soft-tissue mass arising from the anterior surface of the soleus or from the fibula and soleal line of the tibia.[82,83] It can insert into the Achilles tendon or superior aspect of the calcaneal tuberosity. The vast majority of these patients are asymptomatic, although occasionally patients give a history of exertional pain. In the absence of exertional pain, the signal intensity of the accessory muscle is identical to normal muscles. The classic location of this accessory muscle, which obliterates the fat in Kager's triangle, usually permits a simple diagnosis (Figure 6.19).

Other accessory muscles are less frequently identified. The peroneus quartus muscle usually originates on the distal peroneal muscles and has a variable attachment, most commonly on the peroneal tubercle of the calcaneus at the lateral aspect of the foot. Other small accessory muscles, such as the tibial calcaneus internus muscle, peroneal calcaneal internus muscle, and the accessory flexor digitorum longus muscle can also occasionally be encountered.[84]

Tophaceous Gout

Patients presenting with tophi in North America and the Western world in general have become far less frequent in recent years as a result of improvements in medical therapy for this disease. Typically, tophi appear in the chronic phase of the disease.

On MR imaging, tophi are usually of low signal intensity on T1-weighted images (Figure 6.20). On T2-weighted images, a variable increase in the signal intensity of the lesion can be observed.[49,85–88] This latter finding is likely partially dependent on the amount of calcification present in the tophus, with a heavily calcified lesion less likely to show increased signal intensity.[49,87] Patients with tophi may be quite symptomatic, due to both an associated inflammatory reaction, and a compression of adjacent structures by the lesion. Relatively uniform contrast enhancement following administration of intravenous gadolinium has been reported.[88] Adjacent bony erosions and intraosseous tophi may also be present.

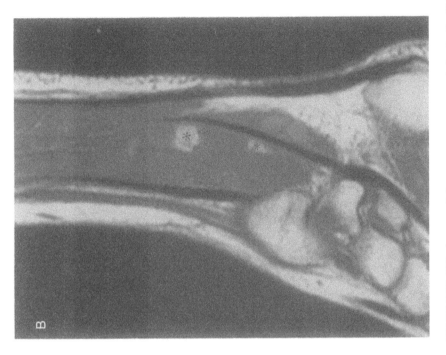

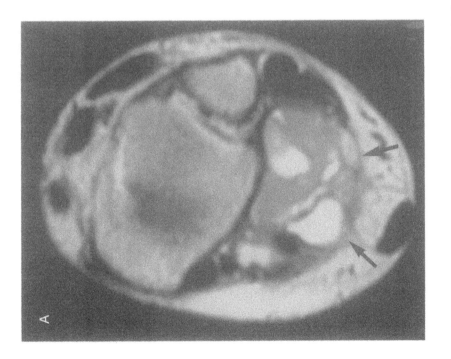

FIGURE 6.18 Ewing's sarcoma. (A) Axial T2-weighted fast spin-echo image (TR4066/TEef90) shows an inhomogeneous mass posterior to the tibia with no evidence of any cortical or medullary change within the bone (arrows). (B) Sagittal T1-weighted fast-spin-echo image (TR416/TEef8) demonstrates the mass is of low signal intensity with high-signal-intensity foci consistent with areas of hemorrhage (asterisks). *(continued)*

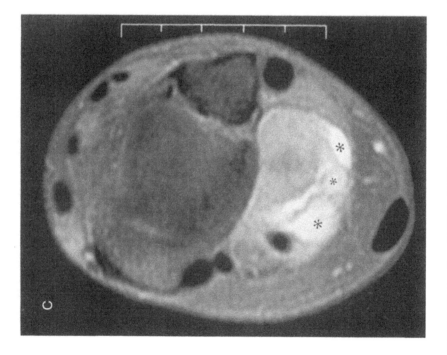

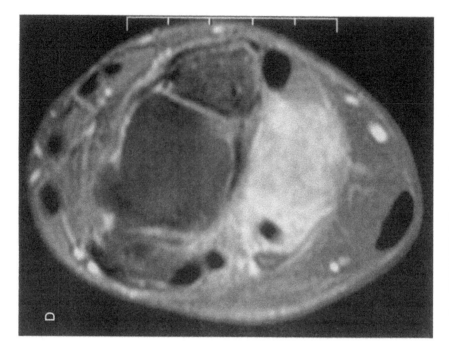

FIGURE 6.18 (continued) (C) Axial T1-weighted fast-spin-echo image with fat saturation (TR900/TEef8.5) reveals hemorrhagic high-signal areas posteriorly (asterisks). (D) Following intraveneous gadolinium only moderate enhancement is noted.

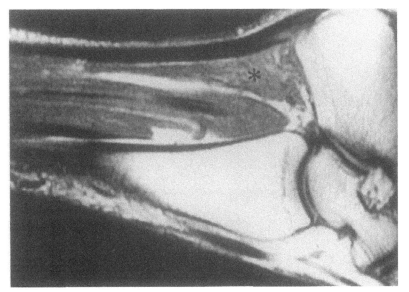

FIGURE 6.19 Accessory soleus muscle. Sagittal spin-echo T1-weighted image shows a typical accessory soleus muscle obliterating Kager's fat pad (asterisk). (Courtesy of A. R. Spouge, M.D., London, Ontario, Canada.)

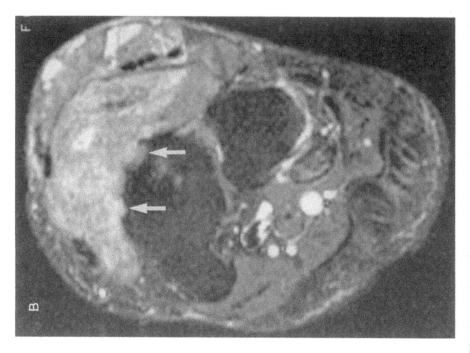

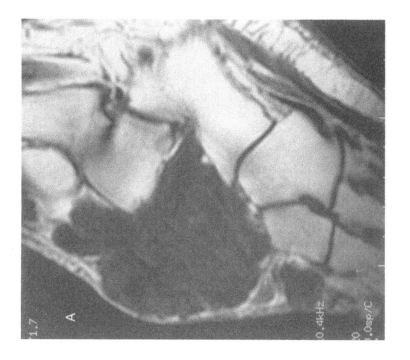

FIGURE 6.20 Tophaceous gout. (A) Sagittal T1-weighted spin-echo image (TR400/TE9) shows a large, homogeneous-appearing low-signal mass anterior to the talus. (B) Axial fat-suppressed fast inversion recovery (TR5550/TI130/TEef30) demonstrates scattered foci of increased signal within the mass. Note the anterior displacement of the tendons and the erosion of the anterior cortex of the talus (arrows).

Soft-Tissue Masses Associated with Underlying Bony Changes

A variety of different lesions originating in bone may present with a soft-tissue mass. Examples of these include stress fractures, bony metastases (Figure 6.21), or osteomyelitis (Figure 6.22).

Occasionally, inflammation around accessory ossicles can occur, which can be pronounced, particularly if a fracture is present. This is especially true in the vicinity of the os trigonum, but can be seen around many other ossicles including the os cuboidium, secundarium, or the accessory navicular. In this situation a small pseudobursa may be present, which shows low signal intensity

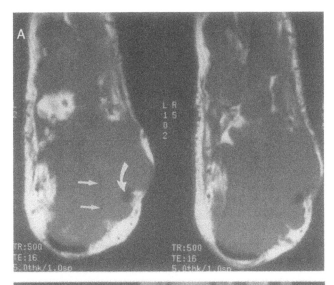

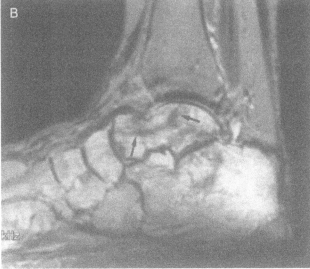

FIGURE 6.21 Diffuse breast metastases to bone. The patient had a history of mastectomy 7 years previously and presented with a soft-tissue mass at the lateral aspect of the foot. (A) Contiguous axial T1-weighted spin-echo images (TR500/TE16) at the level of the calcaneus. Note the bulky mass at the lateral aspect of the foot, with displacement of the peroneal tendon (curved arrow). A remaining shell of cortex at the lateral aspect of the calcaneous can be discerned (arrows). (B) Sagittal T2-weighted spin-echo image (TR2000/TE80) shows diffuse, patchy high signal intensity throughout the bones of the foot, with sparing of the tibia from metastatic breast carcinoma. The pattern would be consistent with a shower of tumor emboli to the foot. Note low-signal lines (arrows) in the talus representing an insufficiency fracture.

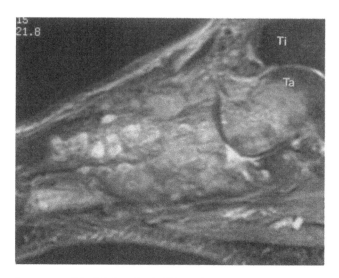

FIGURE 6.22 Chronic osteomyelitis (Madura foot). This patient presented with irregular soft tissue swelling due to chronic osteomyelitis from a mixed fungal infection. Sagittal fast inversion-recovery image (TR4000/TI150/TEef21) shows vague abnormal increased signal intensity in the bones of the foot. The soft tissues, especially dorsally, also show inhomogeneous areas of increased signal intensity. Due to the chronicity of this infection, considerable fibrosis can be present, and therefore the extent of edema is often less impressive than with acute infections. (Ti = tibia; Ta = talus).

on T1-weighted images and high signal intensity on T2-weighted images. In the absence of a bursa, irregular soft-tissue edema can be present in the surrounding soft tissues.

Soft-Tissue Inflammation

In most instances inflammatory change in the soft tissues can be readily identified clinically. On occasion, subacute or chronic changes may mimic a tumor, especially if a clear history is not available. Abscesses, cellulitis, or panniculitis fall into this category[89–93] (Figure 6.23 and 6.24).

Tendon Abnormalities

Patients can sometimes present with post-traumatic or inflammatory changes in or adjacent to a tendon or tendon sheath. A particularly common example of this is a partial or complete tendon tear. Although any tendon can potentially be involved, abnormalities of the Achilles, posterior tibial, and peroneal tendons are particularly common. Abnormal signal intensity in the substance of the low-signal tendon is present on all sequences, and is most prominent on fat-suppressed T2-weighted images[94,95] (Figure 6.25). Fluid in a distended tendon sheath can also be present, manifested by low signal intensity on T1-weighted images and high signal intensity on T2-weighted images. Infectious tenosynovitis produces similar but often more pronounced findings. Although these findings are usually evident on longitudinal images, it is important to obtain axial images of the tendon to assess the tendon adequately.

Varicosities

Occasionally distended veins can produce mass effect and become symptomatic. The appearance on MR imaging can sometimes be accentuated by placing a tourniquet above the ankle to distend the veins further. We have found that T2-weighted spin-echo, STIR, and gradient-echo sequences are particularly helpful in demonstrating the varicosities, which show high signal intensity on these sequences (Figure 6.26).

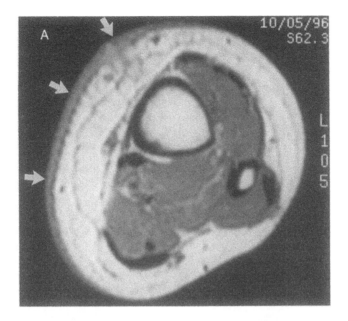

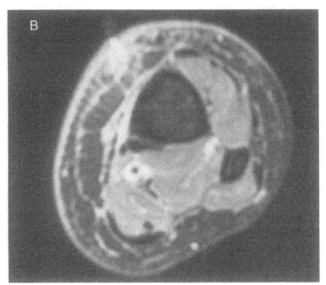

FIGURE 6.23 Panniculitis. The patient presented with ill-defined thickening on clinical examination and a superficial lipoma or other tumor was suspected. (A) Axial proton-density spin-echo image (TR2000/16) just above the level of the ankle joint demonstrates skin thickening medially (arrows) and coarsening of the septa in the subcutaneous tissues. (B) Inversion-recovery image (TR2000/TI150/TE18) demonstrates increased signal in the same structures noted in (A), as well as increased signal in the deep fascia.

SUMMARY

In summary, the foot and ankle can harbor a wide variety of benign and malignant soft-tissue masses. Attention to their location and imaging characteristics or radiographs, CT, and MR imaging should allow one to generate a reasonable differential diagnosis in most cases. In all cases, close cooperation with the referring physician and/or surgeon is critical. Follow-up of the histology of the lesions is also helpful in gaining a better understanding of these lesions.

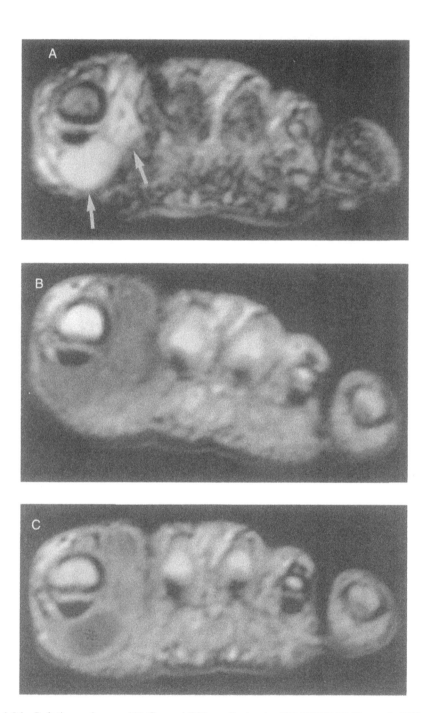

FIGURE 6.24 Soft-tissue abscess. (A) Coronal T2* gradient-echo (TR400/TE 20 flip angle 20°) shows an area of uniform high signal intensity at the plantar aspect of the first toe extending into the first web space (arrows). (B) Precontrast T1-weighted spin-echo image (TR500/TE21) shows the same region is of low signal intensity. (C) Following infusion of intravenous gadolinium an area of rim enhancement is noted surrounding the fluid-filled abscess at the plantar aspect of the toe (asterisk). The area in the web space enhances more diffusely, which indicates that this area represents nonliquefied inflamed tissue.

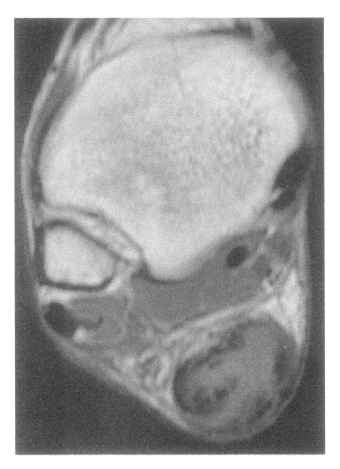

FIGURE 6.25 High-grade partial tear of the Achilles tendon. Axial T1-weighted spin-echo (TR500/TE19) image through the distal tendon demonstrates marked thickening and increased signal intensity of the tendon with a few remaining scattered low-signal-intensity tendon fibers.

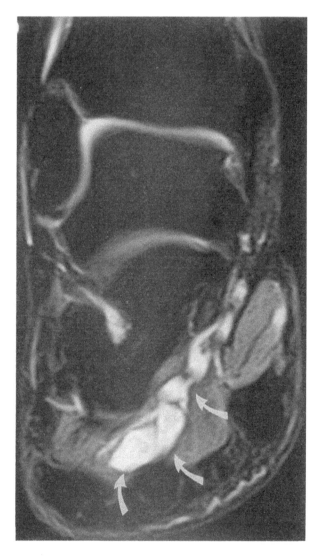

FIGURE 6.26 Varicosities. Coronal inversion-recovery image (TR2247/TI150/TE30) demonstrates high-signal-intensity serpentine structures in the region of the tarsal tunnel (arrows). When sufficiently dilated, these varicosities can produce compression and irritation of adjacent structures.

REFERENCES

1. Sharafuddin, M. J. A. and Sundaram, M., The role of magnetic resonance imaging in the diagnosis of soft tissue lesions, *Crit. Rev. Diag. Imaging*, 35, 379–483, 1994.
2. Demas, B. E., Heelan, R. T., Lane, J., Marcove, R., Hajdu, S., and Brennan, M. F., Soft-tissue sarcomas of the extremities: comparison of MR and CT in determining the extent of disease, *AJR*, 150, 615–620, 1988.
3. Kirby, E. J., A Laboratory Review of 67,000 foot tumors and lesions, *J. Am. Podiatr. Assoc.*, 74, 341–347, 1984.
4. Kransdorf, M. J., Benign Soft-tissue tumors in a large referral population: Distribution of specific diagnoses by age, sex and location, *AJR.*, 164, 395–402, 1995.
5. Zanetti, M., Strehle, J. K., Zollinger, H., and Hodler, J., Morton neuroma and fluid in the intermetatarsal bursae on MR images of 70 asymptomatic volunteers, *Radiology*, 203, 516–520, 1997.
6. Berlin, S. J., A laboratory review of 67,000 foot tumors and lesions, *J. Vasc. Podiatr. Assoc.*, 74, 341–347, 1984.
7. Munk, P. L., Recent advances in magnetic resonance imaging of musculoskeletal tumors, *Can. Assoc. Radiol. J.*, 42, 39–47, 1991.
8. Resch, S., Stenstrom, A., Jonsson, A., and Jonsson, K., The diagnostic efficacy of magnetic resonance imaging and ultrasonography in Morton's neuroma: a radiological–surgical correlation, *Foot Ankle*, 15, 88-92, 1994.
9. Ontell, F. and Greenspan, A., Chondrosarcoma complicating synovial chondromatosis: findings with magnetic resonance imaging, *Can. Assoc. Radiol. J.*, 45, 318–323, 1994.
10. Wetzel, L. H. and Levine, E., Soft-tissue tumors of the foot: value of MR Imaging for specific diagnosis, *AJR*, 155, 1025–1030, 1990.
11. Peabody, T. D. and Simon, M. A., Principles of staging of soft-tissue sarcomas, *Clin. Orthop.*, 289, 19–31, 1993.
12. Stess, R. M., Ariza, J., and Gooding, G. A. W., Preoperative imaging for soft tissue tumors of the foot, *J. Foot Ankle Surg.*, 33, 295–297, 1994.
13. Biondetti, P. R. and Ehman, R. L., Soft-tissue sarcomas: use of textural patterns in skeletal muscle as a diagnostic feature in postoperative MR Imaging, *Radiology*, 183, 845–848, 1992.
14. Vanel, D., Shapeero, L. G., De Baere, T. et al., MR Imaging in the follow-up of malignant and aggressive soft-tissue tumors: results of 511 examinations, *Radiology*, 190, 263–268, 1994.
15. Munk, P. L., Vellet, A. D., Bramwell, V., Bell, R., Hammond, A., and Beauchamp, C., Soft tissue sarcomas: a plea for proper management, *Can. J. Surg.*, 36, 178–180, 1993.
16. Shives, T. C., Biopsy of soft-tissue tumors, *Clin. Orthop.*, 289, 32–35, 1993.
17. Noria, S., Davis, A., Kandel, R., et al., Residual disease following unplanned excision of a soft-tissue sarcoma of an extremity, *J. Bone Joint Surg., (Am.)* 78A, 650–655, 1996.
18. Munk, P. L., Lee, M. J., Janzen, D. L., Poon, P. Y., Connell, D. G., and Bainbridge, T., Lipoma and liposarcoma: evaluation using CT and MR Imaging, *AJR*, 169, 589–594, 1997.
19. Schofield, T. D., Pitcher, J. D., and Youngberg, R., Synovial chondromatosis simulating neoplastic degeneration of osteochondroma: findings on MRI and CT, *Skeletal Radiol.*, 23, 99–102, 1994.
20. Kirby, E. J., Shereff, M. J., and Lewis, M. M., Soft-tissue tumors and tumor-like lesions of the foot, *J. Bone Joint Surg. (Am.)*, 71-A, 621–626, 1989.
21. Crim, J. R., Seeger, L. L., Yao, L., Chandnani, V., and Eckardt, J. J., Diagnosis of soft-tissue masses with MR Imaging: can benign masses be differentiated from malignant ones?, *Radiology*, 185, 581–586, 1992.
22. Sundaram, M. and Sharafuddin, M. J. A., MR Imaging of benign soft-tissue masses, *MRI Clin. North Am.*, 3, 609–626, 1995.
23. Hermann, G., Abdelwahab, I. F., Miller, T. T., Klein, M. J., and Lewis, M. M., Tumor and tumor-like conditions of the soft tissue: magnetic resonance imaging features differentiating benign from malignant masses, *Br. J. Radiol.*, 65, 14–20, 1992.
24. Ma, L. D., McCarthy, E. F., Bluemke, D. A., and Frassica, F. J., Differentiation of benign from malignant musculoskeletal lesions using MR Imaging: pitfalls in MR evaluation of lesions with a cystic appearance, *AJR*, 170, 1251–1258, 1998.

25. Ma, L. D., Frassica, F. J., Scott, W. W., Fishman, E. K., and Zerhouni, E. A., Differentiation of benign and malignant musculoskeletal tumors: potential pitfalls with MR Imaging, *RadioGraphics.*, 15, 349–366, 1995.

26. Verstraete, K. L., Van der Woude, H.-J., Hogendoorn, P. C. W., De Deene, Y., Kunnen, M., and Bloem, J. L., Dynamic contrast-enhanced MR Imaging of musculoskeletal tumors: basic principles and clinical applications, *J. Magn. Reson. Imaging*, 6, 311–321. 1996.

27. Ma, L. D., Frassica, F. J., McCarthy, E. F., Bluemke, D. A., and Zerhouni, E. A., Benign and malignant musculoskeletal masses: MR Imaging differentiation with rim-to-center differential enhancement ratios, *Radiology*, 202, 739–744, 1997.

28. Verstraete, K. L., Dierick, A., De Deene, Y., et al., First-pass images of musculoskeletal lesions: a new and useful diagnostic application of dynamic contrast-enhanced MRI, *Magn. Reson. Imaging*, 12, 687–702, 1994.

29. Verstraete, K. L., De Deene, Y., Roels, H., Dierick, A., Uyttendaele, D., and Kunnen, M., Benign and malignant musculoskeletal lesions: dynamic contrast-enhanced MR Imaging — parametric "first-pass" images depict tissue vascularization and perfusion, *Radiology*, 192, 835–843, 1994.

30. Keigley, B. A., Haggar, A. M., Gaba, A., Ellis, B. I., Froelich, J. W., and Wu, K. K., Primary tumors of the Foot: MR Imaging, *Radiology*, 171, 755–759, 1989.

31. Kier, R., MR Imaging of foot and ankle tumors, *Magn. Reson. Imaging*, 11, 149–162, 1993.

32. Levey, D. S., Park, Y. H., and Sartoris, D. J., Imaging of pedal soft tissue neoplasms, *J. Foot Ankle Surg.*, 4, 411–419, 1995.

33. Zanetti, M., Ledermann, T., Zollinger, H., and Hodler, J., Efficacy of MR Imaging in patients suspected of having Morton's neuroma, *AJR*, 168, 529–532, 1997.

34. Redd, R. A., Peters, V. J., Emery, S. F., Branch, H. M., and Rifkin, M. D., Morton neuroma: sonographic evaluation, *Radiology*, 171, 415–417, 1989.

35. Shapiro, P. P. and Shapiro, S. L., Sonographic evaluation of interdigital neuromas, *Foot Ankle Int.*, 16, 604–606, 1995.

36. Terk, M. R., Kwong, P. K., Suthar, M., Horvath, B. C., and Colletti, P. M., Morton Neuroma: Evaluation with MR Imaging performed with contrast enhancement and fat suppression, *Radiology*, 189, 239–241, 1993.

37. Erickson, S. J., Canale, P. B., Carrera, G. F., et al., Interdigital (Morton) neuroma: high-resolution MR Imaging with solenoid coil, *Radiology*, 181, 833–836, 1991.

38. Lauger, J., Palmer, J., Monill, J. M., Franquet, T., Bague, S., and Roson, N., MR Imaging of benign soft-tissue masses of the foot and ankle, *RadioGraphics*, 18, 1481–1498, 1998.

39. Williams, J. W., Meaney, J., Whitehouse, G. H., Klenerman, L., and Hussein, Z., MRI in the investigation of Morton's neuroma: which sequences, *Clin. Radiol.*, 52, 46–49, 1996.

40. Narra, V. R., Shirkhoda, A., Shetty, A. N., Bis, K. G., Armin, A.-R., and Gurgun, M., Giant cell tumor of the tendon sheath in the ankle: MRI with pathologic correlation, *J. Magn. Reson. Imaging*, 5, 781–783, 1995.

41. Jelinek, J. S., Kransdorf, M. J., Shmookler, B. M., Aboulafia, A. A., and Malawer, M. M., Giant cell tumor of the tendon sheath: MR findings in nine cases, *AJR*, 162, 919–922, 1994.

42. Kirby, E. J., Mesenchymal chondrosarcoma of the soft tissue of the left foot: case report 788, *Skeletal Radiol.*, 22, 300–305, 1993.

43. Ugal, K. and Morimoto, K., Magnetic resonance imaging of pigmented villonodular synovitis in subtalar joint, *Clin. Orthop. Rel. Res.*, 283, 281–284, 1992.

44. Jelinek, J. S., Kransdorf, M. J., Utz, J. A. et al., Imaging of pigmented villonodular synovitis with emphasis on MR Imaging, *AJR*, 152, 337–342, 1989.

45. Hughes, T. H., Sartoris, D. J., Schweitzer, M. E., and Resnick, D. I., Pigmented villonodular synovitis: MRI characteristics, *Skeletal Radiol.*, 24, 7–12, 1995.

46. Kliman, M. E. and Freiberg, A., Ganglia of the foot and ankle, *Foot Ankle*, 3, 45–46, 1982.

47. Lee, T. H., Wapner, K. L., and Hecht, P. J., Plantar fibromatosis, *J. Bone Joint Surg. (Am.)*, 75A, 1080–1084, 1993.

48. Morrison, W. B., Schweitzer, M. E., Wapner, K. L., and Lackman, R. D., Plantar fibromatosis: a benign aggressive neoplasm with a characteristic appearance on MR Images, *Radiology*, 193, 841–845, 1994.

49. Miller, L. J., Pruett, S. W., Losanda, R., Fruauff, A., and Sagerman, P., Tophaceous gout of the lumbar spine: MR findings, *J. Comp. Assist. Tomogr.*, 20, 1004–1005, 1996.
50. Feld, R., Burk, L., McCue, P., Mitchell, D. G., Lackman, R., and Rifkin, M. D., MRI of aggressive fibromatosis: frequent appearance of high signal intensity on T2-Weighted Images, *Magn. Reson. Imaging*, 8, 583–588, 1990.
51. Beggs, I., Imaging of peripheral nerve tumors, *Clin. Radiol.*, 52, 8–17, 1997.
52. Cerofolini, E., Landi, A., DeSantis, G., Maiorana, A., Canossi, G., and Romagnoli, R., MR of benign peripheral nerve sheath tumors, *J. Comp. Assist. Tomogr.*, 15, 593–597, 1991.
53. Peh, W. C. G., Shek, T. W. H., and Yip, D. K. H., Magnetic resonance imaging of subcutaneous diffuse neurofibroma, *Br. J. Radiol.*, 70, 1180–1183, 1997.
54. Varma, D. G. K., Moulopoulos, A., Sara, A. S., et al., MR Imaging of extracranial nerve sheath tumors, *J. Comp. Assist. Tomogr.*, 16, 448–453, 1992.
55. Kransdorf, M. J., Moser, R. P., Meis, J. M., and Meyer, C. A., Fat-containing soft-tissue masses of the extremities, *RadioGraphics*, 11, 81–106, 1991.
56. Maurice, H., Crone, M., and Watt, I., Synovial chondromatosis, *J. Bone Joint Surg.* (Am.), 70-B, 807–811, 1988.
57. Edeiken, J., Edeiken, B. S., Ayala, A. G., Raymond, A. K., Murray, J. A., and Guo S-Q., Giant solitary synovial chondromatosis, *Skeletal Radiol.*, 23, 23–29, 1994.
58. Perry, B. E., McQueen, D. A., and Lim, J. J., Synovial chondromatosis with malignant degeneration to chondrosarcoma, *J. Bone Joint Surg.* (Am.), 70-A, 1259–1261, 1988.
59. Davis, R. I., Hamilton, A., and Biggart, J. D., Primary synovial chondromatosis: a clinicopathologic review and assessment of malignant potential, *Human Pathol.*, 29, 683–688, 1998.
60. Kenan, S., Abdelwahab, I. F., Klein, M. J., and Lewis, M. M., Case report 817: synovial chondrosarcoma secondary to synovial chondromatosis, *Skeletal Radiol.*, 22, 623–626, 1993.
61. Villacin, A. B., Brigham, L. M., and Bullough, P. G., Primary and secondary synovial chondrometaplasia, *Human Pathol.*, 10, 439–451, 1979.
62. Norman, A. and Steiner, G. C., Bone erosion in synovial chondromatosis, *Radiology*, 161, 749–752, 1986.
63. Kramer, J., Recht, M., Deely, D. M. et al., MR appearance of idiopathic synovial osteochondromatosis, *J. Comput. Assist. Tomogr.*, 17, 772–776, 1993.
64. Murphey, M. D., Fairbairn, K. J., Parman, L. M., Baxter, K. G., Parsa, M. B., and Smith, W. S., Musculoskeletal angiomatous lesions: radiologic–pathologic correlation, *RadioGraphics*, 15, 893–917, 1995.
65. Suh, J. S., Hwang, G., and Hahn, S.-B., Soft tissue hemangiomas: MR manifestations in 23 patients, *Skeletal Radiol.*, 23, 621–625, 1994.
66. Jones, B. C., Sundaram, M., and Kransdorf, M. J., Synovial sarcoma: MR Imaging findings in 34 patients, *AJR*, 161, 827–830, 1993.
67. Morton, M. J., Berquist, T. H., McLeod, R. A., Unni, K. K., and Sim, F. H., MR Imaging of synovial sarcoma, *AJR*, 156, 337–340, 1991.
68. Blacksin, M., Siegel, J. R., Benevenia, J., and Aisner, S. C., Synovial sarcoma: frequency of non-aggressive MR characteristics, *J. Comput. Assist. Tomogr.*, 21, 785–789, 1997.
69. Adler, C. P., Mesenchymal chondrosarcoma of the soft tissue of the left foot, *Skeletal Radiol.*, 22, 300–305, 1993.
70. Huvos, A. G. and Marcove, R. C., Chondrosarcoma in the young: a clinicopathologic analysis of 79 patients younger than 21 years of age, *Am. J. Surg. Pathol.*, 11, 930–942, 1987.
71. Wile, A. G., Evans, H. L., and Romsdahl, M. M., Leiomyosarcoma of soft tissue: a clinicopathologic study, *Cancer*, 48, 1022–1032, 1981.
72. Kransdorf, M. J. and Meis-Kindblom, J. M., Dermatofibrosarcoma protuberans: radiologic appearance, *AJR*, 163, 391–394, 1994.
73. Munk, P. L., Sallomi, D. F., Janzen, D. L. et al., Malignant fibrous histiocytoma of soft tissue: imaging with emphasis on MRI, *J. Comput. Assist. Tomogr.*, 22, 819–826, 1998.
74. Murphey, M. D., Gross, T. M., and Rosenthal, H. G., Musculoskeletal malignant fibrous histiocytoma: radiologic–pathologic correlation, *RadioGraphics*, 14, 807–826, 1994.
75. Peterson, K. K., Renfrew, D. L., Feddersen, R. M., Buckwater, J. A., and El-Khoury, G. Y., Magnetic resonance imaging of myxoid containing yumors, *Skeletal Radiol.*, 20, 245–250, 1991.

76. Mahajan, H., Kim, E. E., Wallace, S., Abello, R., Benjamin, R., and Evans, H. L., Magnetic resonance imaging of malignant fibrous histiocytoma, *Magn. Reson. Imaging*, 7, 283–288, 1989.

77. Miller, T. T., Hermann, G., Abdelwahab, I. F., Klein, M. J., Kenan, S., and Lewis, M. M., MRI of malignant fibrous histiocytoma of soft tissue: analysis of 13 cases with pathologic correlation, *Skeletal Radiol.*, 23, 271–275, 1994.

78. Sartoris, D. J., Haghighi, P., and Resnick, D., Clear cell sarcoma plantar aspect right foot: case report 423, *Skeletal Radiol.*, 16, 325–332, 1987.

79. O'Keeffe, F., Lorigan, J. G., and Wallace, S., Radiological features of extraskeletal Ewing sarcoma, *Br. J. Radiol.*, 63, 456–460, 1990.

80. Link, S. C., Erickson, S. J., and Timins, M. E., MR Imaging of the ankle and foot: normal structures and anatomic variants that may simulate disease, *AJR*, 161, 607–612, 1993.

81. Moskovic, E., Serpell, J. W., Parsons, C., Fisher, C., and Thomas, J. M., Benign mimics of soft tissue sarcomas, *Clin. Radiol.*, 46, 248–252, 1992.

82. Brodie, J. T., Dormans, J. P., Gregg, J. R., and Davidson, R. S., Accessory soleus muscle, *Clin. Orthop.*, 337, 180–186, 1997.

83. Lorentzon, R. and Wirell, S., Anatomic variations of the accessory soleus muscle, *Acta Radiol.*, 28, 627–629, 1987.

84. Mellado, J. M., Rosenberg, Z. S., Beltran, J., and Colon, E., The peroneocalcaneus internus muscle: MR Imaging features, *AJR*, 169, 585–588, 1997.

85. Fleet, M. S. and Raby, N., An unusual presentation of gout, *Clin. Radiol.*, 52, 156–158, 1997.

86. Chaoui, A., Garcia, J., and Kurt, A. M., Gouty tophus simulating soft tissue tumor in a heart transplant recipient, *Skeletal Radiol.*, 26, 626–628, 1997.

87. Ruiz, M. E., Erickson, S. J., Carrera, G. F., Hanel, D. P., and Smith, M. D., Monoarticular gout following trauma: MR appearance, *J. Computer Assist. Tomogr.*, 17, 151–153, 1993.

88. Yu, J. S., Chung, C., Recht, M., Dailiana, T., and Jurdi, R., MR Imaging of tophaceous gout, *AJR*, 168, 523–527, 1997.

89. Munk, P. L., Vellet, A. D., Hillborn, M. D., Crues, J. V., Helms, C. A., and Poon, P. Y., Musculoskeletal infection: findings on magnetic resonance imaging, *J. Can. Assoc. Radiol.*, 45, 355–362, 1994.

90. Miller, T. T., Randolph, D. A., Staron, R. B., Feldman, F., and Cushin, S., Fat-suppressed MRI of musculoskeletal infection: fast T2-weighted techniques versus gadolinium-enhanced T1-weighted images, *Skeletal Radiol.*, 26, 654–658, 1997.

91. Hopkins, K. L., Li, K. C. P., and Bergman, G., Gadolinium-DTPA-enhanced magnetic resonance imaging of musculoskeletal infectious processes, *Skeletal Radiol.*, 24, 325–330, 1995.

92. Gordon, B. A., Martinez, S., and Collins, A. J., Pyomyositis: characteristics at CT and MR Imaging, *Radiology*, 197, 279–286, 1995.

93. Rahmouni, A., Chosidow, O., Mathieu, D. et al., MR Imaging in acute infectious cellulitis, *Radiology*, 192, 493–496, 1994.

94. Brandser, E. A., El-Khoury, G. Y., and Saltzman, C. L., Tendon injuries: application of magnetic resonance imaging, *J. Can. Assoc. Radiol.*, 46, 9–18, 1995.

95. Whitehouse, G. H., Magnetic resonance imaging in the diagnosis of muscle and tendon injuries, *Imaging*, 4, 95–105, 1992.

7 Infection of the Ankle and Foot: MR Appearances

Joseph G. Craig and Marnix T. van Holsbeeck

CONTENTS

INTRODUCTION

Assessment of possible infection in the foot and ankle is a common reason to obtain an MR (magnetic resonance) examination. In nondiabetic patients infection is commonly secondary to penetrating trauma, postsurgical sequelae, or hematogenous spread. Infection in the diabetic foot is usually secondary to local soft-tissue infection and remains a difficult diagnostic challenge.[1] MR imaging is of proven value in the assessment of infection in the ankle and foot.[2-7] Although MR imaging shows superb soft-tissue and marrow resolution, the signal changes are not specific. In particular, changes in the marrow may be due to osteomyelitis but also can be reactive marrow edema secondary to infection, trauma, infarction, or neuropathic change, among other entities.

This chapter reviews the MR imaging features of infection in the soft tissues and bones of the foot. Particular emphasis is given to the diabetic foot, as this is often the most common indication for assessment of possible infection.

TECHNIQUE

Optimal results occur with the use of a high-field-strength magnet and dedicated extremity coils. Depending on the clinical indication, the whole foot or only part of the foot may need to be imaged. The site of clinical suspicion for infection as well as the sites of soft-tissue abnormality including ulcers, sinus tracts, and focal inflammatory soft-tissue swelling are useful to know prior to the examination. For imaging of the whole foot, a field of view (FOV) of around 24 cm is used. For more localized abnormalities, an FOV of 10 to 16 cm is typically obtained.

T1-weighted, fast-spin-echo fat-suppressed T2-weighted, and/or fast short tau inversion recovery (STIR) sequences are typically obtained, although the planes of imaging will depend on the clinical problems being addressed. For most examinations, the authors obtain sagittal T1-weighted, sagittal and coronal fast-spin-echo fat-suppressed T2-weighted, and sagittal fast STIR sequences.

Use of gadopentetate dimeglumine (gadolinium) with fat-suppressed T1-weighted imaging has been reported to increase the sensitivity and specificity of the diagnosis of osteomylitis.[8] However, fat-suppressed postgadolinium T1-weighted sequences will not differentiate marrow edema from osteomyelitis and the uptake is not specific.[9] Use of gadolinium may allow better definition of soft-tissue masses including ring enhancement of abscesses (Figure 7.1). Postgadolinium images may also show sinus tracts, and if an intraosseous abscess is present, there will be ring enhancement within the bone[8] (Figure 7.2).

CELLULITIS/SOFT-TISSUE EDEMA

Cellulitis refers to an infection in the deep subcutaneous layer and is usually due to *Staphylococcus* or *Streptococcus* infection.[10] Cellulitis is normally an obvious clinical diagnosis. An MR examination is usually obtained to exclude coexistent osteomyelitis. On MR imaging, cellulitis is seen as an area of decreased signal intensity within the skin and subcutaneous tissue on the T1-weighted image and increased signal intensity on the fast-spin-echo fat-suppressed T2-weighted or fast STIR images (Figure 7.3). The images should also be carefully inspected for an adjacent abscess or osteomyelitis.

In patients with diabetes, edema is commonly seen on the dorsum of the foot (Figure 7.4). This does not necessarily imply a diagnosis of cellulitis. These changes have been examined histologically and only nonspecific edema was found. Edema may also be seen in the plantar compartments that lie between the plantar aponeurosis and the metatarsals[11] (Figure 7.4).

SUBCUTANEOUS ABSCESS

In patients without diabetes, a subcutaneous abscess is usually secondary to penetrating trauma to the foot. In patients with diabetes, a subcutaneous abscess is usually secondary to infection of the soft tissues around a pressure point or ulcer. The exclusion of coexistent osteomyelitis is of primary clinical importance.

SEPTIC TENOSYNOVITIS

Infection in the tendon sheath may be secondary to penetrating trauma or a complication of the diabetic foot. MR imaging evidence of tenosynovitis is increased signal intensity within a distended tendon sheath on T2-weighted or STIR images (Figure 7.5). In the diabetic foot, a distended tendon sheath with increased signal intensity may be seen and this does not necessarily imply sepsis.[12] In diabetes, tendon sheaths may have a small or moderate amount of fluid around them, which is not necessarily characteristic of an abnormality. The exact amount of fluid that characterizes an abnormality has not been defined clearly in the literature.[12] When a distended tendon sheath is seen close to an area of infection, the possibility of septic tenosynovitis should be considered.[11] Percutaneous aspiration with laboratory analysis may be required to confirm the diagnosis.

SEPTIC ARTHRITIS

In the nondiabetic foot, septic arthritis is usually secondary to penetrating trauma. In the patient with diabetes, septic arthritis most often occurs from contiguous spread of localized infection, usually an

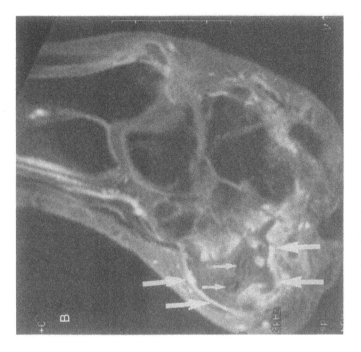

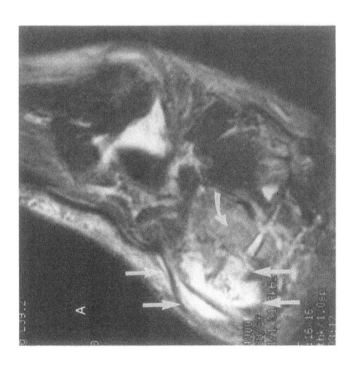

FIGURE 7.1 Gadolinium soft-tissue abscess. A 51-year-old male patient with diabetes and a prior amputation of the forefoot presented with swelling around the ankle. Radiographs showed destruction of the head of the talus consistent with osteomyelitis. The sagittal T1-weighted section through the mid- and hind foot showed an area of decreased signal intensity on the plantar aspect of the foot. (A) Sagittal fast fat-suppressed T2-weighted image (4000, 88 eff, Echo Train 8) shows an irregular area of increased signal intensity anterior to the talus and navicular (straight arrows). Note also the increased signal intensity in the lateral cuneiform (curved arrow) secondary to osteomyelitis/reactive marrow edema. (B) Sagittal postgadolinium fat-suppressed T1-weighted fast multiplanar spoiled GRASS (FMP SPGR) (150, 2.1) image shows peripheral enhancement of an irregular abscess cavity (long arrows) containing pockets of air (short arrows).

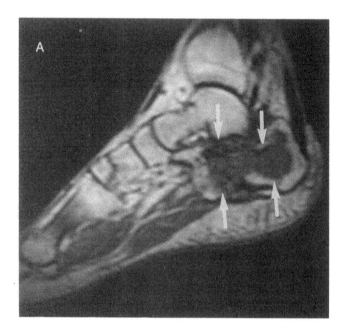

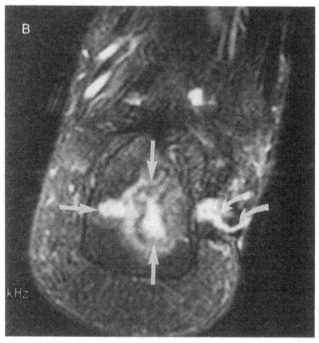

FIGURE 7.2 Intraosseous abscess. A 39-year-old male fell from a roof and sustained a calcaneus fracture, which was treated with open surgical reduction and fixation. The surgical hardware was subsequently removed and he developed a persistent sinus tract at the wound site. (A) Sagittal-spin-echo T1-weighted image shows an irregular area of low signal intensity within the calcaneus (arrows). (B) Coronal fast fat-suppressed T2-weighted image (6000, 90 eff, Echo Train 8) shows an irregular area of increased signal intensity within the calcaneus (straight arrows) and the associated sinus tract (curved arrows).   (*continued*)

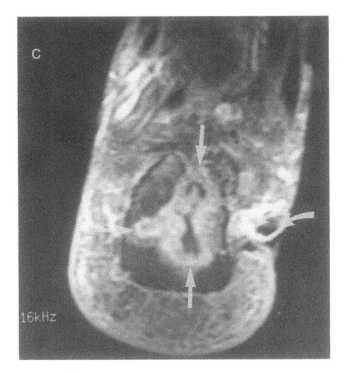

FIGURE 7.2 (continued) (C) Coronal postgadolinium fat-suppressed T1-weighted image (550, 14) at a similar level to (B) shows peripheral enhancement around the abscess (straight arrows), with a central nonenhancing area consistent with pus. Note also the enhancement along the sinus tract (curved arrows). Cultures grew *Enterobacter taylorae.*

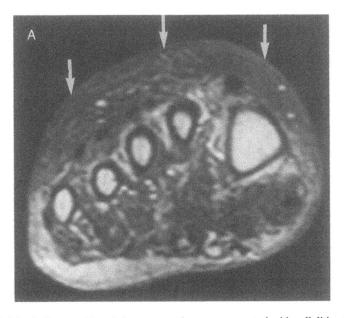

FIGURE 7.3 Cellulitis. A 43-year-old male intravenous drug user presented with cellulitis of the right foot. An MR imaging examination was obtained to exclude an associated osteomyelitis. (A) Coronal T1-weighted (533, 35) image through the forefoot shows prominence of the soft tissues of the dorsum of the foot with diffusely decreased signal intensity of the skin and subcutaneous fat (arrows). Note the normal fatty marrow signal intensity in the metatarsals. *(continued)*

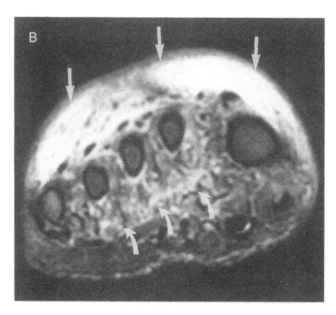

FIGURE 7.3 (continued) (B) Coronal fat-suppressed fast-spin-echo T2-weighted (4400, 80 eff, Echo Train 8) image at the same level shows diffusely increased signal intensity within the skin and subcutaneous tissue (straight arrows). There is also increased signal intensity within the muscles of the plantar aspect of the foot (curved arrows) consistent with reactive edema. Note the normal signal intensity of the metatarsals, excluding osteomyelitis.

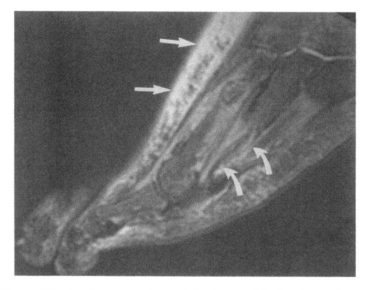

FIGURE 7.4 Edema within the subcutaneous tissue of the dorsum of the foot in a patient with diabetes. An 83-year-old patient with diabetes was evaluated for ulceration of the right great toe. There was no cellulitis clinically. Sagittal fast-spin-echo fat-suppressed T2-weighted image (4000, 84 eff, Echo Train 8) shows increased signal intensity on the dorsum of the foot (straight arrows). The T1-weighted image shows decreased signal intensity. Increased signal intensity on the dorsum of the foot on T2-weighted or STIR images (with decreased signal intensity on the T1-weighted images) is a common finding in patients with diabetes and does not necessarily correlate with cellulitis. Note also the mildly increased signal intensity within the plantar compartment of the foot (curved arrows), also a nonspecific finding in patients with diabetes.

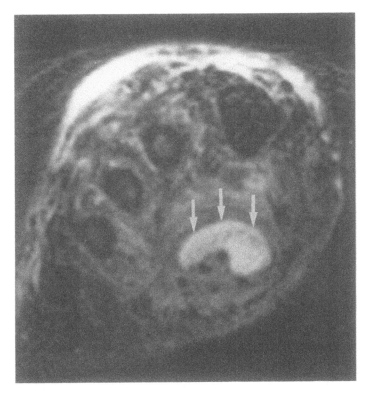

FIGURE 7.5 Septic tenosynovitis. A 28-year-old female patient with diabetes had complaints of fever, chills, malaise, and pain in the right foot. She had an ulcer over the plantar aspect of the right hind foot. Coronal fast-spin-echo fat-suppressed T2-weighted image (5933, 80 eff, Echo Train 8) shows an inhomogeneous distended flexor hallucis longus tendon sheath (arrows). The T1-weighted image shows decreased signal within the tendon sheath. Aspiration of the tendon sheath under ultrasound guidance yielded 2 ml of purulent fluid. There was no associated osteomyelitis.

ulcer or abscess. In pure septic arthritis, the imaging findings are nonspecific and usually consist of an effusion within the joint. A reactive or sympathetic effusion is impossible to differentiate from an infected effusion by MR imaging criteria. In the patient with diabetes this is a common problem and aspiration of the joint with laboratory analysis may be required to provide a definitive answer.

In septic arthritis with associated osteomyelitis the diagnosis is less problematic. Review of the conventional radiographs may show destruction of bone on both sides of the joint, confirming the diagnosis before review of the MR examination. In patients with septic arthritis with associated osteomyelitis, the MR exam shows a joint effusion with associated marrow changes of decreased signal intensity on T1-weighted sequences and increased signal intensity on T2-weighted sequences (Figure 7.6). In the diabetic foot, these changes may be similar to neuropathic changes and knowledge of relevant clinical history and pertinent clinical findings, particularly the site of focal infection, is crucial to allow the radiologist to make a correct diagnosis.

MARROW EDEMA

Signal intensity changes meeting MR imaging criteria for osteomyelitis but with histologic results or clinical follow-up not confirming the diagnosis have been reported previously.[3–6,8,9,13–15] Various explanations have been offered for this discrepancy. In the diabetic foot, cases that meet MR imaging criteria for osteomyelitis but that proved only to have marrow edema at pathologic examination

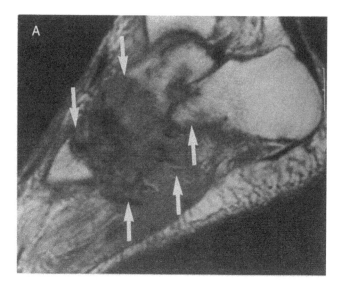

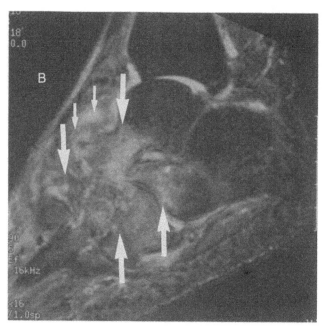

FIGURE 7.6 Septic arthritis/osteomyelitis. A 29-year-old female intravenous drug user presented with a history of increasing pain and swelling in the right foot. Initial radiographs showed bony erosion of bone in the midtarsal joints. An MR imaging examination was obtained to assist in preoperative planning. (A) Sagittal T1-weighted image (450, 27) shows diffusely decreased signal intensity within the mid-foot, anterior talus, and calcaneus (arrows). (B) Sagittal fast STIR image (2616, 38 eff, 160, Echo Train 6) shows increased signal intensity within the mid-foot, anterior talus, and the anterior calcaneus (long arrows). There are also pockets of loculated fluid superiorly (short arrows). The fluid was aspirated under ultrasound guidance. Cultures grew *Staphylococcus aureus.*

have been recently described.[9] On pathologic examination eosinophilic staining material is seen between fat lobules consistent with edema from an inflammatory response. The range of signal intensities for osteomyelitis overlaps the range for marrow edema, but patients with osteomyelitis usually have higher signal intensity.[9]

Marrow edema is a major cause of false-positive diagnoses of osteomyelitis. Edema of the marrow is a nonspecific finding and may be reactive to adjacent infection or secondary to infarct, neuropathic change, and altered gait, among other possibilities (Figure 7.7). Where two or more bones show signal intensity changes suggestive of osteomyelitis, one may be infected but the other(s) may not (Figure 7.8).

In cases with focal soft-tissue infection (usually an infected ulcer or an abscess) with adjacent MR imaging signal intensity changes in the bone marrow, it is often impossible to differentiate reliably marrow edema from osteomyelitis. In general, the more intense the signal intensity changes

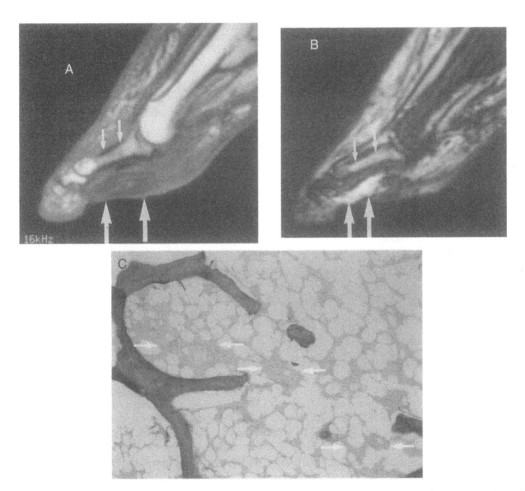

FIGURE 7.7 Marrow edema. A 49-year-old male patient with diabetes presented with increasing pain and swelling in the right second and third toes. (A) Sagittal T1-weighted image (416, 15) through the forefoot shows decreased signal intensity within the soft tissues on the plantar aspect of the foot (long arrows) and decreased signal intensity within most of the proximal phalanx (short arrows) of the second toe. (B) Sagittal fast-spin-echo fat-suppressed T2-weighted image (4750, 95 eff, Echo Train 8) through the same area shows focally increased signal intensity under the proximal phalanx of the second toe consistent with a focal inflammatory soft-tissue mass (long arrows) and increased signal intensity within the proximal phalanx (short arrows). The third toe had a similar appearance. The toes were resected at surgery. (C) Representative histologic section with hematoxylin and eosin (H&E) stain of the resected surgical proximal phalanx specimen shows diffusely eosinophilic pink-staining material (arrows point to representative areas) between the fat lobules consistent with edema of the marrow. The proximal phalanx from the third toe had a similar appearance. There was no evidence of osteomyelitis in either toe.

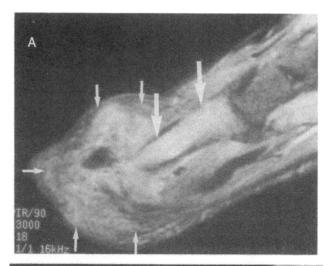

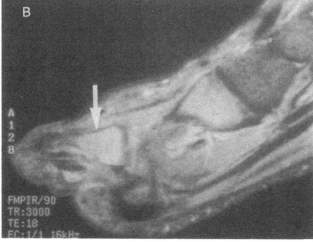

FIGURE 7.8 Marrow edema/osteomyelitis. A 44-year-old male with diabetes presented with a history of increasing pain and swelling of the medial aspect of the right foot. Radiographs showed erosion of the head of the first metatarsal. The T1-weighted images showed diffusely decreased signal along the first ray. (A) Sagittal fast STIR image (3000, 18 eff, 100, Echo Train 6) shows diffusely increased signal intensity along the shaft of the first metatarsal (long arrows) and an adjacent inflammatory mass (short arrows). (B) Sagittal fast STIR image (3000, 18 eff, 100, Echo Train 6) shows increased signal intensity within the proximal phalanx of the great toe (arrow). The signal is of similar intensity to that in the first metatarsal; the distal phalanx had a similar appearance. The patient then proceeded to surgery with amputation of the great toe and first metatarsal.   (*continued*)

on T2-weighted or STIR images, the more likely the diagnosis of osteomyelitis. There is, however, an overlap between marrow edema and osteomyelitis, often making it impossible to differentiate reliably between these two entities.

OSTEOMYELITIS

Osteomyelitis around the foot and ankle may be secondary to penetrating trauma, including post-surgical changes (Figure 7.2), secondary to spread from contiguous infection in the soft tissues (Figure 7.8), or hematogenous in origin (Figures 7.9 and 7.10).

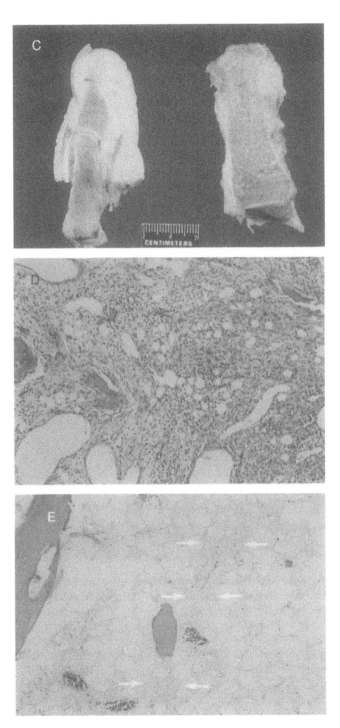

FIGURE 7.8 (continued) (C) The resected first metatarsal and great toe, which have been sectioned in the sagittal plane, are displayed. (D) Representative histologic section (H&E stain) from the first metatarsal shows changes of an acute and chronic inflammatory infiltrate with areas of fibrosis within the bone marrow. These appearances are consistent with acute and chronic osteomyelitis. (E) Representative histologic section (H&E stain) from the proximal phalanx shows diffuse eosinophilic pink-staining material between the fat lobules consistent with edema of the marrow (arrows show representative areas). The distal phalanx had a similar appearance.

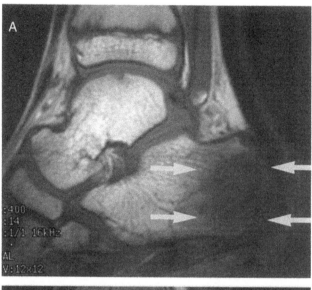

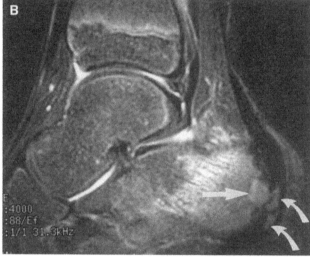

FIGURE 7.9 Hematogeneous osteomyelitis. A 9-year-old boy presented 2 weeks after a fall with increasing pain in the left hind foot. (A) Sagittal T1-weighted image (400, 14) through the ankle and hind foot shows extensive edema within the posterior calcaneus (arrows). (B) Sagittal fast-spin-echo fat-suppressed T2-weighted image (4000, 88 eff, Echo Train 8) shows extensive edema within the calcaneus corresponding to the area of decreased signal intensity on the T1-weighted image. In addition, there is a small, more-focal area of increased signal intensity adjacent to the apophysis (straight arrow) and two areas within the apophysis (curved arrows).   *(continued)*

The standard MR imaging criteria for the diagnosis of osteomyelitis are decreased signal intensity on the T1-weighted sequences and increased signal intensity on T2-weighted sequences within the bone marrow.[4,5,8,15] Other investigators have used a wide range of other criteria including increased signal intensity on T2-weighted sequences,[6,14] increased signal intensity on T2-weighted or STIR sequences,[9] decreased signal intensity on T1-weighted sequences or increased signal intensity on T2-weighted sequences,[13] decreased signal intensity on T1-weighted sequences, increased signal intensity on T2-weighted sequences, and enhancement with gadolinium.[7,8,16] Sensitivities and specificities for osteomyelitis with MR imaging have ranged from 75 to 98% and from 53 to 96%, respectively.[8,13,15] For studies specifically addressing osteomyelitis in the diabetic

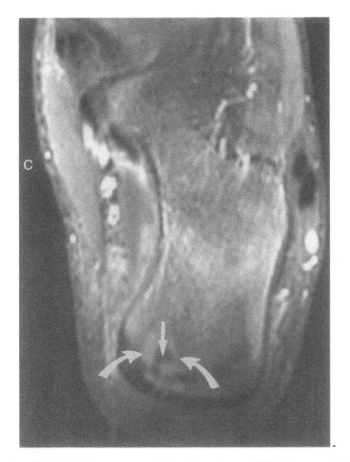

FIGURE 7.9 (continued) (C) Axial fat-suppressed T1-weighted image (433, 14) postgadolinium image shows focal enhancement in same region as in (B) (curved arrows) with a central (straight arrow) nonenhancing area in the calcaneus consistent with ischemia or pus. There is also more diffuse enhancement corresponding to the diffuse edema seen in the calcaneus in (A) and (B). Pathologic examination of biopsy material from this site showed changes of osteomyelitis.

foot, sensitivities and specificities have ranged from 82 to 99% and from 71 to 81%, respectively.[5,7,9] Additional MR imaging findings for osteomyelitis of the foot include cutaneous ulcer, cellulitis, soft-tissue mass, soft-tissue abscess, sinus tract, and cortical interruption.[16] Rim enhancement on fat-suppressed postgadolinium T1-weighted images seen within bone is highly suggestive of osteomyelitis[8] (Figure 7.2).

The majority of cases of possible osteomyelitis in the foot and ankle referred for imaging are patients with diabetes. In this setting, most infection in the bones of the diabetic foot results from direct extension of the infection from the adjacent soft tissues, usually infected ulcers.[1] In the diabetic foot in particular, the importance of the clinical history and relevant clinical findings cannot be overly stressed. It is crucial to know the site of the soft-tissue abnormality whether it be ulcer, suspected abscess, sinus tract, or cellulitis so that the adjacent bone can be carefully reviewed for possible osteomyelitis. Of equal importance is a review of the patient's recent conventional radiographs. If the diagnosis of osteomyelitis can be made on the radiographs, then the MR imaging becomes most important for defining the extent of the bony infection and for displaying the associated soft-tissue abnormality.

Osteomyelitis may occur with only mildly increased signal intensity on T2-weighted images and no change in the signal intensity on T1-weighted sequences.[9,16] Although this is not a

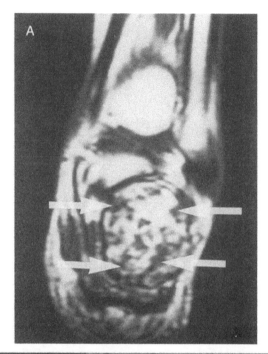

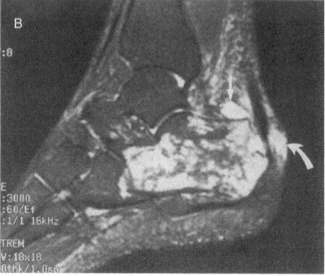

FIGURE 7.10 Hematogeneous osteomyelitis from tuberculosis. A 50-year-old female patient presented with a history of pain in the left hind foot. The initial radiographs showed areas of patchy lucency and sclerosis in the calcaneus. (A) Coronal T1-weighted image (400, 14) shows multiple small areas of decreased signal intensity within the calcaneus (arrows). (B) Fast-spin-echo fat-suppressed T2-weighted image (3000, 60 eff, Echo Train 8) shows multiple corresponding areas of increased signal intensity within the calcaneus. There is also fluid in the retrocalcaneal bursa (straight arrow) and superficial to the Achilles tendon (curved arrow). A bone biopsy was performed and cultures grew *Mycobacterium tuberculosis*.

common finding, such disconcordance in marrow signal intensity has been noted in both the diabetic and nondiabetic foot. With signal intensity changes that meet standard MR imaging criteria for osteomyelitis and an adjacent soft-tissue abnormality, pathologic review of the specimen may reveal only nonspecific marrow edema (Figure 7.7). The range of signal intensities for osteomyelitis overlaps that for marrow edema but patients with osteomyelitis usually have higher signal intensity on MR imaging.[9] The more intense the signal intensity changes on T2-weighted or STIR images, the more likely the diagnosis of osteomyelitis.[9] Signal intensity change in any part of the bone on T2-weighted sequences or STIR images equal to that of fluid in the joints or tendon sheaths is highly suggestive of osteomyelitis.[9] In many instances, however, it is impossible to differentiate reliably between osteomyelitis and marrow edema even with the use of gadolinium. In bone with osteomyelitis, MR imaging will not differentiate between the area of infection and the adjacent reactive edema within the bone. Fortunately this is not an important clinical differentiation.

MR imaging is particularly helpful if there is no signal intensity change within the bone. Normal signal intensity within the bone excludes osteomyelitis. This finding is useful in the preoperative surgical planning, where an MR imaging examination can effectively display the abnormal tissue.

NEUROPATHIC CHANGE

Neuropathic change in the diabetic foot is common. The intertarsal and tarsometatarsal joints are frequently involved. The changes can be very pronounced, particularly in the mid-foot with marked disorganization, fragmentation, subluxation or dislocation, and complete disintegration of bone.[17]

Neuropathic change in the diabetic foot without associated infection has been reported as showing decreased signal intensity on both the T1- and T2-weighted sequences.[6] Although this pattern occasionally occurs, it is uncommon. Neuropathic change is more likely to show decreased signal intensity on T1-weighted images and increased signal intensity on T2-weighted or STIR images, particularly in the mid-foot and hind foot and at the tarsometatarsal junction. These signal intensity changes are not specific and may be due to other causes (Figure 7.11). Furthermore, changes of decreased signal intensity on T1-weighted images and increased signal intensity on T2-weighted or STIR images without radiographic findings of neuropathic change may be seen in the diabetic foot.[9] Whether this represents very early neuropathic change or is due to some other cause has not been determined.[9]

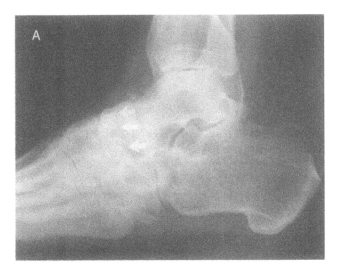

FIGURE 7.11 Neuropathic change. A 29-year-old male with diabetes was assessed for possible osteomyelitis of his right foot. (A) Coned-down lateral radiograph of the foot shows sclerosis of the mid-foot tarsals and dislocation of the head of the talus from the navicular (arrows). *(continued)*

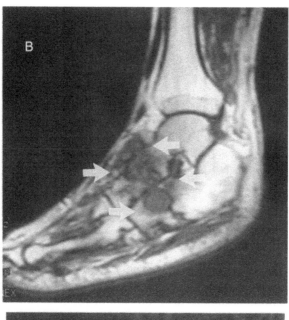

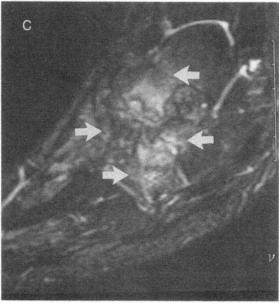

FIGURE 7.11 (continued) (B) Sagittal T1-weighted image (400, 24) through the foot shows disorganization and decreased signal intensity within the mid-foot (arrows). (C) Sagittal fast-spin-echo fat-suppressed T2-weighted image (4500, 95 eff, Echo Train 8) shows disorganization within the mid-foot and increased signal intensity within the tarsal bones (arrows). Note that there is no adjacent soft-tissue irregularity, making the diagnosis of associated osteomyelitis unlikely. These appearances are consistent with neuropathic change and there was no evidence of osteomyelitis at follow-up.

The criteria for osteomyelitis in the vicinity of neuropathic joints are the same for the remainder of the diabetic foot and require the signal intensity changes with an adjacent soft-tissue mass or ulcer[9] (Figure 7.12). In such cases, if the bone adjacent to the soft-tissue abnormality shows signal intensity changes, it should be assumed to be infected. Although it is possible that the bone with the signal intensity changes adjacent to a soft-tissue abnormality simply shows neuropathic or other changes

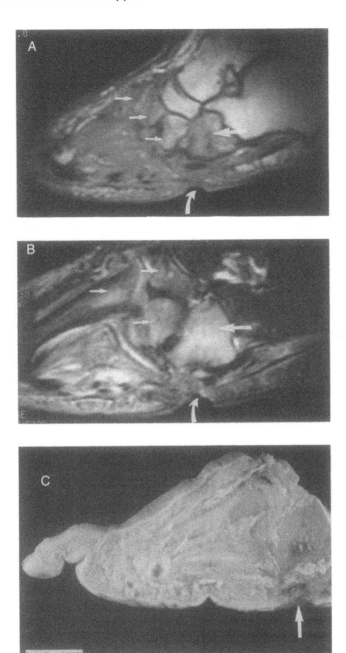

FIGURE 7.12 Neuropathic change and osteomyelitis. A 45-year-old male patient with diabetes with an ulcer on the lateral aspect of his right foot adjacent to the cuboid was evaluated for osteomyelitis. Radiographs showed subtle neuropathic changes in the mid-foot. (A) Sagittal T1-weighted image (400, 27) shows decreased signal intensity within the cuboid (long arrow) and also within the cuneiforms (short arrows). Note also the ulcer (curved arrow). (B) Sagittal fast-spin-echo fat-suppressed T2-weighted image (5133, 95 eff, Echo Train 8) shows increased signal intensity within the cuboid (long arrow) and the navicular, lateral cuneiform, and base of the second metatarsal (short arrows). Note the ulcer (curved arrow). Note also that the cuboid has the highest signal intensity. (C) Sagittal section of the gross anatomic specimen following mid-foot amputation. Note the ulcer (arrow). Cultures from the cuboid grew *Pseudomonas aeruginosa.* *(continued)*

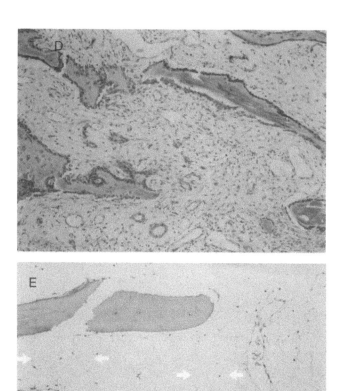

FIGURE 7.12 (continued) (D) Histologic section from the cuboid shows changes of an acute and chronic inflammatory infiltrate with areas of fibrosis within the bone marrow consistent with acute and chronic osteomyelitis. (E) Histologic section (H&E stain) from the navicular bone shows a pale eosinophilic material between fat cells diagnostic of marrow edema (arrows show representative areas). The cuneiforms also showed only marrow edema.

and is not infected, it is difficult, if not impossible, to differentiate from osteomyelitis. If the bone in question adjacent to the soft-tissue abnormality shows higher signal intensity on T2-weighted or STIR images than the adjacent bones, then this is highly suggestive of infection (Figure 7.12).

SUMMARY

Assessment for possible infection is a common reason to obtain MR imaging of the ankle and foot. Cellulitis and subcutaneous abscess are usually straightforward diagnoses, and of primary importance is the exclusion of coexistent osteomyelitis. Fluid may be seen around tendons of the foot and ankle particularly in patients with diabetes. A large amount of fluid around a tendon sheath, particularly if it is close to a region of infection, should raise the possibilty of septic tenosynovitis, and aspiration with laboratory analysis may be required.

Septic arthritis is seen as an effusion within a joint and cannot be differentiated by imaging from a reactive effusion by MR criteria. If there is associated osteomyelitis, signal intensity changes in the bones on both sides of the joint are seen.

Osteomyelitis can be a very difficult diagnosis in the foot, particularly the diabetic foot. Relevant clinical history describing the site of soft-tissue abnormality and review of the patient's conventional radiographs are critical. The signal intensity changes on MR imaging are not specific and may be due to reactive edema of the marrow rather than osteomyelitis. Marrow edema cannot be reliably differentiated from osteomyelitis, but in general the more intense the signal intensity changes on T2-weighted or STIR sequences, the more likely the diagnosis of osteomyelitis. Fat-suppressed T1-weighted postgadolinium imaging will improve the visualization of soft-tissue abnormalities and outline abscesses including intraosseous abscesses, but will not differentiate marrow edema from osteomyelitis. Neuropathic changes are common in the diabetic foot. The criterion for osteomyelitis associated with neuropathic joints is the same for the remainder of the diabetic foot and requires signal associated intensity changes in bone with an adjacent soft-tissue mass or ulcer.

REFERENCES

1. Lipsky, B. A., Pecoraro, R. E., and Wheat, L. J., The diabetic foot: soft tissue and bone infection, *Infect. Dis. Clin. North Am.*, 4, 409, 1990.
2. Tang, J. S. H., Gold, R. H., Bassett, L. W. et al., Musculoskeletal infection of the extremities: evaluation with MR imaging, *Radiology*, 166, 205, 1988
3. Mason, M. D., Zlatkin, M. B., Esterhai, J. L., Dalinka, M. K., Velchik, M. G., and Kressel, H. Y., Chronic complicated osteomyelitis of the lower extremity: evaluation with MR imaging, *Radiology*, 173, 355, 1989.
4. Yuh, W. T. C., Corson, J. D., Baraniewski, H. M., Shamma, A. R., Kathol, M. H., Sato, Y., El-Khoury, G. Y., Hawes, D. R., Platz, C. E., Cooper, R. R., and Corry, R. J., Osteomyelitis of the foot in diabetic patients: evaluation with plain film, ^{99m}Tc-MDP bone scintigraphy, and MR imaging, *AJR*, 152, 795, 1989.
5. Wang, A., Weinstein, D., Greenfield, L., Chiu, L., Chambers, R., Stewart, C., Hung, G., Diaz, F., and Ellis, T., MR imaging and diabetic foot infections, *Magn. Reson. Imaging*, 8, 805, 1990.
6. Beltran, J., Campanini, D. S., Knight, C., and McCalla, M., The diabetic foot: magnetic resonance imaging evaluation, *Skeletal Radiol.*, 19, 37, 1990.
7. Morrison, W. B., Schweitzer, M. E., Wapner, K. L., Hecht, P. J., Gannon, F. H., and Behm, W. R., Osteomyelitis in feet of diabetics: clinical accuracy, surgical utility, and cost effectiveness of MR imaging, *Radiology*, 196, 557, 1995.
8. Morrison, W. B., Schweitzer, M. E., Bock, G. W., Mitchell, D. G., Hume, E. L., Pathria, M. N., and Resnick, D., Diagnosis of osteomyelitis: utility of fat-suppressed contrast-enhanced MR imaging, *Radiology*, 189, 251, 1993.
9. Craig, J. G., Amin, M. B., Wu, K., Eyler, W. R., van Holsbeeck, M. T., Bouffard, J. A., and Shirazi, K., Osteomyelitis of the diabetic foot: MR imaging-pathologic correlation, *Radiology*, 203, 849, 1997.
10. Resnick, D., *Diagnosis of Bone and Joint Disorders*, 3rd ed., W. B. Saunders, Philadelphia, 1995, 2385.
11. Moore, T. E., Yuh, W. T. C., Kathol, M. H., El-Khoury, G. Y., and Corson, J. D., Abnormalities of the foot in patients with diabetes mellitus: findings on MR imaging, *AJR*, 157, 813, 1991.
12. Resnick, D., *Diagnosis of Bone and Joint Disorders,* 3rd ed., W. B. Saunders, Philadelphia, 1995, 3172.
13. Unger, E., Molofsky, P., Gatenby, R., Hartz, W., and Broder, G., Diagnosis of osteomyelitis by MR imaging, *AJR*, 150, 605, 1988.
14. Beltran, J., Noto, A. M., McGhee, R. B., Freedy, R. M., and McCalla, M. S., Infections of the musculoskeletal system: high-field-strength MR imaging, *Radiology*, 164, 449, 1987.
15. Erdman, W. A., Tamburro, F., Jayson, H. T., Weatherall, P. T., Ferry, K. B., and Peshock, R. M., Osteomyelitis: characteristics and pitfalls of diagnosis with MR imaging, *Radiology*, 180, 533, 1991.
16. Morrison, W. B., Schweitzer, M. E., Batte, W. G., Radack, D. P., and Russel, K. M., Osteomyelitis of the foot: relative importance of primary and secondary MR imaging signs, *Radiology*, 207, 625, 1998.
17. Resnick, D., *Diagnosis of Bone and Joint Disorders,* 3rd ed., W. B. Saunders, Philadelphia, 1995, 3426.

8 Arthropathies and Other Synovial-Related Pathology*

Donald J. Flemming

CONTENTS

INTRODUCTION

Evaluation of arthritis of the foot and ankle with MR (magnetic resonance) imaging occurs in three basic clinical scenarios. The most commonly encountered situation is when the diagnosis of arthritis is already established and MR imaging is requested to assess for complications of either the disease or therapy such as tendon rupture, avascular necrosis, fracture, or infection. The appearance of these complications is discussed in detail elsewhere in the book. Such patients may also be referred for MR imaging to document the extent or activity of the disease. This request is uncommon in everyday practice and is more frequently seen in the research or academic setting. On occasion, a patient may be evaluated for pain, possible infection, and/or a mass, and an arthropathy may not have been considered by the referring physician. It is important to recognize the typical MR imaging appearance of arthritides in this setting because arthritis of the foot and ankle is common.

Ideally, musculoskeletal MR images should be interpreted with conventional radiographs. This is especially true when arthropathies are a diagnostic consideration because they typically can be readily diagnosed by X-ray. However, important manifestations of arthopathies such as early erosion, effusion,

---

* The opinions or assertions contained herein are the private views of the author and are not to be construed as official nor as reflecting the views of the Departments of the Navy or Defense.

and tenosynovitis that are difficult to detect on radiography are easily appreciated on MR imaging because of superior contrast resolution and multiplanar imaging. Regardless of etiology, signs suggestive of an arthropathy on MR imaging include effusion, synovial hypertrophy, cartilage defects, and signal changes in subchondral bone on both sides of the joint. These basic findings, with the exception of shallow cartilage defects, are usually appreciated on routine conventional T1-, T2-, or fast-spin-echo (FSE) T2-weighted images. Fat suppression used in conjunction with T2-weighted images improves the detection of subtle marrow change. Differentiation of effusion and synovial hypertrophy may be difficult with routine sequences.[1] Fluid tends to have hyperintense signal in comparison with intermediate signal of hypertrophied synovium on T2-weighted images.[2] This distinction is usually readily appreciated on FSE images with long effective echo times.[3] Additionally, a T1-weighted three-dimensional (3D) fat-suppressed gradient-echo sequence has been recently reported as being able to distinguish between fluid and synovial hypertrophy without the use of intravenous contrast.[4] Synovial hypertrophy is a nonspecific phenomenon that is ubiquitous with the inflammatory arthropathies, but can also be seen in osteoarthritis.

Intravenous gadolinium is useful when evaluating for infection, but is not typically necessary to appreciate the changes of arthritis. Dynamically acquired images of a joint following the administration of intravenous gadolinium have been reported to help delineate the extent of active synovitis.[5-8] Dynamic acquisition is required because the contrast is filtered by the synovium and diffuses rapidly into the joint.[9] This phenomenon is the basis for indirect arthrography, and diffusion of contrast into the joint can occur regardless of the pathologic status of the synovium. Normal synovial enhancement is either not appreciable or minimal if present. Diseased synovium is manifested as enhancement in the periphery of the joint that may range from thin and smooth to thick and irregular. Although this technique has not been widely applied to patients in general practice, it is useful in therapeutic trials where it is especially important to document the extent of disease and response to treatment.

On radiographs, erosions and articular space loss are relatively late manifestations of damage to the articular cartilage. MR imaging offers the opportunity to detect erosions earlier through a combination of multiplanar technique and direct visualization of cartilage. Early detection of disease may direct more aggressive medical therapy or surgical intervention that potentially can alter the clinical outcome of the disorder. Cartilage damage may be imaged using fat-suppressed FSE proton-density-weighted and FSE T2-weighted sequences, but the ideal technique should be fast and should maximize contrast between hyaline cartilage, subchondral bone, and joint fluid. Currently, direct visualization of cartilage is best performed with 3D fat-suppressed spoiled gradient-echo (SPGR) sequences.[10] Normal hyaline cartilage is bright in signal relative to adjacent structures with this technique and, with proper coil selection, the use of 3D SPGR sequences allows for the acquisition of thin-section high-resolution images. SPGR imaging is especially useful in evaluating the cartilage of the talar dome (Figure 8.1) or first metatarsal head that is relatively thick but may be of limited utility in other joints of the foot and ankle because of insufficient spatial resolution.

Although the manifestations of arthropathies tend to be centered on joints by definition, the effects of these diseases on other soft-tissue structures may be readily appreciated on MR imaging. The tendons of the foot and ankle, with the exception of the Achilles tendon, are invested in a sheath that is lined with synovium. These tenosynovial sheaths may become inflamed in systemic diseases such as rheumatoid arthritis (RA). Bursae such as the intermetatarsal or retrocalcaneal bursae may also be involved and be a prominent part of the MR imaging appearance of an arthropathy.

INFLAMMATORY ARTHRITIDES

The inflammatory arthitides encompass a family of disorders that destroy cartilage and subchondral bone through synovial inflammation. The classic inflammatory arthropathy is rheumatoid arthritis (RA). The seronegative spondyloarthropathies, primarily psoriatic and Reiter disease, represent the

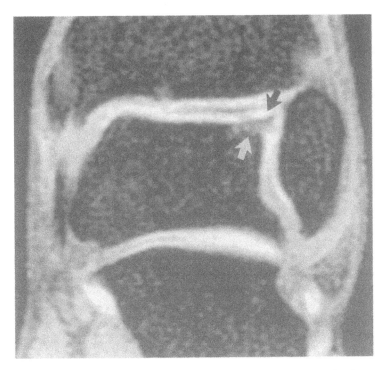

FIGURE 8.1 Articular cartilage flap. A 28-year-old man with persistent pain following an ankle sprain. Coronal fat-suppressed spoiled gradient-echo image shows hyperintense signal of hyaline cartilage with a flap of cartilage (black arrow) elevated from subchondral bone (white arrow) in the lateral talar dome.

second most commonly encountered inflammatory arthritides in the foot and ankle. Although these arthropathies have distinct clinical and radiologic presentations, on MR imaging they may share many similar imaging features and differentiation with this modality may be difficult.

RHEUMATOID ARTHRITIS

Rheumatoid arthritis (RA) is the most commonly encountered erosive arthritis in clinical practice. Patients are typically female with a disease ratio of 2:1 to 3:1 female to male. RA is a common disease with an annual incidence of 0.2 to 0.4/1000 in females.[11] The onset of symptoms is most commonly seen between the ages of 25 and 55 years. Patients usually present with an insidious onset of joint complaints in a polyarticular symmetric distribution and 75 to 80% of patients are rheumatoid factor positive on serum testing.[12]

The foot is commonly affected in RA patients with 80 to 90% of patients demonstrating pedal disease. Foot complaints may be the initial presenting symptom in 10 to 20% of patients and forefoot involvement, particularly the metatarsal–phalangeal (MTP) joints, predominates. Mid-foot and hind foot disease presents as articular space narrowing with minimal erosions that may be underestimated on radiographs.

Foot deformities such as hallux valgus, lateral drift of the toes, and pes planus are common sequelae of the effects of RA on ligaments, tendons, and joints. Clinical and radiographic findings are usually sufficient to establish the diagnosis of RA and MR imaging is typically utilized for detection of complications. MR imaging, however, offers the ability to assess comprehensively the tendons, ligaments, cartilage, and bone of an affected joint. Despite the frequent involvement of the foot in this disease, the majority of MR imaging research efforts has focused on knee and wrist manifestations.

Synovial hypertrophy is one of the most widely investigated MR imaging manifestations of RA. The capsule of diseased joints is distended by a combination of effusion and synovial hypertrophy. Synovial hypertrophy is intermediate in signal on T1-weighted images and is typically higher in signal than adjacent effusion depending on imaging parameters. Synovial hypertophy is best appreciated on T2-weighted images, particularly fat-suppressed FSE T2-weighted sequences. Abnormal synovium is thickened and may demonstrate frondlike projections that are lower in signal than adjacent effusion with long TE images. Dynamically acquired images following intravenous gadolinium administration will demonstrate the extent of synovial hypertrophy on early images as thickened, irregular areas of enhancement (Figure 8.2). The extent of enhancement in a joint may be a more accurate predictor of disease activity than commonly used clinical indicators such as erythrocyte sedimentation rate (ESR) and c-reactive protein levels.[13]

Erosions are detected earlier on MR imaging than on conventional radiographs because of a combination of higher contrast discrimination of subchondral bone and tomographic evaluation of complex anatomy.[14–17] Erosions are manifested as focal round areas of low signal intensity in subchondral bone on T1-weighted images. Erosions may be either intermediate or high signal on T2-weighted images. The appearance on T2-weighted images depends on whether the defect is filled with fluid or hypertrophied synovium. The material in erosions may demonstrate enhancement following intravenous gadolinium administration.[18] Erosions may or may not be associated with edema in the bone marrow immediately adjacent to the defect in subchondral bone. In fact, edema adjacent to erosive change was found to correlate with progressive erosive changes despite clinical improvement following institution of therapy in a published report.[19] Edema in the periarticular soft tissues including the joint capsule and subcutaneous fat may be seen on both T1-weighted and, particularly, fat-suppressed T2-weighted sequences as a reflection of the inflammatory nature of this disease. Focal defects may be seen in cartilage, but hyaline cartilage is typically uniformly thinned in the inflammatory arthropathies, which accounts for the concentric joint space narrowing seen on conventional radiographs later in the disease.

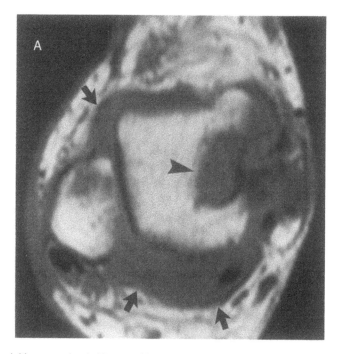

FIGURE 8.2 Synovial hypertrophy. A 43-year-old woman with rheumatoid arthritis and ankle pain. (A) Axial; T1-weighted image without contrast shows intermediate signal distending joint capsule from effusion and synovial hypertrophy (arrows). A subchondral cyst is seen in the talar dome (arrowhead). (Courtesy of David A. Rubin, M.D., St. Louis, Missouri.)   (*continued*)

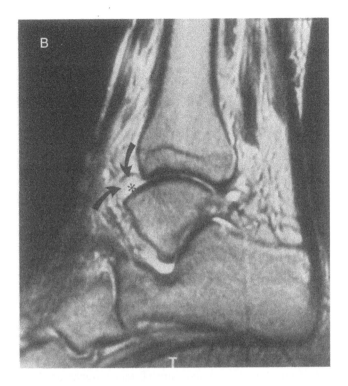

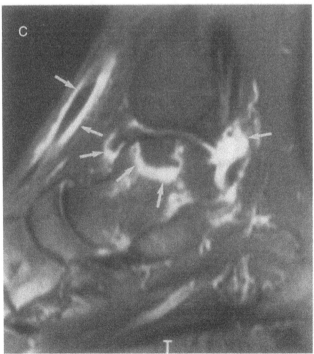

FIGURE 8.2 (continued) (B) Sagittal spin-echo T2-weighted image laterally shows effusion (asterisk). Note synovial hypertrophy in superior aspect of anterior capsule (curved arrow) is slightly lower in signal than the surrounding effusion. (C) Sagittal fat-saturated T1-weighted image following intravenous gadolinium administration demonstrates enhancement in the synovium of the ankle joint, anterior tibialis tendon sheath, and in a subchondral cyst in the talar dome (white arrows). (Courtesy of David A. Rubin, M.D., St. Louis, Missouri.)

Subchondral lucencies may be a prominent radiograph finding in some patients with RA, particularly those with the cystic variant.[20,21] The etiology of these subchondral "cysts" is not clear, but theories of their cause include direct extension of pannus,[22] metabolic bone injury,[23] and intraosseous rheumatoid nodule.[24] Subchondral cysts tend to demonstrate intermediate signal on T1-weighted and increased signal on T2*- or T2-weighted images reflecting their fluid nature. Following intravenous gadolinium administration, most cysts do not enhance;[24] however, rim enhancement may occur occasionally[8] (Figure 8.2).

Tendon sheath disease is an important manifestation of RA and may be the earliest and sometimes only MR imaging finding.[25] Findings of tenosynovitis in the disease include synovial hypertrophy and effusion in a distended tendon sheath. Stranding and edema in the subcutaneous fat surrounding an involved tendon sheath with loss of the interface between the tendon sheath and adjacent fat can also be present. This latter finding is unusual in tenosynovitis that accompanies idiopathic tendon disease such as posterior tibialis tendon tears in high-performance athletes. Synovial hypertrophy may also be seen in bursae of the foot such as the intermetatarsal, retrocalcaneal, and pre-Achilles bursae. Retrocalcaneal disease may lead to erosion of the underlying posterior superior calcaneus.

RA patients are at increased risk for tendon rupture in general and this is particularly evident in the posterior tibialis and Achilles tendons. Rheumatoid tendinopathy is a distinct histopathologic entity and in the Achilles tendon has a different MR imaging appearance in the Achilles tendon than that of degenerative disease.[26] Degenerative tears involving the Achilles tendon typically are manifested by a biconvex configuration on axial images with enlargement in the anteroposterior (AP) diameter. The diseased Achilles tendon in the RA patient, however, tends not to enlarge in the AP diameter but demonstrates increased intrasubstance signal on T1- and/or T2-weighted images. Patients with RA tendinopathy also demonstrated inflammation of the retrocalcaneal bursa that is seen less commonly with idiopathic Achilles tendonopathy.[26]

Other extra-articular MR imaging findings in RA include rheumatoid nodules. Rheumatoid nodules are painless, mobile subcutaneous masses that occur in up to 30% of patients with RA. Patients typically are rheumatoid factor positive and have a well-established diagnosis of RA, but the development of rheumatoid nodules may precede the onset of articular symptoms.[27] These masses occur over pressure points and osseous protuberances and are most commonly seen in the upper extremities. Rheumatoid nodules in the foot are uncommon (1% of patients), but present in the heel pad, adjacent to the Achilles, and under the metatarsal heads when seen. These plantar masses may be painful and require surgical excision. Chronic pressure may result in breakdown of overlying skin and secondary infection.[28] Histologically, rheumatoid nodules demonstrate a central area of necrosis that is surrounded by palisading histiocytes and vascular granulation tissue.[28] MR imaging findings reflect the histology of the lesion. The masses tend to be heterogeneous but predominantly intermediate in signal on T1-weighted images and demonstrate central high signal surrounded by low to intermediate signal on T2-weighted images. A second signal pattern can be present in lesions without classic histologic features, characterized by low to intermediate signal on both T1- and T2-weighted images without central high signal.[30] Heterogeneous enhancement of the nodules occurs following intravenous gadolinium administration.[30] Although a rheumatoid nodule may be confused with a neoplasm, the clinical history and characteristic location of the lesion help lead to the correct MR imaging diagnosis.

The ability to assess synovial hypertrophy and early erosive change on MR imaging accurately is clearly superior to that of conventional radiographs. This important information may lead to earlier and more aggressive therapeutic measures. Accurate depiction of synovial disease also permits an objective method to assess response to therapy. Scoring systems have been proposed to classify and quantify the degree of active disease in the wrist and knee. Decreased volume and enhancement of synovial tissue in the affected joint following intravenous gadolinium administration are indicators of reduced disease activity.[31,32]

SERONEGATIVE SPONDYLOARTHROPATHIES

The seronegative spondyloarthropathies are a family of arthritides including psoriatic arthritis, Reiter disease, ankylosing spondylitis, enteropathic arthritis, and synovitis, acne, pustulosis, hyperostosis, and osteitis syndrome (SAPHO) that share common radiographic and clinical findings. Patients with spondyloarthropathies have a high incidence of HLA B27 compared with the baseline population. Psoriatic and Reiter disease are the spondyloarthropathies that most commonly affect the foot and ankle.

Psoriatic arthritis occurs in approximately 8% of patients with psoriatic skin disease.[33] Patients are typically 20 to 40 years of age and there is no sex predilection. Skin disease, which is usually moderate to severe in extent, precedes the onset of arthritis in 75% of patients; however, in 10% of patients the arthropathy presents prior to the skin involvement.[34] Symptoms are frequently insidious in onset and this arthritis has a predilection for the small joints of the hands and feet.

Reiter disease is an uncommon arthritis, which classically occurs in male patients (up to 50:1 male to female ratio) following a sexually transmitted or enteric infection.[35] The classic triad associated with this disorder is conjuntivitis, urethritis, and arthritis. Various skin manifestations including circinate balanitis, keratoderma blenorrhagicum, and nail changes may also be seen. Reactive arthritis is a term used with increasing frequency by rheumatologists to categorize patients with a clinical and radiographic arthopathy similar to Reiter disease but without the other classic eye, urethral, and skin changes. Reiter disease has a striking predilection for the lower extremities.

Both psoriatic arthritis and Reiter disease typically present with a bilateral asymmetric distribution and frequently involve the distal interphalangeal (DIP) joints in contradistinction to RA. This distribution and the presence of proliferative bone formation, which commonly occur, allow the distinction of these disorders from RA on radiographs.[36] On radiographs, new bone formation can be manifested as periosteal reaction, fluffy excrescences at ligament, tendon, or capsule insertions (also known as enthesis), or fluffy excrescences at sites of articular excavation producing a "brush stroke" appearance to the erosive process. Soft-tissue swelling may be dramatic and involved toes may have a sausage appearance.

The MR imaging appearance of the spondyloarthropathies in small joints is not well documented compared with RA. However, these diseases share many MR imaging features similar to RA.[37] For example, synovial hypertrophy within joints, bursae, and tendon sheaths and erosions have an identical appearance on MR imaging (Figure 8.3). Typical asymmetrical

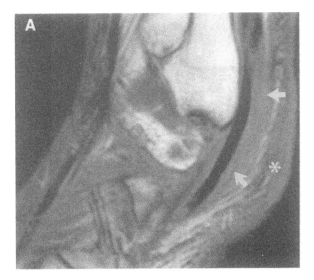

FIGURE 8.3 Tenosynovial hypertrophy. A 56-year-old male with psoriatic arthritis and lateral ankle pain. (A) Sagittal T1-weighted image through the lateral malleolus shows intermediate signal intensity surrounding the peroneal tendons, representing tenosynovial hypertrophy (white arrows).   *(continued)*

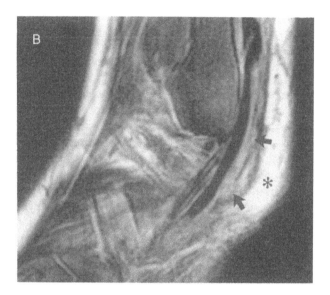

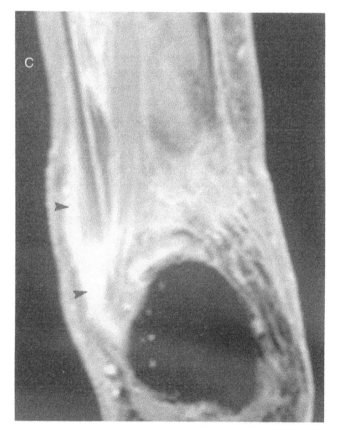

FIGURE 8.3 (continued) (B) Fat-saturated FSE T2-weighted image through same level demonstrates increased signal of hypertrophied synovium typically seen with this sequence (black arrows). Note increased signal within soft tissues adjacent to the tendon sheath representing subcutaneous edema (asterisk). A true abnormality rather than coil artifact is confirmed by intermediate signal replacement in the subcutaneous tissues in (A, asterisk). (C) Postgadolinium fat-saturated T1-weighted image in the coronal plane shows intense enhancement of hypertrophied synovium (arrowheads).

distribution of disease might not be appreciated if both feet are not imaged but DIP joint disease is more commonly seen in the spondyloarthopathies than in RA. Sausage digit soft-tissue swelling is a relatively specific finding associated with spondyloarthropathies and is recognizable on MR images. Investigators attribute the sausage-digit phenomenon to flexor tendon sheath tenosynovitis in the affected toe rather than joint disease[38] (Figure 8.4). Enthes-itis, when recognized on MR imaging, may also be a useful differentiating feature.[37,39] Man-ifestations of enthesitis are best seen on fat-suppressed T2-weighted sequences and include increased signal in tendons and ligaments surrounding a joint and focal increased signal intensity in the bone marrow adjacent to a ligamentous or tendinous insertion (Figure 8.5). Recognizing enthesitis in the small joints of the foot may be difficult and requires small field of view high-resolution images.

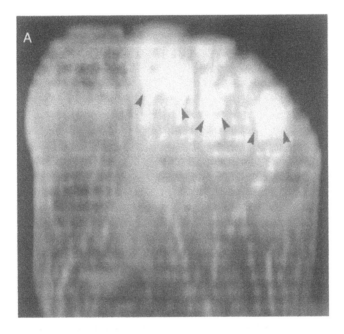

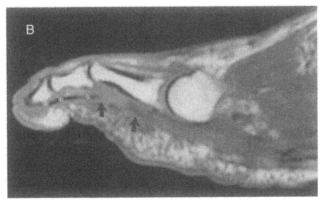

FIGURE 8.4 Sausage digit. A 44-year-old male with psoriatic arthritis and sausage digits. (A) Maximum intensity projection from an axial postgadolinium 3D-spoiled gradient-echo data set shows enhancement of soft tissues surrounding the second, third, and fourth toes (arrowheads). (B) Sagittal T1-weighted image before contrast administration through second digit shows intermediate signal intensity surrounding flexor tendon (aster-isk) representing tenosynovitis (black arrows). *(continued)*

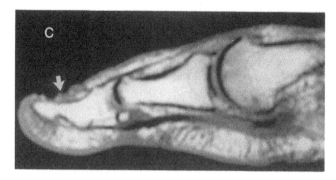

FIGURE 8.4 (continued) (C) The interphalangeal joints are relatively normal. Compare this with the normal tendon sheath in the first toe without a sausage configuration on a sagittal T1-weighted image. Note nail changes in first toe secondary to psoriasis (white arrow).

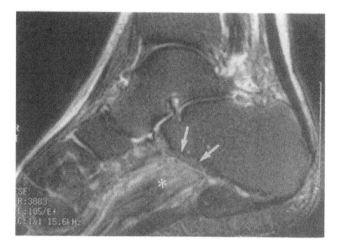

FIGURE 8.5 Enthesitis associated with psoriatic arthritis. A 47-year-old male with psoriatic arthritis. Sagittal fat-suppressed FSE T2-weighted image through the hind foot shows increased signal intensity within the quadratus plantae muscle (asterisk) and its insertion on the plantar aspect of the calcaneus representing enthesitis (arrows).

INFECTION

Septic arthritis is frequently due to a puncture wound and shares many of the MR imaging manifestations of other inflammatory arthritides. However, the findings tend to be more aggressive, particularly in the setting of bacterial infection.[40,41] Synovial hypertrophy, effusion, and destruction of both cartilage and bone are well demonstrated on MR imaging. Soft-tissue edema around the affected joint tends to be very prominent[41] (Figure 8.6). The clinical history, single joint involvement, and dramatic MR imaging findings are usually sufficient to make the diagnosis of septic arthritis. Recognition of normal joint compartmental anatomy in mid-foot and hind foot articulations helps to avoid potential confusion. For example, the anterior subtalar joint is typically in continuity with the talonavicular and calcaneocuboidal joints. Knowledge of this relationship will help the radiologist suggest the correct diagnosis of sepsis when these articulations are recognized as one compartment and no other joints in the foot or ankle are affected.

CRYSTAL DEPOSITION DISEASES

The crystalline arthopathies are a group of diseases reflecting the sequelae of crystal deposition into the soft tissues and joints. The crystal diseases that most commonly affect the foot and ankle

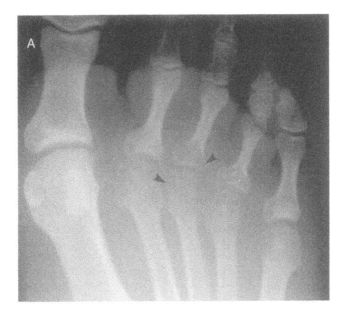

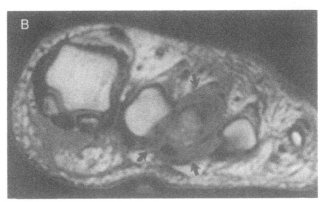

FIGURE 8.6 Septic arthritis. A 36-year-old male with third MTP septic joint 3 weeks after stepping on a nail. (A) AP radiograph of the forefoot shows juxta-articular osteoporosis, articular space narrowing, and erosions involving the third MTP joint (arrowheads). (B) Coronal T1-weighted image through the third MTP joint shows intermediate signal from effusion and synovial hypertrophy surrounding the joint (arrows). *(continued)*

include gout, hydroxyapatite deposition disease (HADD), and calcium pyrophosphate deposition disease (CPPD).

Gout

Gout is a disease caused by the deposition of urate crystals in soft tissues. Typically, patients are hyperuricemic with plasma urate concentrations exceeding 7.0 mg/dl in males and 6.0 mg/dl in females.[42] The risk for developing gout increases with elevated serum levels of urate. Although gout remains a male-predominant disease, it is increasingly common in females with currently reported male-to-female of ratios 2:1 to 7:1, up from previous ratios of 20:1.[43,44] The onset in males is usually over the age of 40 and in females occurs over the age of 60.

Gout tends to involve the lower extremities and the foot and ankle articulations are most commonly affected. The arthropathy presents in the great toe in 50% of patients, and 90% of

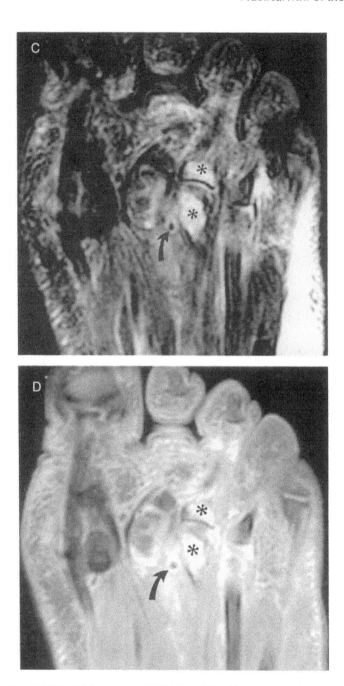

FIGURE 8.6 (continued) (C) Axial fat-saturated FSE T2-weighted image shows increased signal intensity in marrow of the distal third metatarsal and proximal third proximal phalanx (asterisk). Note marked generalized soft-tissue edema in forefoot. (D) Axial postgadolinium fat-saturated T1-weighted image demonstrates enhancement of third MTP joint and involved osseous structures (asterisks). Metallic artifact from puncture wound is seen in (C) and (D) (curved arrow).

patients ultimately have involvement of either the interphalangeal or the metatarsophalangeal joint of the hallux.[43] The tarsal–metatarsal (TMT) joints, retrocalcaneal bursa, and ankle are also frequently involved. Acute attacks present with soft-tissue swelling and redness over the affected joint. Microscopic examination of fluid from joint aspiration demonstrates crystals with a strong negative birefringence under polarized light. There are no published reports in the literature that describe the MR imaging appearance of the synovitis associated with an acute attack of gout prior to the development of tophi. Inflammatory changes such as effusion, inflamed synovium, and soft-tissue edema on MR imaging would be expected, however.

Tophaceous deposits in soft tissues occur in the chronic form of gout. Chronic tophaceous gout is now relatively uncommon due to advances in medical therapy resulting in better control of serum urate levels. It occurs mainly in those patients who are noncompliant or who have uncontrollable hyperuricemia. Typically, patients have recurrent intermittent acute attacks of gout for at least 10 years prior to the development of tophi, but occasionally tophi can be the initial manifestation of the disease.[45]

MR imaging is not usually necessary to evaluate tophaceous gout as the clinical history and radiographs are sufficient for diagnostic purposes. Infrequently, a tophus might be confused with a soft-tissue neoplasm if the history of gouty arthritis is not elicited. Acute symptoms can also be present mimicking septic arthritis. On MR imaging, tophi are intermediate in signal on T1-weighted images and demonstrate variable signal characteristics on T2-weighted images. In one published report, 23% of tophi showed increased signal and 77% demonstrated heterogeneous but generally decreased signal on T2-weighted images[46] (Figure 8.7). Intense homogeneous gadolinium enhancement was present in 89% of tophi in the same series. Edema of the soft tissues is typically present. Hypertrophied synovium, effusion, erosion of underlying bone, and bone marrow edema may also be seen in tophaceous gout. Tophi tend to deposit in and around joints but may be seen in unusual locations such as in the bone or tendons. The MR imaging appearance of tophi is not specific and is indistinguishable from other masses with similar imaging characteristics, including rheumatoid

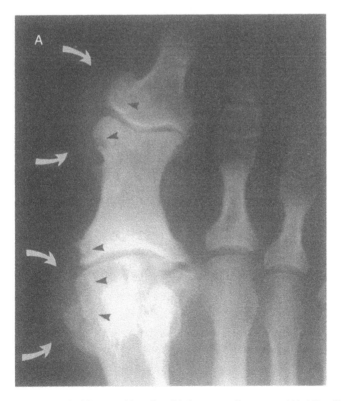

FIGURE 8.7 Tophaceous gout. A 48-year-old male with long-standing gout. (A) AP radiograph of the first toe shows faint soft-tissue density at the medial aspect of the first interphalangeal (IP) and MTP joints due to tophi (curved white arrows). Well-corticated erosions are seen in the underlying bone (arrowheads).

(*continued*)

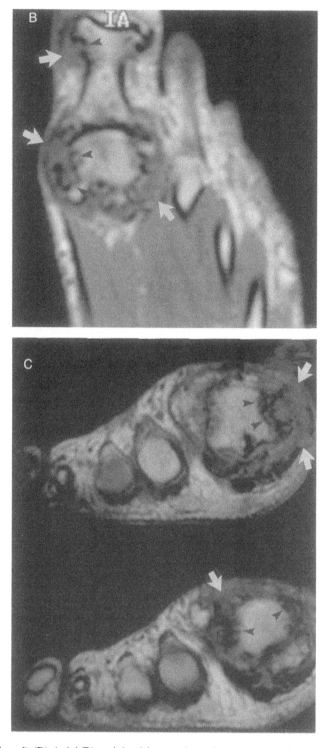

FIGURE 8.7 (continued) (B) Axial T1-weighted image shows heterogeneous but predominantly intermediate-signal-intensity masses representing tophi (white arrows) at medial aspect of the first MTP and IP
joints with erosion (arrowheads) of underlying bone. (C) Coronal T1-weighted images show heterogeneous
but predominantly intermediate-signal-intensity masses representing tophi (white arrows) at medial aspect
of the first MTP and IP joints with erosion (arrowheads) of the underlying bone.   (*continued*)

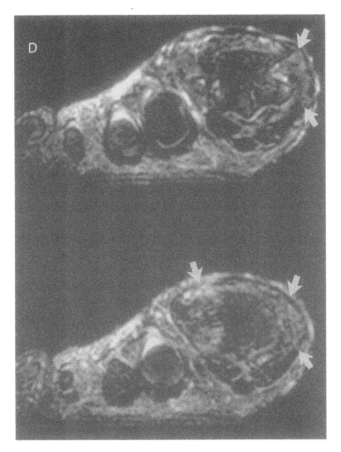

FIGURE 8.7 (continued) (D) The tophi are heterogeneous and predominantly low signal intensity on coronal fat-suppressed FSE T2-weighted images (arrows).

nodules, amyloid, xanthofibromas, and benign fibrous tumors. Polyarticular involvement typically excludes pigmented villonodular synovitis from the differential diagnosis.

HYDROXYAPATITE DEPOSITION DISEASE

Hydroxyapatite deposition disease (HADD), also known as calcific tendonitis, is a very common disease occuring in 2.7% of the population.[47] Calcific deposits are usually demonstrated in the shoulder and may be asymptomatic. The pathogenesis of HADD is not clear. An acute presentation manifested by redness, pain, and swelling can be confused with the diagnosis of infection. Patients are generally middle aged with a slight male predominance. The disorder is characteristically self-limiting.

Involvement of the foot and ankle is uncommon in HADD. The flexor tendons of the foot are most frequently involved in the lower extremity in either the ankle or the forefoot.[48] Other sites of involvement include the medial capsule of the first MTP joint and the distal Achilles tendon. Radiographically, the calcifications associated with HADD tend to be cloudlike or have dense concretions in the periarticular soft tissues, which may assume a comet-tail appearance when intratendinous in location. Multiple radiographic projections may be required to localize small concretions.

MR imaging is not required to make the diagnosis of HADD as radiographs are usually sufficient. There have been no reports of the MR imaging appearance of HADD in the foot and ankle and the appearance is inferred from descriptions of the disease at other locations.[49] Concretions are reportedly low in signal intensity on all pulse sequences and are surrounded by variable amounts of edema, the latter being best visualized on fat-suppressed T2-weighted MR imaging sequences. Without surrounding edema, however, the concretions may be difficult to separate from normal tendon signal.

CALCIUM PYROPHOSPHATE DEPOSITION DISEASE

Calcium pyrophosphate deposition disease (CPPD) is also a common disease. Calcium pyrophosphate crystals are largely responsible for calcification seen in cartilage (chondrocalcinosis) on radiographs. Not all patients with chondrocalcinosis are symptomatic. However, patients with CPPD may experience acute attacks of joint pain, clinically referred to as "pseudogout," due to the deposition of weakly positive birefringent crystals of calcium pyrophosphate in the joint. It is not clear whether deposition of calcium pyrophosphate crystals induces destruction of the articular cartilage or whether defective articular cartilage leads to deposition of crystal.[50] CPPD arthropathy has similar imaging features to osteoarthritis, but is distinguishable based on distribution, severity, and presence of chondrocalcinosis.

Typically patients are older adults and there is no sex predilection. Most cases of CPPD are idiopathic but some patients have other associated diseases, such as hyperparathyroidism or hemochromatosis. The knee, wrist, and pubic symphysis are the most common sites of involvement. Chondrocalcinosis and osteoarthritis are the most common radiographic findings. A distinctive distribution of joint involvement differentiates this disease from primary osteoarthritis including radioscaphoid and severe patellofemoral joint disease in the wrist and knee, respectively. Foot and ankle disease is not uncommon. Arthropathy is most common at the talocalcaneonavicular joint and capsular calcification is the most common finding in the forefoot.[51] Capsule, tendon, and ligamentous calcification may be seen as fine linear areas of density that is distinct from the cloudlike pattern of HADD.[51] Rarely, calcification may occur in a periarticular location due to tophaceous pseudogout, which can be the sole manifestation of the disease.[52]

The MR imaging features of CPPD arthropathy have not been well described. Nonspecific soft-tissue swelling and synovitis may be seen (Figure 8.8). Tophaceous pseudogout may present as a low-signal mass in the soft tissue with variable surrounding soft-tissue edema.

OSTEOARTHRITIS

Osteoarthritis (OA) is a very common heterogeneous disorder that is seen with increasing frequency in patients over 50 years of age. OA can be categorized into primary and secondary forms. OA is classified as secondary when osteophytes, subchondral sclerosis, and subchondral cysts develop in a joint associated with a known underlying disorder such as prior inflammatory arthritis, infection, or trauma. Primary OA is diagnosed when similar radiographic findings develop in the absence of a predisposing condition.

OA of the foot is not uncommon. Primary OA of the foot usually occurs in the first ray related to the demands secondary to the biomechanics of gait. The first TMT and first MTP joints are common sites of OA in the mid-foot and forefoot.[53] Although TMT disease may be relatively asymptomatic, OA of the first MTP joint may be very disabling. Primary disease in the hind foot is uncommon but may be seen at the talonavicular joint. OA of the ankle or other joints of the foot is unusual without antecedent trauma or underlying mechanical deformity.

MR imaging of OA is usually not indicated, as radiographs provide essential diagnostic information in most instances. When performed, MR imaging demonstrates articular space narrowing, osteophyte formation, and subchondral signal changes in the later stages of the disease (Figure 8.9). Subchondral "cysts" are depicted as focal round areas with typical fluid signal (intermediate signal on T1-weighted images and increased signal on T2-weighted images). More diffuse and less well marginated areas of subchondral signal change consistent with fluid in the marrow may also be present in OA on MR imaging. Commonly referred to as "marrow edema," despite no pathologic correlate, the etiology of the more diffuse subchondral signal change is unclear. Thinning of articular cartilage with intrusion of fluid into the subchondral bone is one possible explanation. Alternatively,

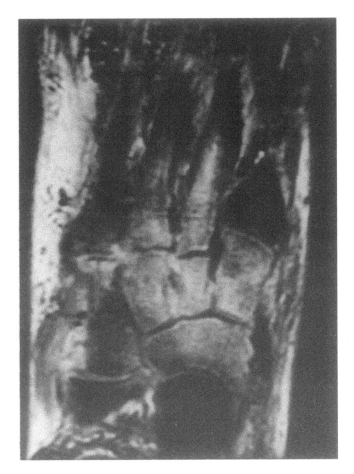

FIGURE 8.8 CPPD arthropathy. Axial inversion recovery images of patient with CPPD arthropathy shows increased signal in tarsal bones and base of metatarsals. (Courtesy of A. R. Spouge, M.D., London, Ontario, Canada.)

"marrow edema" in OA may be due to microfractures of the subchondral bone produced by ineffective cushioning that normal articular cartilage usually provides. The subchondral signal changes tends to be distributed on both sides of the joint. The accompanying osteophytes and lack of pericapsular soft-tissue edema reduces the likelihood of infection in the differential diagnosis as a cause for signal abnormalities. Additional findings in OA include synovial thickening and joint effusion, which vary in size and extent.[10]

MR imaging of suspected OA may be useful in two clinical scenarios. First, the complex anatomy of the foot is not easily evaluated on conventional radiographs. The multiplanar capability of MR imaging permits ready evaluation of the region, and confirmation of degenerative disease can easily be made. Although computed tomography (CT) can also evaluate complex joints, MR imaging has the advantage of imaging the cartilage directly compared with CT, which relies on indirect and relatively late manifestations of abnormal articular cartilage such as changes in sub-chondral bone. Cartilage-specific MR imaging techniques such as fat-suppressed Spoiled Gradient Recalled Echo (SPGR) sequences can directly visualize small cartilage defects prior to the development of radiographically demonstrable OA.[10] For instance, chondral injury of the first metatarsal head may be the initial event that leads to the development of hallux rigidus or hallux limitus. Early detection may direct surgical intervention or alteration in footwear that may delay or prevent the development of OA. Documentation of cartilage defects and their extent may become even more clinically relevant in the future with the advent of cartilage transplantation.

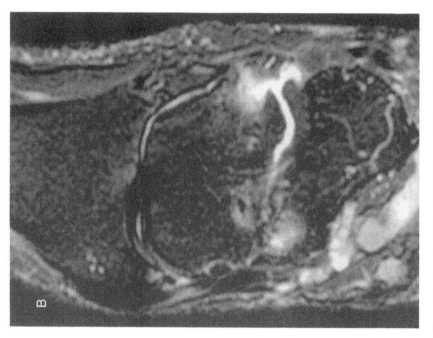

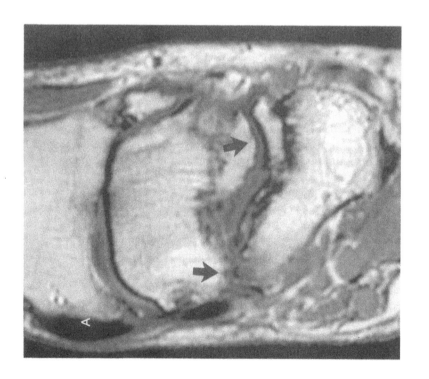

FIGURE 8.9 Osteoarthritis. A 73-year-old male with ankle pain and osteoarthritis. (A) Coronal spin-echo T1-weighted image of the ankle demonstrates severe lateral joint space narrowing with tilting of the talus. Note also subchondral irregularity in the posterior and middle subtalar joints (arrows) with osteophyte formation in the lateral aspect of posterior subtalar joint. (B) Coronal fat-saturated FSE T2-weighted image of the ankle demonstrates severe lateral joint space narrowing with tilting of the talus. Note also subchondral irregularity in the posterior and middle subtalar joints with osteophyte formation in the lateral aspect of posterior subtalar joint (black arrows).

(*continued*)

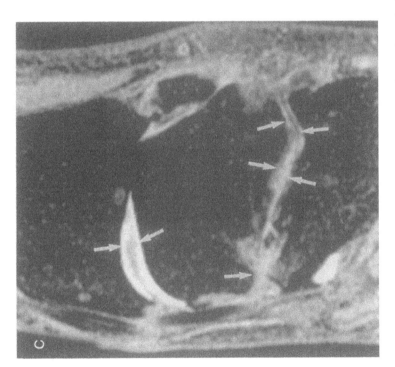

FIGURE 8.9 (continued) (C) Coronal fat-suppressed spoiled gradient-echo image dramatically shows irregularity in the cartilage in the medial aspect of the tibiotalar joint and subtalar joints (arrows).

NEUROPATHIC OSTEOARTHROPATHY

Neuropathic osteoarthropathy is an aggressive destructive arthropathy that occurs in the joints of patients with neuropathic disorders. Charcot was the first to describe the causal relationship between disease of the central nervous system and joints in the year 1868, and this arthropathy still carries his name. The exact reason for development of arthropathy in the setting of neuropathic disease is not known. Although many theories regarding the pathogenesis of this joint disorder have been proposed, trauma and neurovascular insult due to loss of autonomic control of blood flow are the two favored causes. Many disorders of both upper and lower motor neurons can lead to neuropathic osteoarthropathy, including trauma, syphilis, alcoholism, and myelomeningocele, but the most common underlying disease is diabetes mellitus.

The foot is a common site of neuropathic osteoarthropathy, particularly in patients with diabetes. Patients tend to be 50 to 70 years of age without sex predilection and typically have a long-standing history of diabetes. Trauma may be an inciting event.[54] Patients present with painful swelling of the affected joint. Subchondral sclerosis and osteophyte formation is seen radiographically in the hypertrophic form of the disease, but this arthropathy is separated from OA by recognizing framentation, dislocation, fractures, and debris. Bone resorption may be the predominant finding in the atrophic presentation.[55] Disease progression can be dramatic and rapid with dissolution of a joint occurring in a matter of days. The rapid course of joint destruction may raise the question of infection.

The MR imaging appearance of neuropathic osteoarthropathy depends on the stage of disease at the time of imaging. In the chronic form of the disease, fragmentation and dislocation of mid-foot bones are readily appreciated in multiple planes. Low-signal marrow changes on both T1- and T2-weighted images in affected osseous structures can be seen reflecting sclerosis.[56] Subchondral "cysts" may be seen as rounded foci of high signal on T2-weighted images and intermediate signal on T1-weighted images (Figure 8.10). Effusion, particularly in the ankle and subtalar joints, and subcutaneous edema can be demonstrated without infection.[57] Acute disease on MR imaging is reflected by decreased signal on T1-weighted images and increased signal on T2-weighted (particularly fat-suppressed techniques) or inversion-recovery images. Fractures may accompany the marrow changes. Prominent soft-tissue edema is typically seen in the acute form of the disease, as well. The acute findings may be indistinguishable from infection.

Infection in the diabetic foot is a common clinical and radiologic dilemma, and differentiation from neuropathic osteoarthropathy may be difficult. Osteomyelitis is most common over pressure points, particularly in the forefoot of people with diabetes and tends to be associated with skin ulceration. Skin ulcer size and depth affects the probability of underlying osseous infection. Ulcers that involve an area of greater than 2 cm², are deeper than 3 mm, or extend down to bone are more likely to be associated with osteomyelitis.[58,59] On radiographs, infection tends to be associated with ill-defined and irregular margins of involved bone, whereas the osseous margins in an uncomplicated case of neuropathic OA tend to be smooth and well defined. Radiographs may be definitive and are still the most important first examination despite limited sensitivity and specificity.

Scintigraphic evaluation of osteomyelitis in the diabetic foot has been utilized with varying degrees of success. The nuclear bone scan alone tends to be sensitive but not specific.[60] A combination of bone scan with indium-labeled white blood cells (WBC) is most commonly used to evaluate for osteomyelitis with reported sensitivity ranging from 75 to 100% and specificity from 55 to 91%.[61] Potential problems with labeled WBC studies include technical difficulties, time, and expense of labeling the patient's WBC, poor spatial resolution, and poor anatomic localization of soft-tissue abscesses for preoperative planning.[58]

MR imaging has been shown to be a highly effective tool for evaluation of osteomyelitis in the diabetic foot. In this setting, MR imaging allows early diagnosis of osteomyelitis and

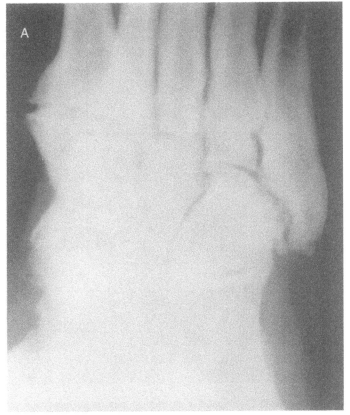

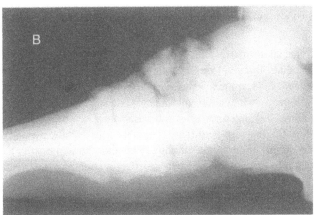

FIGURE 8.10 Neuropathic arthropathy. A 59-year-old male with diabetes with hypertrophic neuropathic osteoarthropathy and concern for osteomylitis. (A) Oblique radiograph shows disorganization of the talonavicular joint associated with a navicular fracture and severe osteoarthritis of the tarsometatarsal joint. (B) Lateral radiograph shows disorganization of the talonavicular joint associated with a navicular fracture and severe osteoarthritis of the tarsometatarsal joint.   (*continued*)

identification of abscesses that can impact on both medical and surgical therapy.[62,63] Some authors have questioned the cost-effectiveness of imaging as opposed to empiric long-term antibiotic therapy,[64] but others have shown MR imaging to be cost-effective.[61] The strength of MR imaging in the evaluation of osteomyelitis is in its strong negative predictive value (91 to 96%). If the bone marrow signal on MR imaging is normal, the diagnosis of osteomyelitis is unlikely.

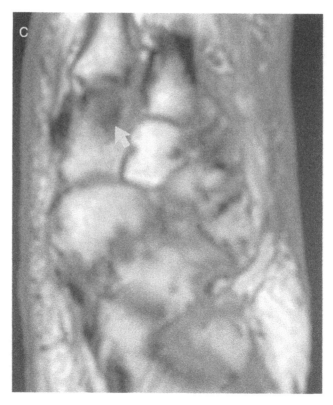

FIGURE 8.10 (continued) (C) Axial T1-weighted image through mid-foot demonstrates subchondral irregular-itity and disorganization throughout the mid-foot articulations. A subchondral cyst is present in the first cuneiform (arrow) without significant generalized marrow abnormality, despite subcutaneous edema. *(continued)*

Bone marrow signal abnormality raises the concern for infection particularly when marrow replacement is intermediate in signal on T1-weighted images and high in signal on T2-weighted images.[65] Fat-suppressed T2-weighted sequences offer the highest sensitivity for detection of marrow abnormality. However, magnetic field heterogeneity may complicate the interpretation of these images as focal areas of incomplete fat saturation may be confused with abnormal marrow. Small structures such as the toes can be difficult to evaluate as volume averaging from surrounding structures may project signal in marrow. Although debatable, fat-suppressed T1-weighted gadolin-ium-enhanced imaging may help delineate areas of infection and, in one report, offered the highest sensitivity and specificity of any sequence.[66] Enhanced images also offer the confident demonstration of abscesses and necrotic tissue that may affect surgical management. When bone marrow signal suggests edema, the differentiation of infection from neuropathic osteoarthropathy may be impossible. Findings that favor osteomyelitis in the setting of neuropathic joint disease include presence of adjacent abscess or sinus tract extending to the affected bone, cortical interruption, and abnormal marrow changes distant to the site of radiographically identifiable neuropathic disease[66] (Figure 8.11). Labeled WBC examination may be necessary to augment investigation of infection, particularly when the site of concern for osteomyelitis is in the same region as acute changes of neuropathic osteoarthropathy.[67]

PROLIFERATIVE SYNOVITIS

Synovial proliferative disorders are uncommon diseases that may affect the synovium of joints, tendon sheaths, or bursae. Intra-articular villonodular synovitis includes pigmented villonodular

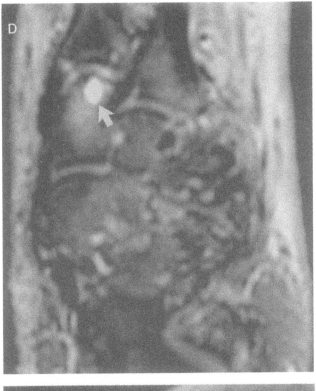

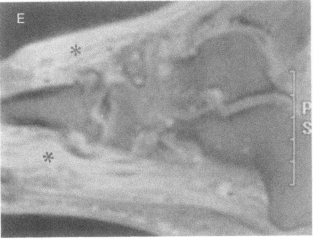

FIGURE 8.10 (continued) (D) Fat-saturated FSE T2-weighted image through mid-foot demonstrates subchondral irregularitity and disorganization throughout the mid-foot articulations. A subchondral cyst is present in the first cuneiform (arrow) without significant generalized marrow abnormality, despite subcutaneous edema. (E) Sagittal fat-saturated T1-weighted image after gadolinium shows lack of significant marrow enhancement and demonstrates soft-tissue enhancement secondary to cellulitis (asterisks). The MR imaging findings are consistent with a neuropathic joint without evidence of infection.

synovitis (PVNS) and synovial chondromatosis (SOC). Each disorder has extra-articular variants that may involve either the tendon sheaths or bursae of the foot and ankle. Giant cell tumor of the tendon sheath (GCTTS) is the extra-articular presentation of PVNS, and tenosynovial chondromatosis is the extra-articular variant of synovial chondromatosis. The MR imaging manifestations of these disorders reflect their histopathology and are frequently highly characteristic.

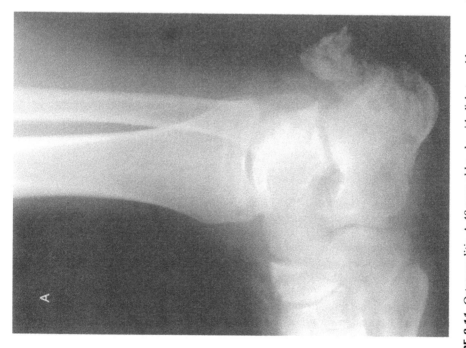

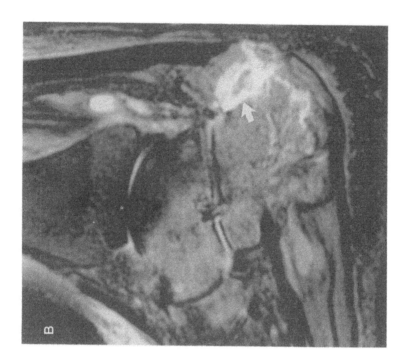

FIGURE 8.11 Osteomyelitis. A 48-year-old male with diabetes with a neuropathic foot and osteomyelitis. (A) Lateral radiograph of the foot shows a comminuted avulsion fracture involving the Achilles insertion. Note the lack of smooth margination to the fracture fragments. (B) Sagittal fat-saturated FSE T2-weighted image shows fluid in the calcaneal fracture (arrow) and an edema-like pattern replacing normal marrow signal in the calcaneus, anterior talus, and tarsal navicular. *(continued)*

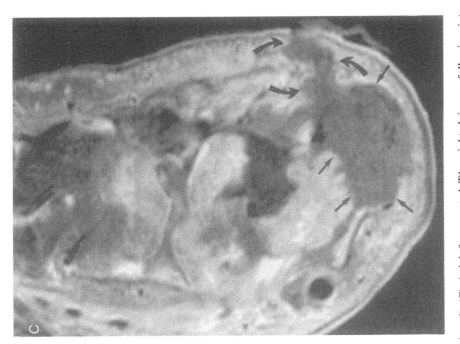

FIGURE 8.11 (continued) (C) Axial fat-saturated T1-weighted image following intravenous gadolinium administration shows a rim-enhancing fluid collection at the fracture site (arrows) with a sinus tract extending out to the skin (curved arrows). *Staphylococcous aureus* infection was confirmed at surgery.

PIGMENTED VILLONODULAR SYNOVITIS

Pigmented villonodular synovitis (PVNS) is an uncommon benign synovial proliferative disorder that most commonly involves the large joints. The knee and hip are involved in 80% of cases. The foot and ankle are the third most common sites of disease and account for 13% of cases.[68] Any articulation may be involved including ankle, subtalar, mid-foot, and MTP joints. PVNS occurs in two forms. The diffuse form of the disease that involves the entire synovial lining of a joint is most common, but a focal nodular or local form can also be seen. The diffuse form of the disease is more likely to be associated with recurrence following treatment. The pathogenesis of this arthropathy is not clear. The proliferating cells are thought to originate from synovial lineage but they express features of osteoclasts or macrophages/histiocytes according to published reports.[69] The cause for proliferation of these cells is not understood, but proposed theories have included trauma and inflammation. More recent work suggests that the proliferation of these cells is a neoplastic event.[68]

Patients tend to be young adults (20 to 30 years old), but the disease has been reported in both very young and old patients. There is no sex predilection. Although usually monoarticular, there are scattered reports of multijoint involvement.[70] Symptoms may be present for months to years prior to presentation. Joint stiffness and swelling is the most common presenting complaint, and pain, if present, is usually a dull ache. A mass, when elicited on physical exam, tends to be soft, and tenderness may be appreciated in 50% of cases.[68] Joint aspiration may reveal brown fluid consistent with old blood but a clear aspirate can also be obtained. Surgery remains the treatment of choice. Intra-articular radiation therapy has been utilized in recurrent disease and as a primary treatment modality. Recurrence rates can approach 50% depending on the series.[71]

The gross pathologic appearance of PVNS has been likened to a "shaggy red beard" reflecting the frondlike projections of synovium seen in this disease. Hemosiderin in the lesion accounts for the reddish discoloration. Microscopically, hyperplastic synovial villi are demonstrated with foamy macrophages and hemosiderin-laden cells.

The radiologic manifestations of PVNS have been well described. Conventional radiographs may demonstrate a soft-tissue swelling or mass. Osseous manifestations, including erosions with sclerotic margins and subchondral lucencies, are seen in only 14% of cases involving the foot and ankle on plain radiographs. Calcification in the mass is very unusual.[72] The joint space is usually preserved until late in the disease. CT may reveal high-attenuation soft tissue in an involved joint and will delineate bone invasion more readily than conventional radiographs in complex joints. Radionuclide bone and thallium-201 scintigraphy can demonstrate increased uptake in an involved joint. Technetium-99m dimercaptosuccinic acid (DMSA) uptake can also be seen.[73]

MR is the imaging modality of choice when PVNS is considered in the differential diagnosis. The characteristic MR imaging appearance of the disease allows noninvasive confirmation of the diagnosis and the ready evaluation of the surgical extent of the disease. On MR imaging, PVNS manifests as multiple masses that are typically heterogeneous but predominantly intermediate and low signal on T1- and T2-weighted images[74] (Figure 8.12). Low signal, felt to reflect hemosiderin in the proliferating synovial tissue, causes more pronounced signal loss on gradient-echo sequences as a result of local field heterogeneity induced by iron deposition. If the hemosiderin is scant, the mass may not be distinguishable from other synovial processes. A variable-sized joint effusion is present. The masses tend to be high in signal on inversion recovery sequences.[75] Diffuse intense enhancement is demonstrated following intravenous gadolinium contrast enhancement[76] (Figure 8.13). Although the appearance of PVNS on MR imaging is distinctive, there are other processes that may mimic the classic pattern of low signal on T1- and T2-weighted images in the synovium, including synovial chondromatosis, amyloidosis, gout, RA, hemangioma, and hemophilia.

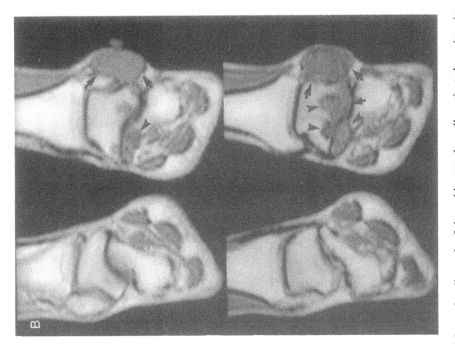

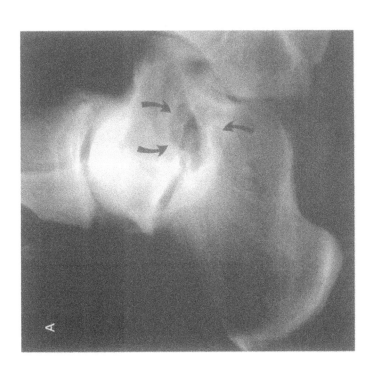

FIGURE 8.12 Pigmented villonodular synovitis. A 28-year-old male with foot pain. (A) Lateral radiograph of the ankle reveals well-corticated erosions involving the sinus tarsi (curved arrows). (B) Coronal spin-echo T1-weighted images demonstrats a predominantly intermediate-signal-intensity lobulated mass replacing the fat of the sinus tarsi in the left hind foot and extending laterally (arrows). Erosions in the talus and calcaneus are seen (arrowheads). (Courtesy of Mark D. Murphey, M.D., Washington, D.C.) *(continued)*

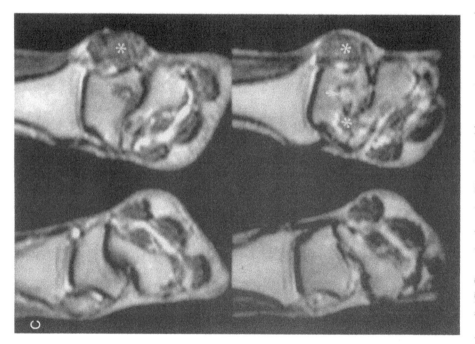

FIGURE 8.12 (continued) (C) Coronal spin-echo T2-weighted images show the mass is predominantly low in signal (asterisks) but also contains on area of high signal (arrow). (Courtesy of Mark D. Murphey, M.D., Washington, D.C.)

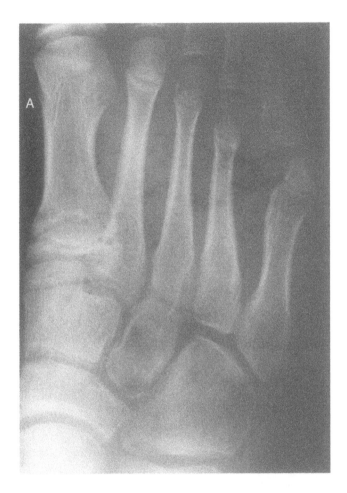

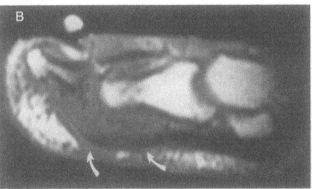

FIGURE 8.13 Diffuse PVNS. A 10-year-old boy with pain in the fifth metatarsal. (A) Dorsoplantar radiograph shows widening of the articular space, medial subluxation of the proximal phalanx, and erosions of the metatarsal head. (B) Sagittal spin-echo T1-weighted image shows an intermediate-signal intensity mass with focal hypotensities centered at the fifth MTP joint. The soft-tissue component is more extensive on the plantar aspect (arrows). (Courtesy of A. R. Spouge, M.D., London, Ontario, Canada.) *(continued)*

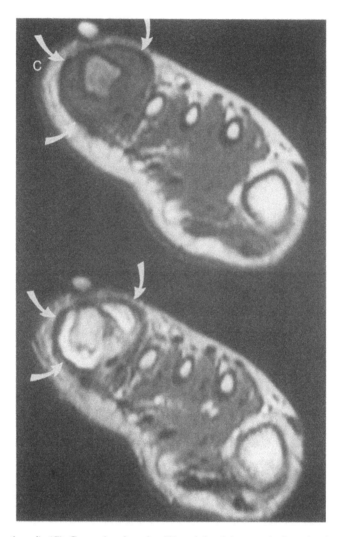

FIGURE 8.13 (continued) (C) Coronal spin-echo T1-weighted images before (top) and after (bottom) gadolinium show diffuse enhancement of the hyperplastic synovium (arrows). PVNS was confirmed histologically. (Courtesy of A. R. Spouge, M.D., London, Ontario, Canada.)

GIANT CELL TUMOR OF THE TENDON SHEATH

Giant cell tumor of the tendon sheath (GCTTS) is the extra-articular form of PVNS and is seen clinically more commonly than PVNS. Most cases (65 to 88%) present in the hand and wrist.[77,78] Foot and ankle involvement represents 5 to 15% of cases and is most commonly seen in the first and second toes. The demographics of affected patients are different from PVNS. Patients are older at presentation with a typical age range of 30 to 50 years and a slight female sex predilection of 1.5:1 to 2:1.[77] The most common clinical presentation is a painless, mobile, nontender mass attached to an underlying tendon. Two forms of the disease have been described. The most common form is localized, which is typically a mass 2 to 4 cm in size involving the digits. The diffuse form of GCTTS presents with a larger mass (up to 9 cm) and may represent extension of PVNS from a joint. Surgical resection is the treatment of choice. As with PVNS, the diffuse form of the disease is more commonly associated with recurrence.

The most common radiographic manifestation of GCTTS is a soft-tissue mass that may be seen in up to 50% of cases.[77] Osseous erosions in adjacent bone may be seen in 21% of cases[78] and periosteal reaction is an uncommon manifestation. Associated calcification leading to concern for synovial chondromatosis can be seen, but is unusual.[77]

Further assessment is often not required but, if it is, MR imaging is the modality of choice. The MR imaging appearance of GCTTS is similar to that described for PVNS and is also dependent on the hemosiderin content in the lesion.[79] On T1-weighted images, the mass tends to be intermediate in signal although low signal may also be seen. Lesions tend to be equal to or lower than muscle in signal on T2-weighted images, although hyperintense signal may be seen. Intense enhancement is usually demonstrated after intravenous gadolinium administration[80] (Figure 8.14). Gradient-echo sequences may demonstrate pronounced signal loss in the mass due to hemosiderin present in the lesion. Lesions that may share similar signal characteristics of GCTTS include fibroma of tendon sheath, plantar fibromatosis, and clear cell sarcoma. A pseudoaneurysm of the dorsalis pedis artery has been reported to be similar in signal to GCTTS.[81]

Synovial (Osteo)chondromatosis

Synovial (osteo)chondromatosis (SOC) is a self-limited metaplastic proliferative disorder of unknown etiology that may be characterized by the formation of cartilage in the synovium of joints, tendon sheaths, or bursae.[82] The cartilage nodules can calcify or ossify and detach from the synovium resulting in loose bodies in the joint. Ossified loose bodies can also occur in OA but SOC is distinguished from this secondary presentation by clinical and histologic findings.

The intra-articular form of SOC typically presents in middle-aged adults, 40 to 50 years of age. This disease is generally considered to be more common in males; however, a female predominance has been noted in one series.[82] No age or sex predilection has been reported for the

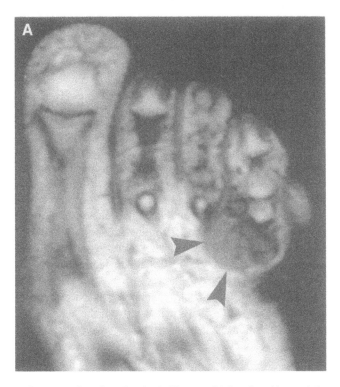

FIGURE 8.14 Giant cell tumor of tendon sheath. A 39-year-old female with a painless mass involving the dorsum of the fourth toe. (A) Axial T1-weighted spin-echo image demonstrates a heterogeneous mass with low and intermediate signal on the dorsum of the fourth toe (arrowheads). (Courtesy of Mark D. Murphey, M.D., Washington, D.C.)

(*continued*)

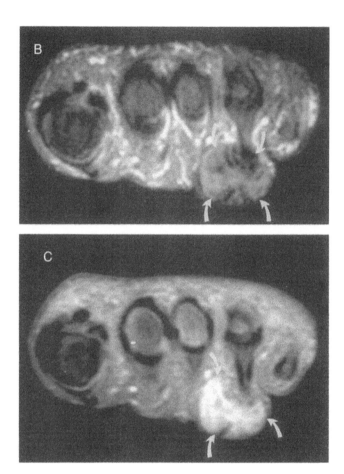

FIGURE 8.14 (continued) (B) Coronal T2-weighted fat-suppressed spin-echo sequence shows the mass is heterogeneous with both low signal and intermediate signal similar to fat (curved arrows). (C) Heterogeneous enhancement is seen within the mass following intravenous gadolinium administration (curved arrows). (Courtesy of Mark D. Murphey, M.D., Washington, D.C.)

extra-articular form of the disease.[83] A familial form of SOC has been reported.[84] The most common presenting complaint is pain followed by swelling and locking. Although any synovial-lined structure may be involved, the most common site of disease is the knee joint, which accounts for over 50% of cases. Monoarticular disease is most common with occasional reports of multifocal involvement.[84] Foot and ankle disease is uncommon, accounting for approximately 11% of cases. Typical locations involved in the foot and ankle include the ankle, subtalar, and hallux interphalangeal joints as well as retrocalcaneal bursa and the flexor hallucis tendon sheath.

SOC has been divided histologically into three categories by Milgram.[85] In Stage I, there is metaplasia of the synovium with cartilage nodules that remain attached to the synovium. In Stage II, metaplasia is again noted but the nodules have detached from the synovium and loose bodies are present. Loose bodies, which are often calcified in the absence of synovial metaplasia, represent Stage III or "burned-out" disease pathologically. The pattern of ossification and the number of loose bodies help distinguish primary from secondary disease.[85] Ossified nodules may demonstrate a central fatty marrow. SOC may show atypical histology raising the diagnostic possibility of chondrosarcoma. However, documented cases of chondrosarcoma in SOC are extremely rare. Synovectomy is the treatment of choice and recurrence rates are relatively low compared with PVNS.

Demonstration of calcified loose bodies is the most important diagnostic radiographic feature. Loose bodies can be identified in up to 79% of cases; they tend to be small, ranging in size from

3 mm to 3 cm.[82] Articular space narrowing with osteophyte formation can be seen but tends to be a late finding. Well-demarcated erosions are more commonly seen in joints with tight capsules rather than capacious joints such as the knee. Radionuclide bone scanning agents may demonstrate radiotracer uptake at involved sites. CT may be helpful in identifying calcifications and in determining the extent of the soft-tissue mass, particularly in complex anatomic areas.

Three signal patterns have been described on MR imaging.[86] The most common pattern is a lobulated intrasynovial mass that is predominantly isointense to muscle on T1-weighted images and hyperintense to muscle on T2-weighted images with central round low-signal foci on both sequences. The central signal void corresponds to calcification on both CT and radiographs. The intrasynovial mass tends to demonstrate low-signal septa on T2-weighted images that separate the lesion into lobules. The second most common pattern on MR imaging is a lobular mass without focal areas of signal void and no radiographically identifiable calcifications. The third pattern on MR imaging consists of central fat signal surrounded by a rim of low signal consistent with enchondral ossification, corresponding to loose bodies seen on radiographs. Heterogeneous, predominantly septal enhancement is seen following intravenous gadolinum contrast administration, which is characteristic of tissue of chondroid derivation[86] (Figure 8.15).

SUMMARY

In summary, while radiographs remain the primary means of imaging rheumatologic disorders, MR imaging can play a complementary role, particularly in the detection of early erosive change and the evaluation of complications of the disease. The findings on MR may also aid the clinician in better staging of these diseases and deciding on therapy.

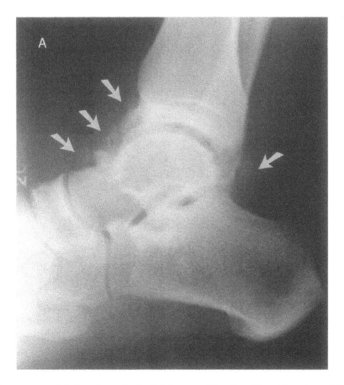

FIGURE 8.15 Primary synovial chondromatosis. A 25-year-old male with ankle pain and locking. (A) Lateral radiograph demonstrates multiple tibiotalar joint bodies anteriorly and to a lesser extent posteriorly (arrows). (From Musculoskeletal Case 4. Presentation, *CJS*, 42 (3), 170, 1999. With permission.)   (*continued*)

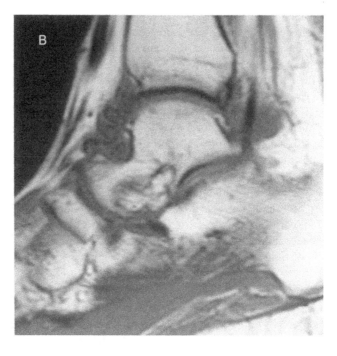

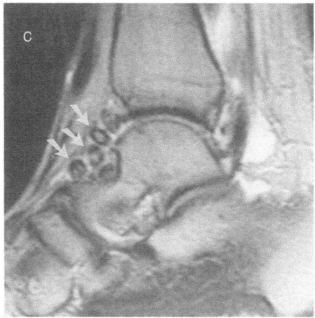

FIGURE 8.15 (continued) (B) Sagittal spin-echo T1-weighted and (C) conventional spin-echo T2-weighted images confirm the cartilaginous nature of the bodies, manifested by central intermediate signal intensity on T1-weighted images and intermediate to high signal intensity on the T2-weighted images. A rim of low-signal calcification is present on both the T1- and T2-weighted images. The uniformity of size, mutiplicity of bodies, and absence of significant underlying osteoarthrosis supports the diagnosis of primary synovial chondromatosis. Innumerable intra-articular bodies were found at operation. (From Musculoskeletal Case 4. Presentation, *CJS*, 42 (3), 170, 1999. With permission.)

REFERENCES

1. Beltran, J., Caudill, J. L., Herman, L. A. et al., Rheumatoid arthritis: MR imaging manifestations, *Radiology*, 165, 153, 1987.
2. Singson, R. D. and Zalduondo, F. M., Value of unenhanced spin echo MR imaging in distinguishing between synovitis and effusion of the knee, *AJR*, 159, 569, 1992.
3. Winalski, C. S., Palmer, W. E., Rosenthal, D. I., and Weissman, B. N., Magnetic resonance imaging of rheumatoid arthritis, *Radiol. Clin. North Am.*, 34, 243, 1996.
4. Rand, T., Imhof, H., Czerny, C. et al., Discrimination between fluid, synovium, and cartilage in patients with rheumatoid arthritis: contrast enhanced spin echo versus non-contrast-enhanced fat-suppressed gradient-echo MR imaging, *Clin. Radiol.*, 54, 107, 1999.
5. Konig, H., Sieper, J., and Wolf, K., Rheumatoid arthritis: evaluation of hypervascular and fibrous pannus with dynamic MR imaging enhanced with Gd-DTPA, *Radiology*, 176, 473, 1990.
6. Kursunoglu-Brahme, S., Riccio, T., Weisman, M. H. et al., Rheumatoid knee: role of gadopentetate-enhanced MR imaging, *Radiology*, 176, 831, 1990.
7. Bjorkengren, A. G., Geborek, P., Rydhom, U., Holtas, S., and Petterson, H., MR imaging of the knee in acute rheumatoid arthritis: synovial uptake of gadolinium-DOTA, *AJR*, 155, 329, 1990.
8. Adam, G., Dammer, M., Bohndorf, K., Christoph, R., Fenke, F., and Gunther, R. W., Rheumatoid arthritis of the knee: value of gadopentenate dimeglumine-enhanced MR imaging, *AJR*, 156, 125, 1991.
9. Herve-Somma, C. M. P., Sebag, G. H., Prieur, A. M. et al., Juvenile rheumatoid arthritis of the knee: MR evaluation with Gd-DOTA, *Radiology*, 182, 92, 1992.
10. McCauley, T. R. and Disler, D. G., MR imaging of articular cartilage, *Radiology*, 209, 629, 1998.
11. MacGregor, A. J. and Silman, A. J., *Rheumatology*, 2nd ed., Mosby, London, 1998, Chap. 5.2.
12. Williams, D. G., *Rheumatology*, 2nd ed., Mosby, London, 1998, Chap. 5.9.
13. Sugimoto H., Takeda, A., Masuyama, J., and Furuse, M., Early-stage rheumatoid arthritis: diagnostic accuracy of MR imaging, *Radiology*, 198, 185, 1996.
14. Gilkeson, G., Pollison, R., Sinclair, H. et al., Early detection of carpal erosions in patients with rheumatoid arthritis: a pilot study of magnetic resonance imaging, *J. Rheumatol.*, 15, 1361, 1988.
15. Foley Nolan, D., Stack, J. P., Ryan, M. et al., Magnetic resonance imaging in the assessment of rheumatoid arthritis. A comparison with plain film radiographs, *Br. J. Rheumatol.*, 30, 101, 1991.
16. Jorgensen, C., Cyteval, C., Anaya, J. M., Baron, M. P., Lamarque, J. L., and Sany, J., Sensitivity of magnetic resonance imaging of the wrist in very early rheumatoid arthritis, *Clin. Exp. Rheumatol.*, 11, 163, 1993.
17. McQueen, F. M., Stewart, N., Crabbe, J. et al., Magnetic resonance imaging of the wrist in early rheumatoid arthritis reveals a high prevalence of erosions at four months after symptom-onset, *Ann. Rheum. Dis.*, 57, 350, 1998.
18. Rominger, M. B., Bernreuter, W. K., Kenney, P. J., Morgan, S. L., Blackburn, W. D., and Alarcon, G. S., MR imaging of the hands in early rheumatoid arthritis: preliminary results, *Radiographics*, 13, 37, 1993.
19. McQueen, F. M., Stewart, N., Crabbe, J. et al., Magnetic resonance imaging of the wrist in early rheumatoid arthritis reveals progression of erosions despite clinical improvement, *Ann. Rheum. Dis.*, 58, 156, 1999.
20. Gubler, F. M., Maas, M., Dijkstra, P. F., and de Jongh, H. R., Cystic rheumatoid arthritis: description of a nonerosive form, *Radiology*, 177, 829, 1990.
21. Resnick, D., Niwayama, G., and Coutts, R. D., Subchondral cysts (geodes) in arthritic disorders: pathologic and radiolographic appearance of the hip joint, *AJR*, 128, 799, 1977.
22. Soila, P., The causal relations of rheumatoid disintegration of juxta-articular bone trabeculae, *Acta Rheumatol. Scand.*, 9, 231, 1963.
23. Rennel, C., Mainzer, F., Mulitz, C. V., and Genant, H. K., Subchondral pseudocysts in rheumatoid arthritis, *AJR*, 129, 1069, 1977.
24. Gubler, F. M., Algra, P. R., Maas, M., Dijkstra, P. F., and Falke, Th. H. M., Gadolinium-DTPA enhanced magnetic resonance imaging of bone cysts in patients with rheumatoid arthritis, *Ann. Rheum. Dis.*, 52, 716, 1993.

25. Rubens, D. J., Blebea, J. S., Totterman, S. M., and Hooper, M. M., Rheumatoid arthritis: evaluation of wrist extensor tendons with clinical examination versus MR imaging — a preliminary study, *Radiology,* 187, 831, 1993.

26. Stiskal, M., Szolar, D. H., Stenzel, I. et al., Magnetic resonance imaging of Achilles tendon in patients with rheumatoid arthritis, *Invest. Radiol.,* 32, 602, 1997.

27. Askari, A., Moskowitz, R. W., and Goldberg, V. M., Subcutaneous rheumatoid nodules and serum rheumatoid factor with arthritis, *JAMA,* 229, 319, 1974.

28. Kaye, B. R., Kaye, R. L., and Bobrove, A., Rheumatoid nodules, *Am. J. Med.,* 76, 279, 1984.

29. Moore, C. P. and Wilkens, R. F., The subcutaneous nodule: its significance in the diagnosis of rheumatic disease, *Semin. Arthritis Rheum.,* 7, 63, 1977.

30. El-Noueam, K. I., Giuliano, V., Schweitzer, M. E., and O'Hara, B. J., Rheumatoid nodules: MR/pathological correlation, *JCAT,* 21, 796, 1997.

31. Ostergaard, M., Gideon, P., Sorensen, K. et al., Scoring of synovial membrane hypertrophy and bone erosions by MR imaging in clinically active and inactive rheumatoid arthritis of the wrist, *Scand. J. Rheumatol.,* 24, 212, 1995.

32. Takeuchi, K., Inoue, H., Yokoyama, Y. et al., Evaluation of rheumatoid arthritis using a scoring system devised from magnetic resonance imaging of rheumatoid knees, *Acta Med. Okayama,* 52, 211, 1998.

33. Wright, V. and Moll, J. M. H., *Seronegative Polyarthritis.,* North Holland Publishing Company, Amsterdam, 1976.

34. Helliwell, P. S. and Wright, V., *Rheumatology,* 2nd ed., Mosby, London, 1998, Chap. 6.

35. Resnick, D., *Diagnosis of Bone and Joint Disorders,* 3rd ed., W.B. Saunders, Philadelphia, 1995, Chap. 30.

36. Brower, A. C., *Arthritis in Black and White,* 2nd ed., W.B. Saunders, Philadelphia, 1997, Chap. 10.

37. Jevtic, V., Watt, I., Rozman, B., Kos-Golja, M., Desmar, F., and Jarh, O., Distinctive radiological features of small hand joints in rheumatoid arthritis and seronegative spondyloarthropathies demonstrated by contrast enhanced (Gd-DTPA) magnetic resonance imaging, *Skeletal Radiol.,* 24, 351, 1995.

38. Olivieri, I., Barozzi, L., Pierro, A., De Matteis, M., Padula, A., and Pavlica, P., Toe dactylitis in patients with spondyloarthropathy: assessment by magnetic resonance imaging, *J. Rheumatol.,* 24, 926, 1997.

39. McGonagle, D., Gibbon, W., O'Connor, P., Green, M., Pease, C., and Emery, P., Characteristic magnetic resonance imaging entheseal changes of knee synovitis in spondyloarthopathy, *Arthritis Rheum.,* 41, 694, 1998.

40. Lee, S. K., Suh, K. J., and Kim, Y. W., Septic arthritis versus transient synovitis at MR imaging: preliminary assessment with signal intensity alterations in bone marrow, *Radiology,* 211, 459, 1999.

41. Strouse, P. J., Londy, F., DiPietro, M. A., Teo, E. L., Chrisp, C. E., and Doi, K., MRI evaluation of infectious and non-infectious synovitis: preliminary studies in a rabbit model, *Pediatr. Radiol.,* 29, 367, 1999.

42. Cohen, M. G. and Emmerson, B. T., in *Rheumatology,* 2nd ed., Mosby, London, 1998, Chap. 8.

43. Rubenoff, R., Gout and hyperuricemia, *Rheum. Dis. Clin. North Am.,* 16, 539, 1990.

44. Yu, T.-F., Some unusual features of gouty arthritis in females, *Semin. Arthritis Rheum.,* 6, 247, 1977.

45. Shmerling, R. H., Stern, S. H., Gravallese, E. M., and Kantrowitz, F. G., Tophaceous deposition in the finger pads without gouty arthritis, *Arch. Intern. Med.,* 148, 1830, 1988.

46. Yu, J. S., Chung, C., Recht, M., Dailiana, T., and Jurdi, R., MR imaging of tophaceous gout, *AJR,* 168, 523, 1997.

47. Bosworth, B. M., Calcium deposits in the shoulder and subacromial bursitis: a survey of 12122 shoulders, *JAMA,* 116, 2477, 1941.

48. Holt, P. D. and Keats, T. E., Calcific tendonitis: a review of the usual and unusual, *Skeletal Radiol.,* 22, 1, 1993.

49. Ramon, F. A., Degryse, H. R., De Schepper, A. M., and Van Marck, E. A., Calcific tendinitis of the vastus lateralis muscle, *Skeletal Radiol.,* 20, 21, 1991.

50. Bjelle, A., Cartilage matrix in hereditary pyrophosphate arthropathy, *J. Rheumatol.,* 8, 959, 1981.

51. Steinbach, L. S. and Resnick, D., Calcium pyrophosphate dihydrate crystal deposition disease revisited, *Radiology,* 200, 1, 1996.

52. Ling, D., Murphy, W. A., and Kyriakos, M., Tophaceous pseudogout, *AJR,* 138, 162, 1982.

53. Resnick, D. and Niwayama, G., *Diagnosis of Bone and Joint Disorders,* 3rd ed, W.B. Saunders, Philadelphia, 1995, 1263.

54. Slowman-Kovacs, S. D., Braunstein, E. M., and Brandt, K. D., Rapidly progressive charcot arthropathy following minor joint trauma in patients with diabetic neuropathy, *Arthritis Rheum.,* 33, 412, 1990.
55. Brower, A. C., The acute neuropathic joint, *Arthritis Rheum.,* 31, 1571, 1988.
56. Beltran, J., Campanini, S., Knight, C., and McCalla, M., The diabetic foot: magnetic resonance imaging evaluation, *Skeletal Radiol.,* 19, 37, 1990.
57. Marcus, C. D., Ladam-Marcus, V. J., Leone, J., Malgrange, D., Bonnet-Gausserand, F. M., and Menanteau, B. P., MR imaging of osteomyelitis and neuropathic osteoarthropathy in the feet of diabetics, *Radiographics,* 16, 1337, 1996.
58. Newman, L. G., Waller, J., Palestro, C. J. et al., Unsuspected osteomyelitis in diabetic foot ulcers: diagnosing and monitoring by leukocyte scanning with indium In111 oxyquinalone, *JAMA,* 266, 1246, 1991.
59. Grayson, M. L., Gibbons, G. W., Balogh, K., Levin, E., and Karchmer, A. W., Probing to bone in infected pedal ulcers. A clinical sign of underlying osteomyelitis in diabetic patients, *JAMA,* 273, 721, 1995.
60. Levine, S. E., Neagle, C. E., Esterhai, J. L., Wright, D. G., and Dalinka, M. K., Magnetic resonance imaging for the diagnosis of osteomyelitis in the diabetic patient with foot ulcer, *Foot Ankle,* 15, 151, 1994.
61. Morrison, W. B., Schweitzer, M. E., Wapner, K. L., Hecht, P. J., Gannon, F. H., and Behm, W. R., Osteomyelitis in feet of diabetics: clinical accuracy, surgical utility, and cost effectiveness of MR imaging, *Radiology,* 196, 557, 1995.
62. Edelman, D., Hough, D. M., Glazebrook, K. N., and Oddone, E. Z., Prognostic value of the clinical examination of the diabetic foot ulcer, *J. Gen. Intern. Med.,* 12, 537, 1997.
63. Cook, T. A., Rahim, N., Simpson, H. C. R., and Galland, R. B., Magnetic resonance imaging in the management of diabetic foot infection, *Br. J. Surg.,* 83, 245, 1996.
64. Eckman, M. H. et al., Foot infections in diabetic patients. Decision and cost-effectiveness analysis, *JAMA,* 273, 712, 1995.
65. Craig, J. G., Amin, M. B., Wu, K. et al., Osteomyelitis of the diabetic foot: MR imaging–pathologic correlation, *Radiology,* 203, 849, 1997.
66. Morrison, W. B., Schweitzer, M. E., Batte, W. G., Radack, D. P., and Russel, K. M., Osteomyelitis of the foot: relative importance of primary and secondary MR imaging signs, *Radiology,* 207, 625, 1998.
67. Lipman, B. T., Collier, B. D., Carrera, G. F. et al., Detection of osteomyelitis in the neuropathic foot: nuclear medicine, MRI, and conventional radiography, *Clin. Nucl. Med.,* 23, 77, 1998.
68. Rao, A. S. and Vigorita, V. J., Pigmented villonodular synovitis (giant cell tumor) of the tendon sheath and synovial membrane, *J. Bone Joint Surg.,* 66A, 76, 1984.
69. Darling, J. M., Goldring, S. R., Harada, Y., Handel, M. L., Glowacki, J., and Gravallese, E. M., Multinucleated cells in pigmented villonodular synovitis and giant cell tumor of the tendon sheath express features of osteoclasts, *Am. J. Pathol.,* 150, 1383, 1997.
70. Vendatam, R., Strecker, W. B., Schoenecker, P. L., and Salinas-Madrigal, L., Polyarticular pigmented villonodular synovitis in a child, *Clin. Orthop. Relat. Res.,* 348, 208, 1998.
71. Byers, P. D., Cotton, R. E., Deacon, O. W. et al., The diagnosis and treatment of pigmented villodular synovitis, *J. Bone Joint Surg.,* 50B, 290, 1968.
72. Baker, N. D., Klein, J. D., Weidner, N., Weissman, B. N., and Brick, G. W., Pigmented villonodular synovitis containing coarse calcifications, *AJR,* 153, 1228, 1989.
73. Kobayashi, H., Kotura, Y., Hosono, M. et al., Case report: uptake of pentavalent technetium-99m dimercaptosuccinic acid by pigmented villonodular synovitis: comparison with computed tomography, magnetic resonance imaging and gallium-67 scintigraphy, *Br. J. Radiol.,* 67, 1030, 1994.
74. Hughes, T. H., Sartoris, D. J., Schweitzer, M. E., and Resnick, D. L., Pigmented villonodular synovitis: MRI characteristics, *Skeletal Radiol.,* 24, 7, 1995.
75. Lin, J., Jacobson, J. A., Jamadar, D. A., and Ellis, J. H., Pigmented villonodular synovitis and related lesions: the spectrum of imaging findings, *AJR,* 172, 191, 1999.
76. Bessette, P. R., Cooley, P. A., Johnson, R. P., and Czarnecki, D. J., Gadolinium enhanced MRI of pigmented villonodular synovitis of the knee, *JCAT,* 16, 992, 1992.
77. Karasick, D. and Karasick, S., Giant cell tumor of tendon sheath: spectrum of radiologic findings, *Skeletal Radiol.,* 21, 219, 1992.

78. Ushijima, M., Hashimoto, H., Tsuneyoshi, M., and Enjoji, M., Giant cell tumor of the tendon sheath. A study of 207 cases to compare the large joint group with the common digit group, *Cancer*, 57, 875, 1986.

79. Jelenik, J. S., Kransdorf, M. J., Shmookler, B. M., Aboulafia, A. A., and Malawer, M. M., Giant cell tumor of the tendon sheath: MR findings in nine cases, *AJR*, 162, 919, 1994.

80. Kransdorf, M. J. and Murphey, M. D., *Imaging of Soft Tissue Tumors*, W. B. Saunders, Philadelphia. 1997, 275.

81. Millett, P. J., Potter, H., and O'Malley, M. J., Idiopathic pseudoaneurysm of the dorsalis pedis artery mimicking pigmented villonodular synovitis, *Foot Ankle Int.*, 20, 42, 1999.

82. Maurice, H., Crone, M., and Watt, I., Synovial chondromatosis, *J. Bone Joint Surg.*, 70, 807, 1988.

83. Karlin, C. A., De Smet, A. A., Neff, J., Lin, F., Horton, W., and Wertzberger, J. J., The variable manifestations of extraarticular synovial chondromatosis, *AJR*, 137, 731, 1981.

84. Felbel, J., Gresser, U., Lohmoller, G., and Zollner, N., Familial synovial chondromatosis combined with dwarfism, *Hum. Genet.*, 88, 351, 1992.

85. Milgram, J. W., Synovial osteochondromatosis: a histopathological study of thirty cases, *J. Bone Joint Surg.*, 59A, 792, 1977.

86. Kramer, J., Recht, M., Deeley, D. M. et al., MR appearance of idiopathic synovial osteochondromatosis, *JCAT*, 17, 772, 1993.

9 Miscellaneous Conditions of the Foot and Ankle

Alison R. Spouge

CONTENTS

INTRODUCTION

There are a variety of conditions of the foot and ankle that can be classified as "miscellaneous." These conditions do not fit nicely into any of the other categories discussed in this book and are therefore outlined in this chapter. Examples of these conditions include the following: compression neuropathies, disorders of the plantar fascia, impingement, and reflex sympathetic dystrophy.

COMPRESSION NEUROPATHIES

TARSAL TUNNEL SYNDROME

Tarsal tunnel syndrome results from compression of the posterior tibial nerve and/or its branches in the tarsal tunnel. The syndrome was initially described in 1962 by Keck[1] and Lam.[2] The clinical presentation of tarsal tunnel syndrome depends on the location of the pathology causing the nerve compression in relation to the branching pattern of the posterior tibial nerve. The syndrome has a slight female predominance and is characterized by dysesthesia, anesthesia, or paresthesia in the distribution of the posterior tibial nerve, which is aggravated by weight bearing. The nerve symptoms can radiate proximally into the calf or distally along the course of the terminal divisions of the posterior tibial nerve in the foot.[3] Sensory deficit is a late complication, and motor impairment rarely develops in association with the syndrome. On physical examination, findings suggestive of the diagnosis include local tenderness in the distribution of the posterior tibial nerve (Valleix phenomenon) and a positive Tinel's sign (percussion of the posterior tibial nerve resulting in paresthesia along the distribution of the nerve).[4] Tarsal tunnel syndrome is often misdiagnosed as one of a number of conditions that have an overlapping clinical presentation. These include interdigital neuroma, plantar fasciitis, lumbar radiculopathy, peripheral vascular disease, diabetic neuropathy, and rheumatoid disorders.[4,5] Electrodiagnostic studies can confirm the diagnosis, but also may be falsely negative.[6] The presence of delayed motor latency on nerve conduction studies and fibrillation potentials with sharp positive wave spikes on electomyography are consistent with the diagnosis of tarsal tunnel syndrome.[6]

The tarsal tunnel is a fibro-osseous channel composed of several structures (Figure 9.1). The roof of the tunnel starts 10 cm proximal to the medial malleolus and extends distally to the sustentaculum tali of the calcaneus. The posterior part of the roof is formed by the deep fascia of the calf and the flexor retinaculum (previously called the laciniate ligament), a fibrous band that is attached superiorly to the medial malleolus and inferiorly to the calcaneal body.[4] Fibrous septa extend vertically from the undersurface of the flexor retinaculum and attach to the calcaneal periosteum, further compartmentalizing the tunnel. Some of the septa also attach to the posterior tibial neurovascular bundle, resulting in traction on the nerve when the foot moves. The abductor hallucis muscle forms the anterior part of the roof of the tarsal tunnel. Some authors restrict the boundaries of the tarsal tunnel to the proximal and distal borders of the flexor retinaculum.[7] Other authors, however, believe that the tunnel extends beyond the borders of the flexor retinaculum, both proximally into the lower calf and distally into the hind foot beneath the abductor hallucis muscle. The proximal and distal portions of the tunnel have been referred to as the tibiotalar and talocalcaneal tarsal tunnels, respectively.[8] The floor of the tunnel is formed by the medial talus and calcaneus. The tarsal tunnel contains the tibialis posterior tendon, flexor digitorum longus tendon, the posterior tibial neurovascular bundle (artery, nerve, and vein), and flexor hallucis longus tendon from anterior to posterior, respectively. The posterior tibial nerve has three terminal divisions in

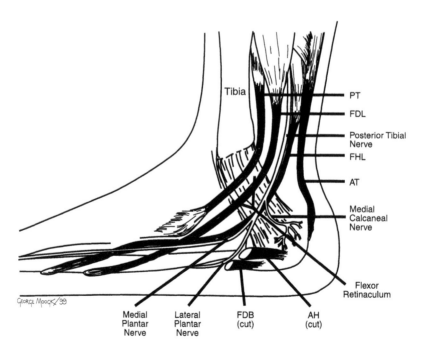

FIGURE 9.1 Anatomy of the tarsal tunnel. View from the medial side of the ankle and foot. PT = posterior tibial tendon, FDL = flexor digitorum longus tendon, FHL = flexor hallucis longus tendon, AT = Achilles tendon, AH = abductor hallucis muscle/tendon, FDB = flexor digitorum brevis muscle/tendon.

the foot. It usually divides into the medial and lateral plantar nerves beneath the flexor retinaculum, although branching can occur proximal to the retinaculum in approximately 5% of patients.[7] The medial plantar nerve provides sensory innervation to the medial 31/2 toes and the lateral plantar nerve supplies the lateral 11/2 toes. The medial calcaneal branch of the posterior tibial nerve is the third terminal division of the posterior tibial nerve. It provides sensory innervation to the heel and has variable anatomy, either arising as a single nerve proximal to, or under, the flexor retinaculum, in 40 and 60% of patients, respectively.[7,9] In approximately 25% of patients, the medial calcaneal nerve consists of multiple branches instead of a single branch.[7]

The superior inherent soft-tissue contrast and detailed anatomy depicted on MR (magnetic resonance) imaging provides excellent delineation of the normal anatomy (Figure 9.2) and pathologic conditions causing tarsal tunnel syndrome.[8,10] High-resolution technique is necessary for optimal evaluation of the region and includes a 512×224 matrix, 8 to 12 cm field of view confined to the affected side, and thin slices in conjunction with axial T1- and T2-weighted sequences. To obtain high-quality images, a local coil is essential and suitable coils include the extremity coil, paired 3-in. circular coils, and a small flexible wraparound coil.

A variety of pathologies, extrinsic or intrinsic to the tarsal tunnel, can produce compression of the posterior tibial nerve and/or its branches resulting in tarsal tunnel syndrome.[4,11] Cimino[4] carried out a comprehensive review of the literature that included 122 patients from 24 published reports and found that idiopathic causes represented the single most common etiology in up to 20% of

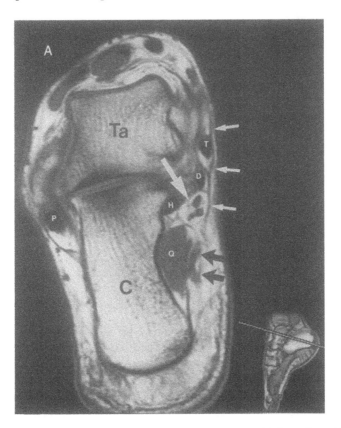

FIGURE 9.2 MR imaging anatomy of the tarsal tunnel. Oblique coronal SE T1-weighted image of the tarsal tunnel in the (A) proximal hind foot. The posterior tibial nerve has divided into the medial (large white arrow) and lateral (black arrows) plantar nerves. Flexor retinaculum (small white arrows); T = posterior tibial tendon; D = flexor digitorum longus tendon; H = flexor hallucis longus tendon; Ta = talus; C = calcaneus; Q = quadratus plantae; P = peroneal tendons. *(continued)*

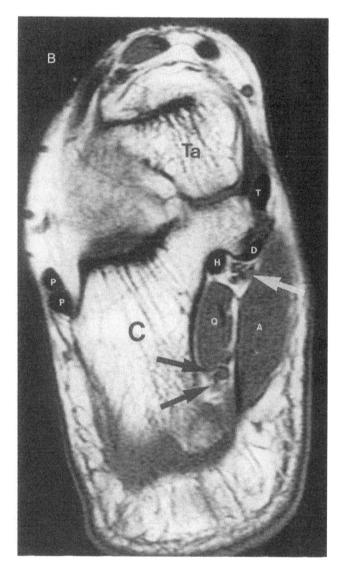

FIGURE 9.2 (continued) Oblique coronal SE T1-weighted image of the tarsal tunnel in the (B) distal hind foot. The posterior tibial nerve has divided into the medial (white arrow) and lateral (black arrows) plantar nerves. T = posterior tibial tendon; D = flexor digitorum longus tendon; H = flexor hallucis longus tendon; A = abductor hallucis muscle; Ta = talus; C = calcaneus; Q = quadratus plantae; P = peroneal tendons.

patients. Traumatic pathology accounted for the syndrome in 17% of patients in Cimino's review, mainly secondary to hind foot and ankle fractures sustained in motor vehicle and industrial accidents.[4] Of the traumatic etiologies, 23% were also found to result from iatrogenic injuries associated with operative procedures, including arthrodesis.[11] Other causes of tarsal tunnel syndrome include varicosities (13% of patients) (Figure 9.3), fibrosis (9% of patients) (Figure 9.4), heel varus malalignment (8% of patients), soft tissue ganglia (Figures 9.5 and 9.6), inflammatory arthropathies, diabetes, obesity, lipomas, an accessory flexor digitorum longus muscle, and hypertrophy of the abductor hallucis muscle.[4]

    Use of orthotics and other conservative measures are usually unsuccessful in treating tarsal tunnel syndrome, and surgical release of the flexor retinaculum and decompression of the posterior tibial nerve are often necessary for successful therapy.

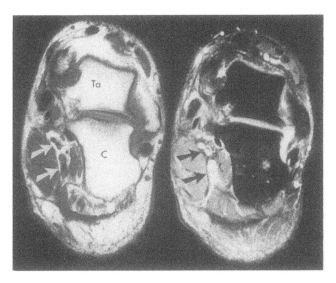

FIGURE 9.3 Varix causing tarsal tunnel syndrome. Coronal SE T1-weighted (left) and inversion recovery (IR) (right) images in the mid- to lower portion of the tarsal tunnel reveal distension of the plantar vessels (arrows) which are high signal intensity on the IR image in this surgically proven case of tarsal tunnel syndrome. Ta = talus; C = calcaneus.

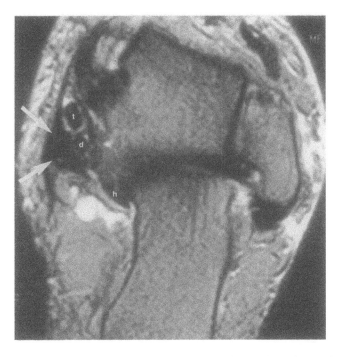

FIGURE 9.4 Scar causing tarsal tunnel syndrome. Oblique axial fast SE T2-weighted fat-suppressed image in a 50-year-old woman who presented with recurrent tarsal tunnel symptoms following a previous surgical release. Low-signal-intensity tissue consistent with scarring (arrows) is evident in the vicinity of the posterior tibial nerve that was surgically confirmed. t = tibialis posterior, d = flexor digitorum longus, h = flexor hallucis longus. (Courtesy of David A. Rubin, M.D., St. Louis, Missouri.)

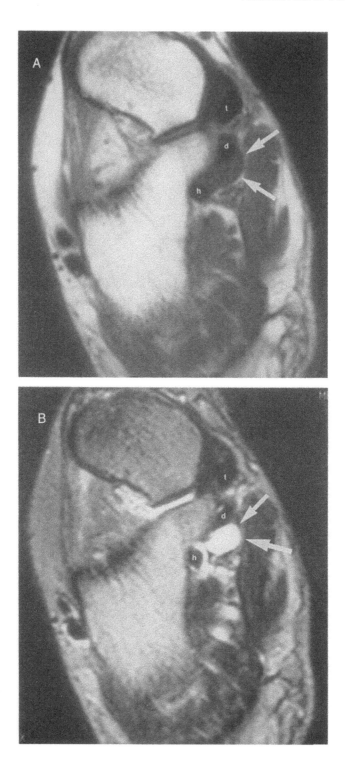

FIGURE 9.5 Ganglion causing tarsal tunnel syndrome. (A) Oblique coronal SE T1- and (B) T2-weighted images in a 37-year-old female presenting with tarsal tunnel syndrome demonstrate a spherical fluid-signal intensity mass between the flexor digitorum and hallucis longus tendons (arrows). A ganglion arising from the flexor hallucis tendons was confirmed at operation. t = tibialis posterior, d = flexor digitorum longus, h = flexor hallucis longus. (Courtesy of David A. Rubin, M.D., St. Louis, Missouri.)

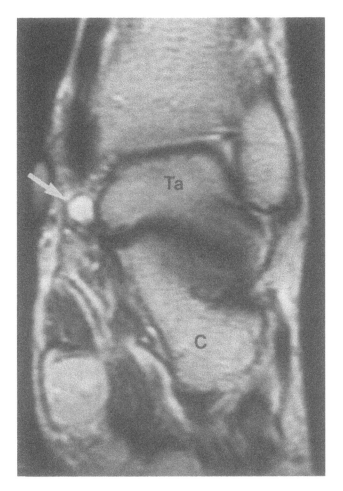

FIGURE 9.6 Ganglion causing tarsal tunnel syndrome. A 37-year-old female with foot paresthesia. Coronal SE T2-weighted image in the hind foot shows a focal high signal intensity lesion in the tarsal tunnel, which was subsequently proved to represent a ganglion (arrow). Ta = talus; C = calcaneus.

MORTON NEUROMA

Morton neuroma has been described in other chapters covering pediatric conditions and soft-tissue tumors and tumorlike lesions. Although not widely recognized as a compression neuropathy, this lesion is believed to develop in response to repetitive compression of the plantar interdigital nerves against the deep transverse metatarsal ligament from dorsiflexion of the toes.[12] It most commonly occurs between the third and fourth metatarsal heads.[12]

ANTERIOR TARSAL TUNNEL SYNDROME

Anterior tarsal tunnel syndrome is caused by compression of the deep peroneal nerve in the space between the talus and navicular bones and the overlying inferior extensor retinaculum.[13] This rare syndrome presents with sensory abnormalities over the dorsum of the foot, often in the region of the first and second toes. It can be caused by a number of conditions including talonavicular osteoarthrosis, ganglia, fractures, pes cavus, and tight footwear. If radiographs do not show any obvious osseous abnormality, MR imaging can be useful in assessing for and evaluating the extent of soft-tissue pathology in patients with the syndrome.[13]

BURSAE

Bursae are synovial-lined sacs that serve to reduce friction and facilitate motion between tightly opposed structures such as tendons and adjacent bones. They are commonly encountered in the foot and ankle.[14] Bursae usually contain a small amount of fluid that is typically not visualized on MR imaging under normal circumstances.[14] The bursae of the foot have received little discussion in the radiologic literature. In general, bursae may be classified as either anatomic or adventitial.[12] Anatomic bursae, although not present at birth, form in response to normal friction between tendons and other structures including adjacent fascia, bones, or other tendons. There are many anatomic bursae in the foot[12] that can occasionally be identified in patients on MR imaging, such as the bursae located on the medial and lateral plantar surfaces of the first and fifth metatarsals[15] (Figure 9.7). Anatomic bursae may become inflamed from a variety of causes including abnormal pressure, trauma, and inflammatory arthropathies.[12] Adventitial bursae develop secondary to abnormal pressure on soft tissues of the foot and ankle and are often related to an osseous abnormality or deformity. The most common adventitial bursae are found in these locations: over a bunion or hammer toe, on the plantar surface of a prominent metatarsal head, around the proximal interphalangeal joint of the fifth toe (referred to as the tailor's bunion bursa), or over an exostosis.[12] Patients usually present with a soft-tissue mass over a pressure point in the foot. Radiographs may show localized soft-tissue swelling at the site of the bursa, which occasionally, in long-standing cases, can undergo calcification or ossification. MR imaging may be requested in atypical clinical presentations when other soft-tissue lesions are

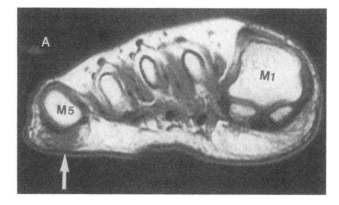

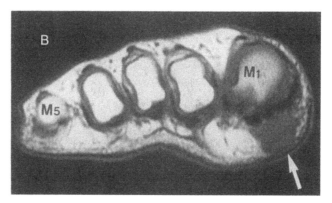

FIGURE 9.7 Plantar bursae. (A) Coronal SE T1-weighted images, proximal and (B) slightly more distal show small bursae on the plantar aspect of the hallux and fifth metatarsal heads (arrows). This 19-year-old patient had no symptoms referable to the areas. M1 = first metatarsal; M5 = fifth metatarsal.

considered in the differential diagnosis. The literature is scant regarding the MR imaging appearance of bursae in the foot. However, the signal characteristics are presumed to resemble bursae located elsewhere in the body: low to intermediate signal intensity on T1-weighted sequences and high signal intensity on T2-weighted sequences.[14,16] The location of the abnormal soft tissue over a pressure point or bone deformity in the region of an anatomic bursa should suggest the diagnosis (Figures 9.8 and 9.9). Conservative therapy, which can consist of anti-inflammatory medication, orthotics, and modified physical activity, is often sufficient to allievi-ate the symptoms. Operative therapy may be necessary to correct an underlying bone or joint abnormality associated with an adventitial bursae.[12]

The bursae around the Achilles tendon are well described in the radiology literature and include the retrocalcaneal bursa (also termed the sub-Achilles or retro-Achilles bursa) in Kager's fat pad and the pre-Achilles bursa (also known as the superficial Achilles bursa)

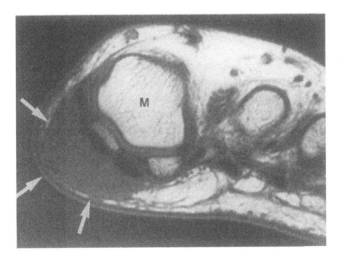

FIGURE 9.8 Hallux bursitis. A 14-year-old boy with a slightly tender mass over the medial aspect of the first metatarsal head. Coronal SE T1-weighted image shows an intermediate signal intensity mass in the plantar soft tissues (arrows). A diffusely thickened bursa was found at surgery. M = first metatarsal.

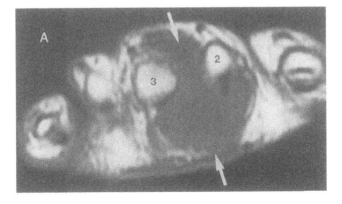

FIGURE 9.9 Intermetatarsal bursitis. This 32-year-old female presented with an enlarging painful mass over the dorsum of her foot. (A) Coronal fast SE T2-weighted MR image shows an irregular fluid-signal intensity mass insinuated between the second and third metatarsal heads (arrows). 2 = 2nd metatarsal; 3 = 3rd metatarsal.   (*continued*)

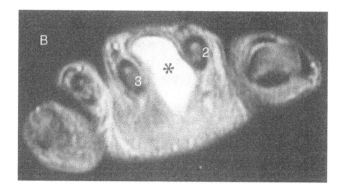

FIGURE 9.9 (continued) (B) Fast SE T2-weighted image slightly distal to (A) shows diffuse increased signal intensity (asterisk) consistent with fluid or synovial thickening. Rim enhancement was present following IV gadolinium (not shown). An inflamed intermetatarsal bursa was confirmed surgically. 2 = 2nd metatarsal; 3 = 3rd metatarsal.

posterior to the Achilles tendon.[16] Inflammation of these bursae is typically related to excessive activity and overuse of the Achilles tendon, but can also be associated with inflammatory arthropathies such as rheumatoid arthritis, psoriasis, and Reiter syndome.[17] On MR imaging, the Achilles bursae show fluid-like signal intensity that is low to intermediate on T1-weighted sequences and high on T2-weighted sequences, consistent with either synovial thickening and/or effusion (Figure 9.10).

DISORDERS OF THE PLANTAR FASCIA

The plantar fascia is a multilayered fibrous aponeurosis that assists in the push-off phase of gait, maintains the medial longitudinal arch, and absorbs forces transmitted through the mid-tarsal joints.[17,18] It consists of a thick central and thinner medial and lateral bands and is normally visualized as a thin linear low-signal-intensity structure on both T1- and T2-weighted sequences contiguous to the flexor and abductor digitorum brevis and abductor digiti minimi muscles (Figure 9.11). It arises

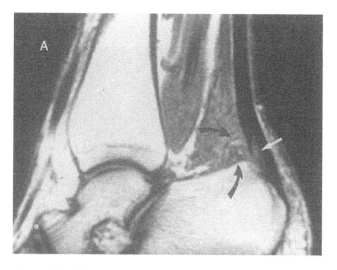

FIGURE 9.10 Retrocalcaneal bursitis. (A) Sagittal SE T1-weighted image shows intermediate signal intensity obliterating Kager's fat pad (black arrows). Focal increased signal intensity is also noted in the adjacent Achilles tendon (white arrow).   (*continued*)

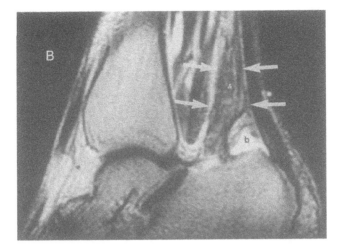

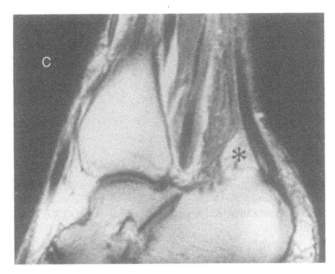

FIGURE 9.10 (continued) (B) Sagittal conventional SE T2-weighted image reveals a localized area of central high signal with a rim of slightly lower signal consistent with retrocalcaneal bursitis (b). The larger intermediate-signal-intensity tissue represents an accessory soleus muscle (A) (arrows). (C) Sagittal post-gadolinium SE T1-weighted image shows diffuse enhancement of the bursa consistent with diffuse thickening of the synovium from bursitis (asterisk).

from the medial aspect of the calcaneal tuberosity and attaches distally to the flexor tendon sheaths and bases of the proximal phalanges.[12,19] The thickness of the fascia is variable in asymptomatic individuals, but usually measures less than or equal to 2 mm in the dorsoplantar dimension and is considered to be abnormally thickened when it measures greater or equal to 5 mm.[20] Conditions affecting the plantar fascia of the foot include plantar fasciitis, acute rupture, and plantar fibromatosis.

PLANTAR FASCIITIS

Plantar fasciitis, one of several causes of heel pain syndrome, most commonly occurs from chronic, repetitive, low-grade trauma, which results in a chronic inflammatory and degenerative response in the aponeurosis. Athletes, particularly runners, are typically affected by this condition, but it can also occur in association with prolonged standing and some inflammatory arthropathies including Reiter syndrome, ankylosing spondylitis, and psoriasis.[17,20] Activity-related pain localized to the region of the plantar

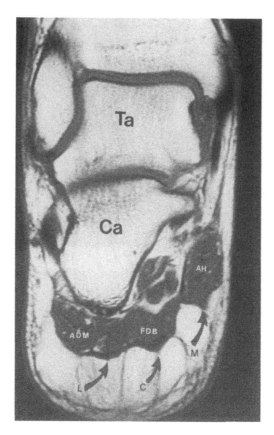

FIGURE 9.11 Plantar fascia anatomy. Coronal SE T1-weighted MR image through the hind foot shows the three components of the plantar fascia (arrows). The central part is the thickest. L = lateral; C = central; M = medial; Ta = talus; Ca = calcaneus; AH = abductor hallucis brevis; FDB = flexor digitorum brevis; ADM = abductor digiti minimi.

surface of the calcaneal tuberosity is the common presenting symptom. The clinical diagnosis is usually straightforward but can be confused with other entities including tarsal tunnel and sinus tarsi syndrome, bursitis, and calcaneal stress fractures.[20] If the clinical symptoms are nonspecific, the diagnosis can be established with MR imaging or ultrasound, although ultrasound remains more operator dependent.[19–21] On MR imaging, plantar fasciitis is manifested by increased signal on both T1- and T2-weighted sequences and thickening of the fascia up to 6 to 10 mm with the greatest involvement closest to the calcaneal attachment[16,19] (Figure 9.12). Inflammatory change in the surrounding subcutaneous tissue can also be present on MR imaging and is manifested by diminished and increased signal intensity on T1- and T2-weighted sequences, respectively. Treatment of plantar fasciitis consists of conservative measures such as orthotics, physiotherapy, steroid injections, and/or anti-inflammatory drugs.[18]

RUPTURE

Acute rupture of the plantar fascia is a rare occurrence. This injury is most often seen in atheletes who have undergone repeated fascial steroid injections for heel pain (Figure 9.13).[12]

PLANTAR FIBROMATOSIS

Plantar fibromatosis is a benign proliferative disorder of the plantar fascia that has been discussed in detail in Chapter 6. The key to differentiating this entity from plantar fasciitis is the more nodular appearance of the mass and the lack of a consistent relationship to the plantar fascia[22] (Figure 9.14).

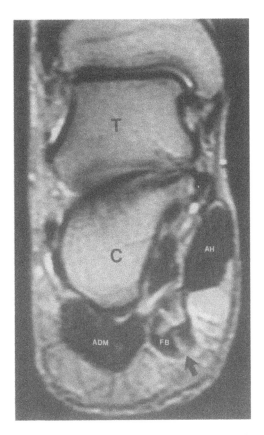

FIGURE 9.12 Plantar fasciitis. Coronal conventional SE T2-weighted MR image in the hind foot shows focal thickening and increased signal intensity in the central component of the plantar fascia consistent with the clinical diagnosis of plantar fasciitis (arrow). T = talus; C = calcaneus; AH = abductor hallucis muscle; FB = flexor digitorum brevis muscle; ADM = abductor digiti minimi muscle.

IMPINGEMENT

Ankle impingement is caused by abnormal soft tissue or bone impeding motion at the tibiotalar joint and has been discussed in Chapter 5. Anterolateral impingement occurs in patients with chronic ankle sprains due to scar tissue in the anterolateral gutter.[23] Posterior impingement is typically caused by a plantar flexion injury with entrapment of the flexor hallucis longus tendon or the posterior ankle capsule in the joint and is often associated with an os trigonum and a prominent or fractured posterior process of the talus.[24]

REFLEX SYMPATHETIC DYSTROPHY

Reflex sympathetic dystrophy (RSD) is a pain dysfunction syndrome not infrequently seen in the foot and ankle. Several terms have been applied to this condition and include causalgia, Sudeck atrophy, reflex neurovascular dystrophy, reflex algodystrophy, and shoulder–hand syndrome.[25] Transient osteoporosis of the hip and regional migratory osteoporosis may also represent forms of RSD.[26] The primary cause of this condition is believed to be related to an overactive sympathetic nervous system, precipitated by a noxious event such as surgery or trauma to the affected extremity. Patients present clinically with a stiff and swollen extremity and pain that is disproportionate to the inciting cause.[25] The clinical presentation is divided into three stages.[27] Initially, the inflammatory stage is manifested by pain and swelling. Then, the dystrophic stage follows next with

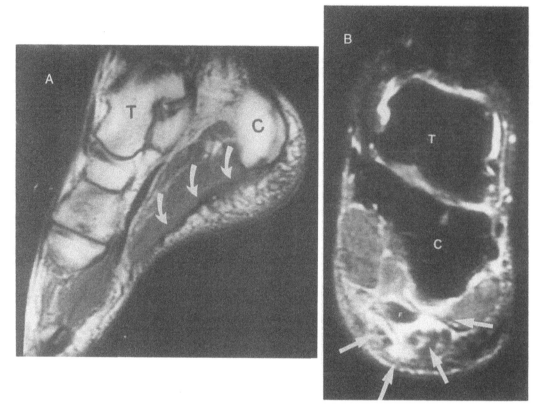

FIGURE 9.13 Acute rupture of the plantar fascia. Varsity basketball player with sudden heel pain during a game. (A) Sagittal SE T1-weighted image shows increased signal, redundancy, and thickening of the plantar fascia (arrows), which is detached from the calcaneus. T = talus; C = calcaneus. (B) Coronal FIR shows extensive edema in the soft tissues surrounding the thickened fascia (arrows). T = talus; C = calcaneus; F = fascia.

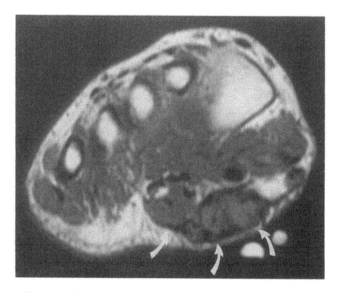

FIGURE 9.14 Plantar fibromatosis. Coronal SE T1-weighted image in the mid-foot shows a bulky intermediate signal intensity mass arising contiguous with and involving the deep surface of the plantar fascia (arrows).

activity-related pain and hypersensitivity of the skin to temperature and pressure changes. The third stage is characterized by skin and muscle atrophy. Sympathetic blockade is an invasive procedure but is the most reliable means of establishing the diagnosis.[25] On radiographs, diffuse osteopenia may be present, particularly in the later stage of the condition.[29] Scintigraphy is highly sensitive but lacks specificity.[30] Power Doppler sonography can show increased soft-tissue blood flow with side-to-side asymmetry in RSD with a reported sensitivity of 73% and specifity of 92%.[31] MR imaging may be useful in excluding other causes of foot and ankle pain and can confirm the diagnosis of RSD in the minority of cases. On MR imaging, the osseous structures of the foot and ankle are frequently normal although diffuse edema-like signal in the bone marrow can be present.[27] The variable findings reported in the bone marrow of the lower extremity in general on MR imaging may relate to the controversial inclusion of transient osteoporosis of the hip and regional migratory osteoporosis as a form of RSD and physiologic differences related to variations in regional anatomy of the lower extremity.[27] The soft-tissue changes associated with RSD on MR imaging are variable depending on the stage of the condition. MR imaging is most useful in the first stage of the disease when the clinical diagnosis is in question. Enhancement of the subcutaneous or periarticular soft tissues with gadolinium and thickening of the skin are usually present in stage 1. Muscle and fascial edema may also be present in this stage. In stages 2 and 3, muscle atrophy can be present on MR imaging; however, the soft tissues are otherwise unremarkable in the later stages of the syndrome and show no enhancement with gadolinium.[32]

SUMMARY

There are a variety of less well-known miscellaneous conditions of the foot and ankle that may cause diagnostic dilemmas when first encountered by physical examination. MR imaging may help isolate many of these conditions and is a very appropriate next imaging step in a diagnostic work-up of the patients with foot and ankle pain.

REFERENCES

1. Keck, C., The tarsal tunnel syndrome, *J. Bone Joint Surg.*, 44A, 180, 1962.
2. Lam, S. J. S., Tarsal tunnel syndrome, *Lancet*, 2, 1354, 1962.
3. Edwards, W. G., Lincoln, C. R., Bassett, F. H., and Goldner, J. L., The tarsal tunnel syndrome: diagnosis and treatment, *JAMA*, 207, 716–720, 1969.
4. Cimino, W. R., Foot Fellows Review. Tarsal tunnel syndrome: review of the literature, *Foot Ankle*, 11 (No. 1), 47–51, 1990.
5. Lam, S. J. S., Tarsal tunnel syndrome, *J. Bone Joint Surg. [Br.]*, 49:87–92, 1967.
6. Stern, D. S. and Joyce, M. T., Tarsal tunnel syndrome: A review of 15 surgical procedures, *J. Foot Surg.*, 28(4):290–294, 1989.
7. Dellon, A. L. and Mackinnon, S. E., Tibial nerve branching in the tarsal tunnel, *Arch., Neurol.*, 41:645–646, 1984.
8. Kerr, R. and Frey, C., MR imaging in tarsal tunnel syndrome, *J. Comp. Assist. Tomogr.*, 15(2), 280–286.
9. Havel, P. E., Ebraheim, N. A., Clark, S. E., Jackson, W. T., and DiDio, L., Tibial nerve branching in the tarsal tunnel, *Foot Ankle*, 9(3), 117–119, 1988.
10. Erickson, S. J., Quinn, S. F., Kneeland, J. B., Smith, J. W., Johnson, J. E., Carrera, G. F., Shereff, M. F., Hyde, J. S., and Jesmanowics, A., MR imaging of the tarsal tunnel and related spaces: normal and abnormal findings with anatomic correlation, *AJR*, 155, 323–328, 1990.
11. Grumbine, N. A., Radovic, P. A., Parsons, R., and Scheinin, G. S., Tarsal tunnel syndome: comprehensive review of 8 cases, *J. Am. Podiatric Med. Assoc.*, 80 (9):457–460, 1990.
12. Jahss, M. H., Miscellaneous soft-tissue lesions, in *Disorder of the Foot and Ankle*, Vol. 2, 2nd ed., W. B. Saunders, Philadelphia, chap. 51, 1533–1539, 1991.
13. Crimm, J. R., Cracchiolo, A., Hall, R. L., Eds., Anatomy in *Imaging of the Foot and Ankle*, Lippincott-Raven, New York, 1996, chap. 1, 1–13.

14. Bureau, N. J., Kaplan, P. A., and Dussault, R. G., MRI of the knee: a simplified approach, in *Curr. Probl. Diagn. Radiol.*, Vol. 24, Jan./Feb. 1995, 1–52.
15. Hartmann, G., The tendon sheaths and synovial bursae of the foot, *Foot Ankle*, 1, 247–269, 1981.
16. Kier, R., Magnetic resonance imaging of plantar fasciitis and other causes of heel pain, in *Magnetic Resonance Clinics of North America: The Foot and Ankle*. W. B. Saunders, Philadelphia, 1994, 97–107.
17. Kwong, P. K., Kay, D., Voner, R. T., and White, M. W., Plantar fasciitis: mechanics and pathomechanics of treatment, *Clin. Sports Med.*, 7, 119–127, 1988.
18. Schepsis, A. A., Leach, R. E., and Gorzyca, J., Plantar fasciitis: etiology, treatment, surgical results, and review of the literature, *Clin. Orthop.*, 266, 185–196, 1991.
19. Grasel, R. P., Schweitzer, M. E., Kovalovich. A. M., Karasick, D., Wapner, K., Hecht, P., and Wander, D., MR imaging of plantar fasciitis: edema, tears and occult marrow abnormalities correlated with outcome, *AJR*, 173, 699–701, 1999.
20. Berkowitz, J. F., Kier, R., and Rudicel, S., Plantar fasciitis: MR imaging, *Radiology*, 179, 665–667, 1991.
21. Gibbon, W. W. and Long, G., Ultrasound of the plantar aponeurosis (fascia), *Skeletal Radiol.*, 28, 21–26, 1999.
22. Morrison, W. B., Schweitzer, M. E., Wapner, K. L., and Lackman, R. D., Plantar fibromatosis: a benign aggressive neoplasm with a characteristic appearance on MR images, *Radiology*, 193, 841–845, 1994.
23. Rubin, D. A., Tishkoff, N. W., Britton, C. A., Conti, S. F., and Towers, J. D., Anterolateral soft-tissue impingement in the ankle: diagnosis using MR imaging, *AJR*, 169, 829–835, 1997.
24. Hendrick, M. R. and McBryde, A. M., Posterior ankle impingement, *Foot Ankle*, 15, 2–8, 1994.
25. Lindenfeld, T. N., Bach, B. R., and Wojtys, E. M., Reflex sympathetic dystrophy and pain dysfunction in the lower extremity, *JBJS*, 78-A(12), 1996.
26. Resnick, D. and Niwayama, G., Transient osteoporosis of the hip, in Resnick, D. and Niwayama, G., Eds., *Diagnosis of Bone and Joint Disorders*, 2nd ed., W. B. Saunders, Philadelphia, 1988, 2034–2053.
27. Koch, E., Hofer, H. O., Sialer, G., Marincek, B., and von Schulthess, G. K., Failure of MR imaging to detect reflex sympathetic dystrophy of the extremities, *AJR*, 156, 113–115, 1991.
28. Roberts, W. J., An hypothesis on the physiological basis for causalgia and related pains, *Pain*, 24, 297–311, 1986.
29. Genant, H. K., Kozin, F., Bekerman, C., McCarty, K. J., and Sims, J., The reflex sympathetic dystrophy syndrome: a comprehensive analysis using fine-detail radiography, photon absorptiometry, and bone and joint scitigraphy, *Radiology*, 117, 21–32, 1975.
30. Holder, L. E., Cole, L. A., and Myerson, M. S., Reflex sympathetic dystrophy in the foot: clinical and scintigraphic criteria, *Radiology*, 184, 531–535, 1992.
31. Nazarian, L. N., Schweitzer, M. E., Mandel, S., Rawool, N. M., Parker, L., Fisher, A. M., Feld, R. I., and Needleman, L., Increased soft-tissue blood flow in patients with reflex sympathetic dystrophy of the lower extremity revealed by power Doppler sonography, *AJR*, 171, 1245–1250, 1998.
32. Schweitzer, M. E., Mandel, S., Schwartzman, R. J., Knobler, R. L., and Tahmoush, A. J., Reflex sympathetic dystrophy revisited: MR imaging findings before and after infusion of contrast material, *Radiology*, 195, 211–214, 1995.

10 The Pediatric Foot and Ankle

E. Michel Azouz, Kamaldine Oudjhane, and Cindy R. Miller

CONTENTS

INTRODUCTION

The foot of a child looks different from that of an adult. Age-related physiologic variations occur in shape through normal growth and development. Some foot deformities may be considered a manifestation of muscle imbalance due to an underlying neuromuscular condition (cerebral palsy, tethered cord, or myelomeningocele). Foot and ankle abnormalities may result in abnormal gait and impaired function of the lower limbs and spine. Radiologic evaluation of the foot and ankle has relied on radiographs obtained in the weight-bearing position that constitute a baseline for further comparative assessment.[1] However, radiography is limited because of the incomplete ossification of the bones in children. Since the advent of magnetic resonance (MR) imaging, progress has been made regarding the understanding of normal maturation of the foot and ankle. The evaluation of the soft-tissue structures and cartilage takes advantage of the different signal intensities of muscle, fat, bone, hyaline and articular cartilage, tendons, and vessels in the available MR imaging sequences. Acquired disorders such as trauma, arthritides, infection, and neoplasms benefit from the multiplanar imaging capabilities and the soft-tissue contrast resolution offered by MR imaging.

TECHNICAL CONSIDERATIONS

Adequate preparation of the pediatric patient must precede sedation and immobilization. Review of radiographs of the foot, ankle, and other segments of the limbs narrows the potential differential diagnosis. Abnormalities may be underestimated by conventional radiography.[2] Tailoring of MR imaging sequences optimizes the evaluation of the young skeleton and soft tissues.

PATIENT PREPARATION AND SEDATION

The parents and child benefit from seeing the scanning machine and should be informed of the noise during the examination. The importance of avoiding motion cannot be stressed enough. Earplugs or earphones for listening to music are offered. Usually, a child older than 6 years does not need sedation. For patients less than 6 years old, sedation is provided.[3] Preprocedure fasting for about 3 hours before the examination is recommended if sedation and intravenous contrast is required. Sedation is administered by nurses supervised by the radiologist if the child's medical condition falls within the Class I or II of the American Society of Anesthesia (ASA). Patients in ASA Class III can receive sedation by the radiologist. All other children need sedation provided by anesthesiologists.

Oral chloral hydrate can be given to infants age 12 months or younger (initial dose of 50 mg/kg) with additional doses repeated every 30 min to a maximal dose of 100 mg/kg. An intravenous (IV) access can be secured if an MR contrast enhancement agent is needed. EMLA cream (lidocaine 2.5% and prilocaine 2.5%, Astra Laboratories) is applied 1 hour prior to puncture over the IV site, which is then covered by an occlusive dressing. IV sedation is delivered in patients more than 1 year of age using pentobarbital sodium (Nembutal, Abbott Laboratories) at a dose of 2 to 3 mg/kg (maximum 50 mg), through slow injection. A repeat dose, if needed, can be given a minute or two after the initial dose but the total dose must not exceed 6 mg/kg. If additional sedation is indicated, IV Fentanyl citrate (Abbott Laboratories) can be given with a dose titration of 1 µg/kg every 5 min until adequate sedation is reached; its maximal cumulative dose is 3 µg/kg. The corollary of a sedation protocol is the continuous and rigorous monitoring of the child by the staff in medical imaging who must be familiar with dealing with the side effects of sedation including respiratory depression. The patient under examination in the MR unit is monitored through the recording of pulse oxymetry (heart rate, respiratory rate, O_2 saturation) via a probe usually placed at the finger. Following the MR study, the patient is monitored in the recovery unit via a pulse oxymeter and vital signs are recorded every 15 min. The patient is discharged when fully awake or easily arousable, with adequate O_2 saturation (95 to 100%).

PATIENT POSITIONING

The objective of pediatric MR imaging is to obtain diagnostic images in the shortest time possible with the fewest artifacts. A cooperative, unsedated patient needs to be comfortable on the table with adequate immobilization (tape, sponges, Velcro® straps). The foot needs to be positioned parallel to one of the orthogonal planes in reference to the bore of the magnet. A sedated infant, who sleeps in the supine position with the knee flexed, will have his or her foot placed in such a position that the plantar aspect is parallel to the coronal plane of the magnet. The foot rests on a sponge placed over the coil. Such an alignment is then secured with tape. Older children may have their foot on a footplate, which straightens the anatomic region, simulating the plantar flexion.

COIL AND PULSE SEQUENCES SELECTION

In general, the smallest surface coil that can cover the area of clinical concern is chosen. The goal is to obtain optimal spatial resolution and signal-to-noise ratio. A small flexible coil (such as the adult wrist coil) is generally used — large adolescents may require a knee coil. The imaging protocol includes different sequences: T1-weighted conventional spin-echo (SE), proton-density and T2-weighted SE or fast SE (FSE) with fat suppression, FSE inversion-recovery (IR), and gradient-recalled-echo (GRE) images with or without spoiling (SPGR or MPGR).[2] For localization, fast GRE sequences may be used when the anatomy of interest is in a plane nonorthogonal to the axes of the magnet. T1-weighted sequences provide little difference in tissue contrast between muscle and cartilage. T2-weighted FSE, IR, and GRE sequences will offer better differentiation between muscle and cartilage. Detection of bone marrow abnormalities is optimized by the use of fat-suppression techniques. In the case of congenital vascular anomalies, FSE T2-weighted sequences help define the size of the lesion. IV injection of gadolinium allows the opacification and demonstration of the vascular malformation itself. Two-dimensional (2D) time of flight (TOF) MR angiography (MRA) sequence shows the vascular anatomy. MR venography (MRV) depicts both the superficial and deep venous structures of the lower limbs.[4]

USE OF GADOLINIUM ENHANCEMENT

The use of gadolinium is generally considered safe and the standard IV dose is 0.1 mmol/kg. Nausea and vomiting are occasional side effects that may be alleviated by preprocedure fasting. Many indications for contrast enhancement exist in the field of foot/ankle imaging, which include bone ischemia and necrosis, musculoskeletal infection and inflammation, especially active ankle arthritis, calcaneal enthesitis, osteomyelitis, and soft-tissue abscess. The evaluation of pediatric bone tumors is generally not optimized with additional enhanced sequences. IV gadolinium characterizes soft-tissue masses as cystic or solid lesions.

NORMAL GROWTH, DEVELOPMENT, AND VARIANTS

GROWTH AND DEVELOPMENT OF THE TARSAL BONES

The radiographic appearance of the mature skeleton of the foot and ankle is well documented. The different structures are underestimated by plain radiography of the infant and child feet and ankles. Tarsal and metatarsal bones, as well as the phalanges, develop by endochondral ossification. Onset of ossification occurs in the second through the fourth fetal months for the metatarsal bones, between 25 and 31 weeks of gestation for the talus, between 22 and 25 weeks of gestation for the calcaneus, between 37 weeks of gestation and 3 weeks after birth for the cuboid and between 2 and 5 years for the navicular bone. Most tarsal ossification occurs after birth; the calcaneus is approximately 60% ossified at 3 months of age. T1-weighted imaging allows a comprehensive evaluation of the development of these small bones.[5] Ossification centers are not mere miniatures of the cartilaginous anlages. Early ossification of the talus is centered in the neck region (Figures 10.1 and 10.2). The long axes of the cartilaginous anlage of the talus and its ossification center differ in orientation, in the coronal and sagittal planes[6] (Figure 10.3). Early calcaneal ossification is centered in the distal two thirds of the cartilaginous anlage. Early ossification of the cartilaginous anlage is centered in the central or lateral third of the navicular and in the middle of the cuboid anlage. Radiographic measurement of the talocalcaneal angles, which classically decrease with age, reflect the change in axis of the talar ossification center.

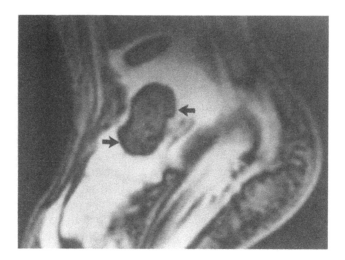

FIGURE 10.1 Normal talus (15-month-old girl). Sagittal GRE image (TR 266/TE 11, flip angle 30°) of the talus shows an ossification center surrounded by a rim of low signal intensity corresponding to the zone of provisional calcification (arrows). The peripheral cartilaginous anlage of the talus (and the whole navicular) have a high signal intensity on this GRE sequence.

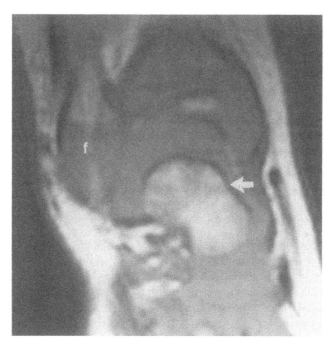

FIGURE 10.2 Normal talus (1-year-old girl). Coronal T1-weighted image (TR 400/TE 18) of the talus shows the homogeneous intermediate signal intensity of cartilage and a central nucleus of fatty marrow transformation with high signal intensity. This area is bordered by a line of low signal intensity related to the zone of provisional calcification (arrow). f = fibular epiphysis.

GROWTH AND DEVELOPMENT OF THE DISTAL TIBIA AND FIBULA

Age-related changes of the physes and epiphyses occur in the distal tibia and fibula. The distal tibial epiphyseal ossification and physeal closure begins anteromedially and progresses

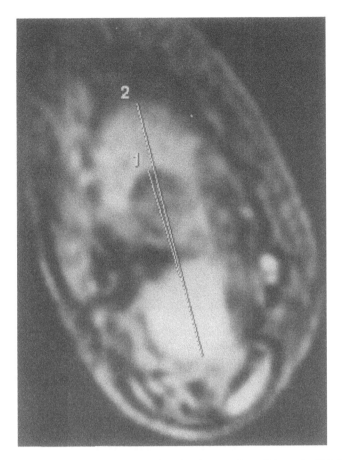

FIGURE 10.3 Normal talus ossification center and cartilaginous anlage (11-week-old infant). Coronal GRE image (TR 183/TE 11, flip angle 30°). Note the difference in orientation of the axis of the ossification nucleus (1) and the axis of the cartilage component (2).

posteriorly and laterally. The anterolateral portion of the physis is the last area to fuse. The distal fibula lengthens more than the distal tibia. Physeal integrity is best evaluated with imaging sequences that maximize the contrast between bone and cartilage. Cartilage has a very high signal intensity and its adjacent bone is hypointense on fat-suppressed proton-density-weighted SE and GRE sequences. Before completion of ossification of the epiphysis, T2-weighted imaging is best for differentiation between the epiphyseal cartilage (low signal) and hyperintense physeal cartilage.[7] The distal tibial physis develops an anteromedial undulation before closure. Normal growth and ossification of epiphyses are intimately related to vascularity of the epiphyseal and physeal cartilages.[8] Gadolinium enhancement is greater in the physis than in the vessels and the epiphyseal cartilage shows the least enhancement (Figure 10.4). Five stages of epiphyseal vascularity development have been identified.[7] Vascularity is characterized by parallel vascular channels in the unossified epiphysis; the vascular pattern becomes radial after growth of the ossification center. Physeal enhancement decreases with physeal closure. In the bone marrow of the extremities, the enhancement ratio after gadolinium injection is greater in the hemato-poietic metaphysis than in the fatty epiphysis. Gadolinium administration obscures the changes in the marrow signal intensity, which is seen secondary to fatty conversion. Fat-suppression techniques in enhanced MR sequences improve the visualization of the differential enhancement of hematopoietic and fatty marrow.[9]

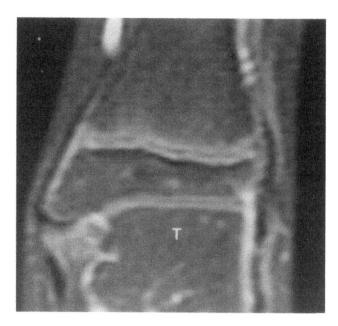

FIGURE 10.4 Normal distal tibial epiphysis and metaphysis (8-year-old girl). Coronal T1-weighted SE image (TR 400/TE 12) with fat suppression obtained after IV gadolinium injection. There is enhancement of the physis and in the epiphyseal vessels (focal bright dots). T = talus.

NORMAL VARIANTS

The secondary ossification centers of the metatarsals and phalanges develop between 6 and 24 months after birth and the calcaneal apophysis develops between 5 and 12 years of age. Both secondary and primary ossification centers initially contain hematopoietic marrow and then rapidly convert to fatty marrow.

Common accessory bones occur, including the accessory navicular, the os trigonum at the proximal talus, and the os vesalianum pedis at the base of the fifth metatarsal. There are three types of accessory navicular bones: the os tibiale externum (type 1), the accessory navicular bone (type 2), and the prominent navicular tuberosity or cornuate navicular (type 3), which is a fused type 2. When an accessory navicular is symptomatic, bone marrow edema is present, which can be visualized on T1-weighted and fat-suppressed T2-weighted images. The edema is related to chronic stress and/or osteonecrosis.[10]

Epiphyseal ossification irregularities constitute a normal radiographic variant in the pediatric patient and can cause diagnostic problems on plain radiographs and on computed tomography (CT) and MR images. Irregularity of contour of the ossification center, with normal signal intensity of overlying cartilage and the absence of bone marrow edema, favors normal variants and generally excludes osteochondrosis dissecans. An accessory muscle can present as a soft-tissue mass in the ankle area. The accessory soleus muscle is a rare variant that usually manifests as an asymptomatic swelling in the posteromedial part of the ankle, but may be painful with exercise. It arises from the anterior surface of the soleus or from the fibula and the soleal line of the tibia. It inserts onto the Achilles tendon or onto the calcaneus, inferior, anterior, and medial to the Achilles tendon insertion. (Figure 10.5A). MR imaging confirms the isointense signal of muscle (Figure 10.5B to D). Pain may be relieved by surgery (fasciotomy). The peroneus quartus muscle is a more common anatomic variant, seen in up to 20% of the population. It arises from the muscular part of the peroneus brevis muscle and inserts onto the peroneal tubercle of the calcaneus.[11] Tendons may show intermediate signal intensity on T1-weighted sequences due to the "magic angle" effect.

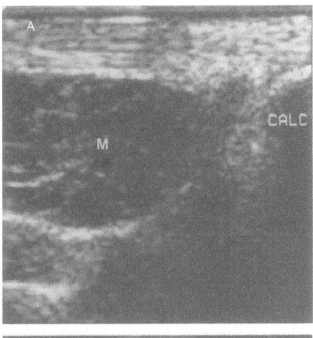

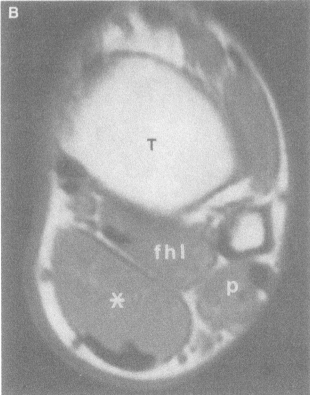

FIGURE 10.5 Accessory soleus muscle (16-year-old boy). (A) Sagittal ultrasound from a posteromedial approach demonstrates the hypoechoic muscle (M), above the level of calcaneus (CALC). (B) Axial T1-weighted SE MR image (TR 500/TE 11) shows the accessory muscle (asterisk) of similar signal intensity to the flexor hallucis longus (fhl) and peroneal (p) muscles. T = tibia. *(continued)*

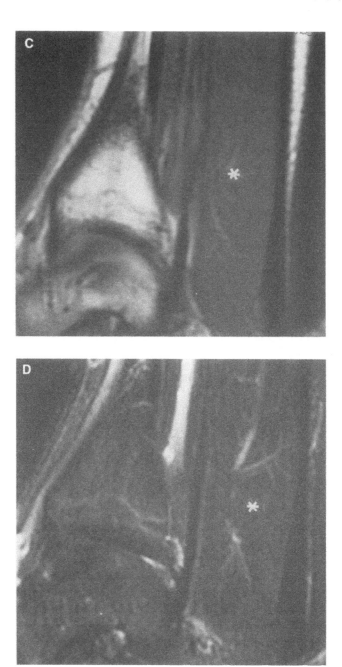

FIGURE 10.5 (continued) (C) Sagittal T1-weighted SE MR image (TR 500/TE 11) and (D) Sagittal T1-weighted SE MR image (TR 500/TE 11) with fat suppression, after IV gadolinium reveals the normal signal intensity of the accessory muscle (asterisk).

CONGENITAL ANOMALIES

Foot deformities at birth can be positional in nature (uterine packing phenomena) or true genetic anomalies. Clinical evaluation of the neonatal foot is crucial. Radiographs are not very helpful in infants and young children because many bones are still cartilaginous. Coexistent hip dysplasia and foot deformity is reported to range from 2 to 10%.[12] Sonography may provide a dynamic assessment of the navicular relationship to the talus in club foot;[13] however, MR imaging provides a more global assessment of foot deformities.

CLUB FOOT (CONGENITAL TALIPES EQUINOVARUS)

This common foot deformity occurs in 1 in 1000 live births. It constitutes an enigma concerning its cause and pathologic anatomy. It continues to present a challenge to the orthopedic surgeon regarding its general management and surgical correction. The deformity is characterized by plantar flexion of the ankle with subtalar inversion and medial subluxation of the navicular, which is often in close proximity to the medial malleolus. Soft-tissue contractures are commonly associated and can be due to fibrosis of the distal calf muscles, abnormal tibialis posterior and peroneal muscles, and hypoplasia of the anterior tibial artery.[14] The classic radiographic signs include a cavus foot, decrease of the talocalcaneal angle on anteroposterior (AP) and lateral radiographs (varus deformity), equinus deformity of the hind foot and adduction of the forefoot. Because the bones of the infant foot are small, it is difficult to obtain optimal imaging planes in the deformed foot, and therefore MR imaging has not been used widely in the preoperative assessment of club foot. In addition, MR imaging may produce partial volume averaging artifacts. CT scanning with 3D reconstruction has shown an abnormal talar pronation (intorsion or medial tilt).[15] MR imaging studies demonstrate the pathologic anatomy, including the abnormal alignment between the anterior calcaneus and the cuboid bone, the medial subluxation of the cuboid,[16] the talonavicular and the calcaneocuboid deformities, and are best assessed on the coronal plane with GRE imaging sequences.[17] Classification of the severity of club foot deformity was studied recently by Wang et al.[18] using MR imaging with multiplanar reconstruction. Cahuzac et al.[19] have recently shown that the volume of the hind foot bones is approximately 20% smaller in club foot than in the normal foot. With 3D MR imaging, the volume of the ossification center of the calcaneus is shown to be reduced by 40%, and the longitudinal axis of the talus ossific nucleus is more medial than the axis of its cartilaginous anlage. This difference in orientation is greater in club foot than in a normal foot. Such a study shows the limits of plain radiographic assessment with regard to the actual interosseous relationships. MR imaging is also useful in the evaluation of recurrent deformity following soft-tissue release surgery, since the bones are still incompletely ossified.

CONGENITAL VERTICAL TALUS

Congenital vertical talus constitutes a severe form of congenital flat foot and is characterized by a vertically oriented talus and a fixed dorsal dislocation of the navicular bone. In 60% of patients it is associated with neurologic impairment due to myelomeningocele or arthrogryposis. The navicular bone is wedge shaped and the talar head is flattened. MR imaging may help to delineate the deformity and position of the nonossified navicular and talus and demonstrate the abnormal calcaneocuboid and subtalar joints.

SKEW FOOT

This deformity consists of metatarsus adductus with supination of the forefoot, valgus deformity of the hind foot, and a mid-foot deformity which is best appreciated clinically as a soft-tissue step-off along the medial aspect of the foot between the head of the talus and the base of the first metatarsal. The lateral radiograph of the foot shows an increased talocalcaneal angle and abnormal alignment between the talus and the head of the first metatarsal with or without a rocker-bottom deformity of the foot. MR imaging demonstrates the plantar and lateral displacement of the navicular on the head of the talus. The mid-talar axis lies in line or medial to the base of the first metatarsal. This is not seen with isolated metatarsus adductus deformity, which is usually corrected with serial casting.[20]

Tarsal Coalition

Tarsal coalition consists of a congenital fibrous, cartilaginous, or bony fusion between two or more tarsal bones. The fusion most frequently involves the calcaneus and navicular, the talus and calcaneus, or the talus and navicular. It typically presents in adolescent boys with painful spastic flat foot, and the pain usually increases when the coalition ossifies. The time when the coalition ossifies varies according to the location; calcaneonavicular occurs between 8 and 12 years of age, talocalcaneal between 12 and 16 years of age, and talonavicular between 3 and 5 years of age. Radiographs may demonstrate a bony bar on the oblique view at the calcaneonavicular level. A sclerotic C-shaped line of degenerative changes on the lateral view of the ankle can develop in response to a subtalar coalition.[21] CT scanning clarifies the extent of a bony fusion but cannot accurately define a fibrous coalition.

MR imaging depicts all coalitions, including the fibrous type (Figure 10.6), which reveals zones of intermediate or low signal intensity at the site of the fusion.[22] It plays a role in excluding tarsal coalition and identifying other causes of subtalar joint pathology including juvenile rheumatoid arthritis manifested by synovitis and pannus demonstrated on IV gadolinium-enhanced fat-suppressed T1-weighted sequences.

Bone Dysplasias, Syndromes, and Foot Deformity

Foot deformities can be associated with many congenital systemic disorders. Tarsal coalitions associated with syndromes usually involve the cuneiform bones and only become radiographically

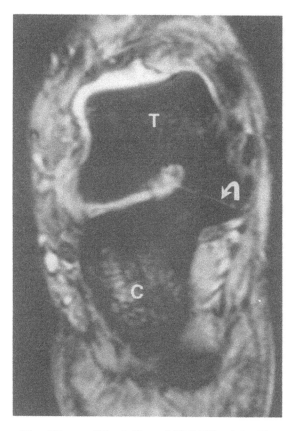

FIGURE 10.6 Fibrous coalition (16-year-old boy). Coronal GRE T2*-weighted image shows a thin low signal cleft (curved arrow) replacing the normal articular cartilage of the middle facet of the subtalar joint consistent with a fibrous coalition. T = talus; C = calcaneus. (Courtesy of A. R. Spouge, M.D., London, Ontario, Canada.)

detectable in late adolescence. Tarsal fusion may be seen in symphalangism, arthrogryposis, and acrocephalosyndactyly. Digital anomalies (polydactyly, syndactyly, symphalangism) may be syndromic. MR imaging may help define metatarsal fusion in unossified bone structures (Figure 10.7). Bracket epiphysis in the toes is best demonstrated by MR imaging on GRE sequences manifested by the presence of physeal cartilage signal (Figure 10.8).[23]

Asymmetry in the size and length of the lower extremities is seen in hemihypertrophy syndromes, including Beckwith–Wiedemann syndrome. Silver syndrome is an asymmetric form of short stature. Absence, deformity, and fusion of portions of the foot and ankle may be seen in conjunction with longitudinal lower limb anomalies such as fibular or tibial hemimelia.[24]

Trevor disease (dysplasia epiphysealis hemimelica) is a nongenetic growth disorder seen in children and young adults. Its clinical features include pain, swelling, and deformity. These findings are unilateral, occur more frequently in the lower than in the upper limb, and the talus is a site of predilection. The radiographic appearance of Trevor disease is a lobulated osseous mass, resembling an osteochondroma.[25] MR imaging delineates the anomaly and its relationship to the tarsal bones in different planes (Figure 10.9).

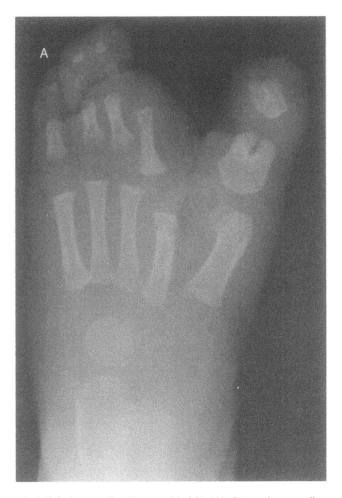

FIGURE 10.7 Congenital digital anomalies (1-year-old girl). (A) Dorsoplantar radiograph of the right foot shows soft-tissue syndactyly of the third and fourth toes, absence of the middle and distal phalanges of the second toe, hypoplasia of the second metatarsal, attempted duplication of the phalanges of the great toe, and a wide first interdigital space.   (*continued*)

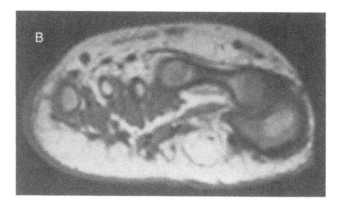

FIGURE 10.7 (continued) (B) Coronal T1-weighted SE MR image (TR 500/TE 20) at the level of the head of the first metatarsal identifies interposed bone in a transverse orientation with some fatty diaphyseal marrow and cartilaginous epiphyses.

Localized gigantism may be related to soft-tissue or bone overgrowth. MR imaging provides tissue characterization of the enlarged ankle or foot by identifying the signal intensity of fat or the presence of vascular or other anomalies. The differential diagnosis of localized gigantism includes neurofibromatosis, macrodystrophia lipomatosa, hemangiomatosis, lymphangiomatosis, Klippel–Trenaunay syndrome, Parkes–Weber syndrome, Bannayan–Zonana syndrome, Sturge–Weber syndrome, epidermal nevus syndrome, and Proteus syndrome. The latter includes regional gigantism

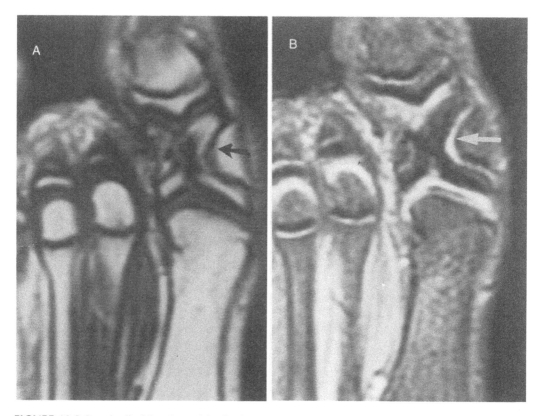

FIGURE 10.8 Longitudinal bracket epiphysis (9-year-old girl). (A) Axial T1-weighted SE MR image (TR 400/TE 11) shows the bracket epiphysis (arrow) in the proximal phalanx of the great toe. (B) Axial GRE image (TR 500/TE 13.3, flip angle 30°) confirms the cartilage signal at the bracket epiphysis (arrow).

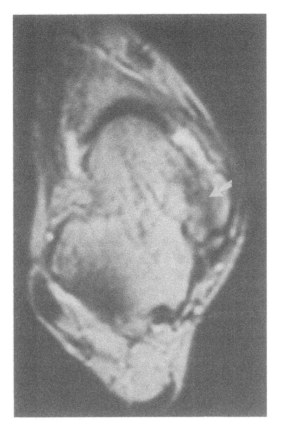

FIGURE 10.9 Trevor disease (dysplasia epiphysealis hemimelica) (14-year-old girl). Axial T2-weighted SE image (TR 3300/TE 95) depicts the medial bony overgrowth attached to the talus (arrow).

of the extremities, e.g., macrodactyly, lymphangiomatous hamartomas or lipomatosis, genu valgum, leg length discrepancy, hind foot deformity, exostoses, and scoliosis.[26] Plain radiographs evaluate the leg length discrepancy and the bone changes. MR imaging delineates the lipomatous or the vascular (venous or lymphatic) masses.

TRAUMATIC INJURIES

Trauma to the foot and ankle is very common, and the "ankle sprain" is the most common traumatic injury to the musculoskeletal system. Acute injuries may result from falls, playground, bicycle or motor vehicle accidents, and sports injuries. Chronic repetitive trauma may result in stress fractures, especially in the distal tibia, fibula, calcaneus, talus, navicular, or metatarsal. As in adults, bone demineralization such as seen in osteoporosis or chronic disease may result in insufficiency fractures of the foot and ankle.[5] In children, osteoporosis is present in osteogenesis imperfecta, myelomeningocele, and cerebral palsy. In osteopetrosis and its variants, dense bones are brittle and may fracture easily. Most foot and ankle fractures can be easily evaluated with radiographs and are treated conservatively. Complex and severely comminuted fractures may need CT with multiplanar reformatting for better assessment. Subtle fractures may be detected on scintigraphy and further evaluated with MR imaging which will also demonstrate coexisting soft-tissue injuries. In adolescents, fractures of the distal tibial growth plate and epiphysis are relatively common and may be part of a distal tibial triplane fracture. The juvenile Tillaux fracture is a Salter–Harris type III fracture of the lateral part of the distal tibial epiphysis in which the fragment is displaced laterally by the distal tibiofibular ligament and may be rotated. These fractures occur through the lateral part of the distal tibial epiphysis when the posterior and medial parts of the growth plate have fused and the anterior and lateral parts of the physis are still open. Occult fractures and bone contusions (bone bruises) are better evaluated by MR imaging.[27] Radiographs are normal in such instances but the child complains of persistent foot or ankle pain and swelling and bone scintigraphy shows increased uptake in the region of the occult trabecular or cortical fracture. Close proximity of the osseous injuries to the physis may render interpretation of the bone scan more challenging.

Bone contusions (bone bruises) may occur as isolated lesions following trauma, or may be associated with other fractures or dislocations. They are attributed to occult trabecular microfractures and are not radiographically visible, but are easily detected on MR imaging. They are typically homogeneous or reticular low-signal-intensity areas within the marrow fat on T1-weighted images, with the edema or hemorrhage demonstrated as high signal intensity on fat-suppressed T2-weighted and IR sequences (Figure 10.10). There may be an associated joint effusion. An intense marrow edema pattern may also develop in the adolescent athlete as a result of chronic repetitive low-grade mechanical stress.[27]

Osteochondral impaction injuries of the talar dome are often seen in young athletes. They may be radiographically occult, especially if an isolated transchondral injury is present. The fracture involves the medial or lateral aspects of the articular surface of the talus equally and may be seen on radiography, CT, or MR imaging. The osteochondral fragment can be assessed on MR imaging with proper selection of a pulse sequence that optimally demonstrates both cartilage and bone, usually a gradient-echo sequence in both the axial and coronal planes. Associated effusion or hemarthrosis is seen on the T2-weighted SE or FSE images as high-signal-

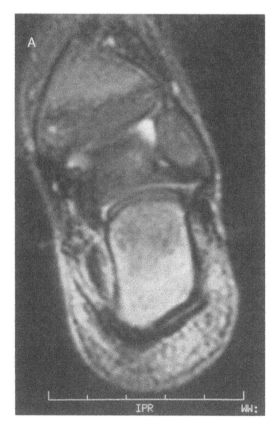

FIGURE 10.10 Calcaneal contusion (6-year-old girl). This patient complained of bilateral severe heel pain 2 weeks after excessive jumping. Stress fractures were suspected clinically. Plain radiographs (not shown) were normal. (A) Coronal T2-weighted SE MR image (TR 4000/TE 100) with fat suppression.   *(continued)*

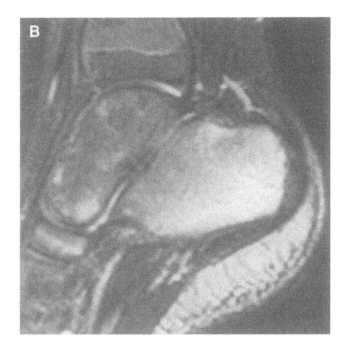

FIGURE 10.10 (continued) (B) Sagittal T2-weighted SE image (TR 3000/TE 100) with fat suppression demonstrates high signal intensity narrow edema in the calcaneus consistent with a bone contusion. There is also high signal intensity in the adjacent soft tissues, likely representing edema, due to repetitive low-grade trauma (jumping).

intensity fluid in the affected joint. The tarsal navicular and metatarsal heads are less frequent sites of osteochondral fractures.

Fatigue-type stress fractures result from prolonged and repetitive muscular activity in normal bone. They are usually diagnosed and followed by radiographs and bone scintigraphy, but CT or MR imaging may be needed if the radiographic diagnosis is equivocal. Radiographs may be negative initially or show only soft-tissue swelling but later on reveal the fracture line and/or periosteal reaction. MR imaging has been shown to be highly sensitive for detecting stress fractures,[28] demonstrating low-intensity band-like linear or irregular low-signal-intensity marrow on T1-weighted images that usually extend to the cortex. Intraosseous increased signal intensity likely corresponding to marrow edema is often seen adjacent to the fracture line on fat-suppressed T2-weighted images and IR images. At times, complex oblique imaging planes are needed for optimal assessment of stress fractures of the foot.[29]

MR imaging may be used to investigate acute complex physeal and epiphyseal injuries as radiographs often underestimate the extent and displacement of the physeal fracture.[30,31] Petit et al.[32] found that gradient-echo MR imaging allows accurate assessment of these injuries because of the high contrast between the fracture line and the background bone provided by this sequence.[32] However, radiographs remain the primary imaging modality for the evaluation of uncomplicated epiphyseal injuries and MR imaging should be reserved for complex fractures.[33] Post-traumatic bone bridging or bars may be the sequelae of physeal trauma especially in the distal tibia or fibula and may result in subsequent growth arrest, angular deformity, or shortening.[34] They are best investigated with MR imaging, which will show the normal bone, cartilage, and the bone bridge across the physis[35] (Figure 10.11). With MR imaging, epiphyseal fractures and dislocations may be detected, properly evaluated, and followed, even prior to the onset of ossification in the epiphysis.

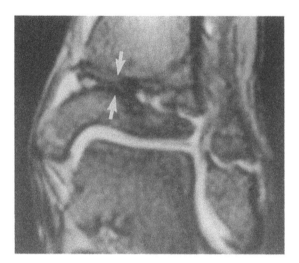

FIGURE 10.11 Distal tibial physeal bone bridge (12-year-old boy). A Salter III epiphyseal injury was sustained 1 year earlier. Coronal GRE image of the ankle shows interruption of the high signal intensity of the cartilaginous physis in the region of the bone bridge (arrows). The articular cartilage also shows high signal intensity on this sequence. (Courtesy of Diego Jaramillo, M.D., Children's Hospital, Harvard Medical School, Boston, MA.)

Imaging of ligament and tendon injuries in children and adolescents is similar to that in adults. Detailed anatomy and pathology of the tendons have been dealt with in preceding chapters, to which the reader is referred for further information.

OSTEOCHONDROSIS DISSECANS AND AVASCULAR NECROSIS

The term osteochondritis dissecans implies an inflammatory process and since this condition is likely post-traumatic in origin, the term osteochondrosis dissecans (OCD) is more appropriate. Its end result is separation of a fragment of subchondral bone and overlying articular cartilage. The medial and lateral articular surfaces of the talar dome are common sites for OCD. There is usually a history of a significant ankle sprain with chronic residual pain. MR is the imaging modality of choice for diagnosis, staging, and follow-up of these lesions as it can provide information regarding the status of the fragment/bone interface, underlying parent bone, overlying articular cartilage and can demonstrate loose bodies resulting from detachment of the fragment into the joint. A high-signal-intensity interface deep to the osteochondral fragment on IR or T2-weighted images suggests instability[27,36] (Figure 10.12). A rim of fluid signal surrounding the lesion is consistent with detachment of the fragment.[37] Sclerosis and cystic change in the lesion is also associated with an unstable fragment. Unstable fragments are treated surgically by either removal or fixation. Intact overlying articular cartilage, contrast enhancement of the lesion, and absence of cystic change imply a stable lesion and justify conservative therapy.[38]

Avascular (ischemic) necrosis (AVN) may be multifocal and secondary to metabolic, collagen vascular disease, or iatrogenic causes. The most common iatrogenic cause is high-dose corticosteroid medication,[39] especially in children with systemic lupus erythematosus or after organ transplantation. The common clinical symptom is pain. The bone changes are bilateral, and often symmetrical (Figure 10.13). Localized foot pain and limp in a child or adolescent can be secondary to AVN of a metatarsal head (Freiberg disease), the tarsal navicular (Köhler disease) (Figure 10.14), or the posterior calcaneal apophysis (Sever disease). AVN of a cuneiform bone has also been described.[40]

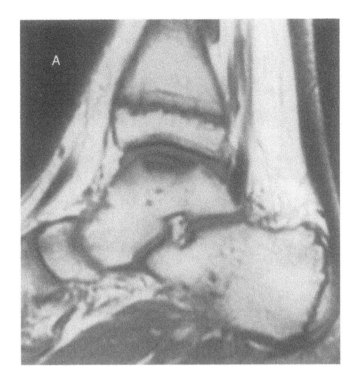

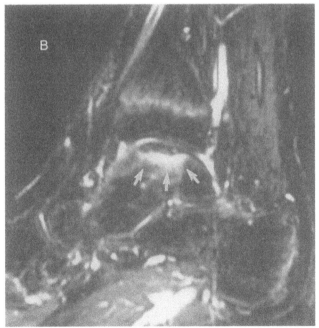

FIGURE 10.12 Osteochondral lesion of the talar dome (13-year-old boy). This previously athletic boy sustained an episode of severe ankle trauma 7 months earlier. (A) Sagittal T1-weighted SE image (TR 650/TE 11). (B) Sagittal IR sequence (TR 5000/TE 32/TI 160) show impaction of the talar dome with an irregular band of high signal intensity surrounding the impacted fragment indicative of instability (arrows).

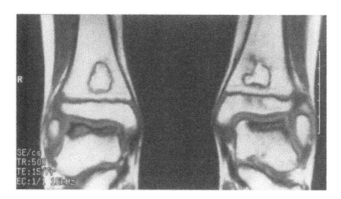

FIGURE 10.13 Bone infarcts (11-year-old boy). This boy was on long-standing steroid treatment for leukemia. Coronal T1-weighted SE images of the ankle (TR 500/TE 15) show the geographic serpentine pattern of bone infarcts in the distal tibial metaphyses. Changes are also seen in the central part of the distal tibial epiphysis on the left side. The infarcted talar domes show low signal, denoting sclerosis and impaction.

Freiberg disease is rare in the pediatric age group. It occurs more frequently in girls and, as in adults, involves the second or third metatarsal head. Köhler disease is more frequent in boys, usually less than 7 years of age. The navicular bone is the last tarsal bone to ossify and its arterial supply originates from a single nutrient artery. The condition is usually self-limited with gradual partial or complete reconstitution of the dense fragmented tarsal navicular. On MR imaging, avascular necrosis shows early bone marrow edema with decreased signal intensity on T1-weighted images and high signal on T2-weighted images. In systemic diseases causing avascular necrosis the bone changes are well defined, serpentine, and geographic.[41] Bone may collapse and areas of impaction will appear as low signal intensity on all sequences.[42] Vascularized granulation tissue is seen in the revascularization phase, with the help of contrast-enhanced MR images obtained

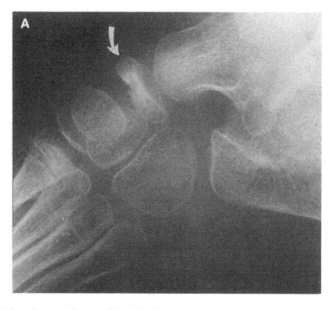

FIGURE 10.14 Köhler disease (5-year-old girl). This patient complained of localized pain on the dorsal aspect of the mid-part of the left foot. (A) Oblique radiograph of the foot shows central irregular sclerosis and flattening of the navicular bone (arrow).   (*continued*)

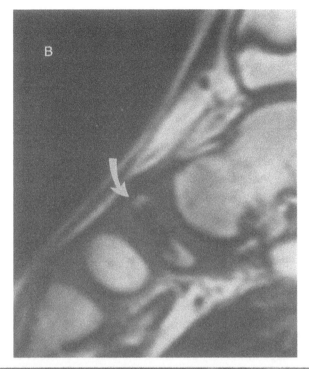

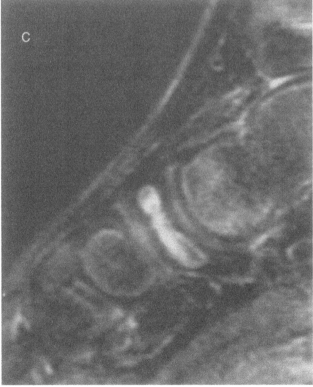

FIGURE 10.14 (continued) (B) Sagittal T1-weighted SE image (TR 400/TE 11) demonstrates extensive low signal intensity in the flattened navicular bone, denoting a possible combination of marrow edema, bone sclerosis, and impaction (arrow). (C) Sagittal IR image (TR 4000/TE 38/TI 160) reveals high signal intensity in the navicular bone marrow consistent with edema.

after IV gadolinium. Residual alteration in the alignment, contour, and general shape of the bone favors the development of early degenerative arthritis. A pattern of bone marrow edema has been described in the symptomatic accessory navicular bone, which is likely secondary to trauma, chronic stress, or avascular necrosis.[10]

INFLAMMATORY DISORDERS

There are two major chronic inflammatory noninfectious arthritides in the pediatric age group: juvenile rheumatoid arthritis (JRA), also called juvenile idiopathic or chronic arthritis, and seronegative juvenile spondyloarthropathies or the enthesitis-related arthritides.[43] Both types result in a painful chronic inflammatory disorder of the involved synovial joints. In JRA, ankles, subtalar joints, and toes are usually involved, particularly in the polyarticular form. MR imaging sequences that optimize the demonstration of the articular cartilage and subchondral bone are crucial for assessment and can be achieved with gradient-echo or fat-saturated FSE. The inflamed hypervascular synovium and pannus may be visualized on IV gadolinium-enhanced fat-suppressed T1-weighted images, and show marked increased signal intensity.[44] Imaging should be completed immediately after gadolinium administration to avoid diffusion of contrast into the joint fluid (Figure 10.15). In the authors' experience, normal synovium shows no apparent enhancement after IV gadolinium administration. A joint effusion is usually present and is hyperintense on T2-weighted images. Inflamed synovial cysts or bursae may be present and show hyperintense signal on T2-weighted sequences (Figure 10.16A). Young children have thick abundant articular cartilage in the foot and ankle and osseous erosions develop late in chronic inflammatory arthritis. MR imaging is therefore crucial for direct imaging of early cartilage changes in this age group.

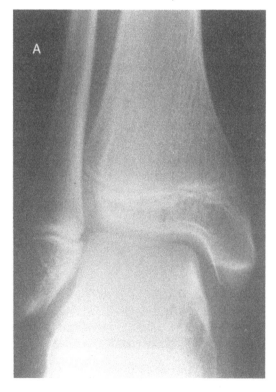

FIGURE 10.15 Juvenile rheumatoid arthritis (13-year-old girl). This patient with known polyarticular JRA presented with right ankle pain. (A) Anteroposterior radiograph of the right ankle is normal.   (*continued*)

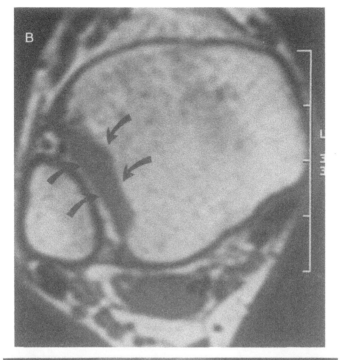

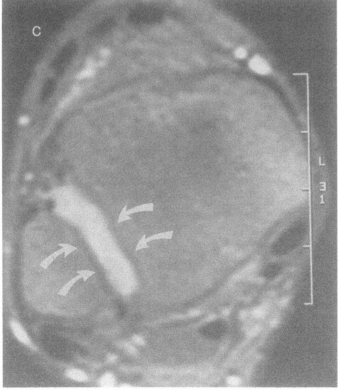

FIGURE 10.15 (continued) (B) Axial T1-weighted SE image (TR 400/TE 11) shows a low signal crescent-shaped effusion in the distal tibiofibular joint (arrows). (C) Enhanced axial T1-weighted SE image (TR 400/TE 11) with fat suppression following IV injection of gadolinium shows the effusion is of high signal intensity due to relatively late scanning and diffusion of gadolinium into the joint (arrows).

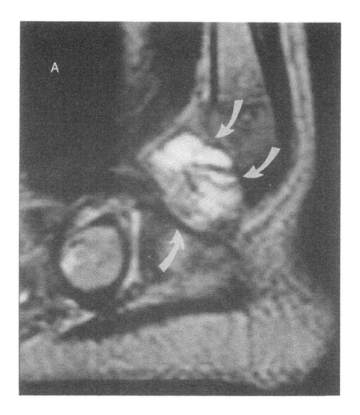

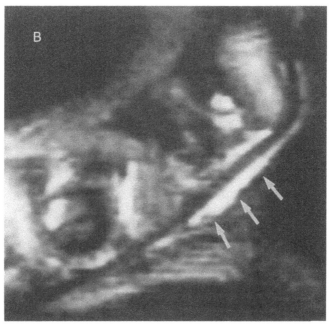

FIGURE 10.16 Inflamed bursa (3-year-old boy). This patient presented with a painful lateral ankle and hind foot swelling. (A) Sagittal fat-suppressed SE T2-weighted image (TR3000/TE105). Loculated high-signal fluid is present in an inflamed bursa (arrows). (B) Sagittal IR image (TR 3000/TE 21/TI 160) shows adjacent peroneal tenosynovitis with high-signal fluid in the distended tendon sheath of the peroneus brevis (arrows). The cause of the bursitis and tenosynovitis was unknown. Needle aspiration and culture of the bursal fluid revealed no organism.

Tenosynovitis may occur secondary to acute trauma, overuse, infection, or arthritis. On MR imaging, tenosynovitis can demonstrate increased size and signal intensity of the tendon and/or excessive fluid in the tendon sheath (Figure 10.16B). Chronic active inflammation and hyperemia are confirmed by the presence of enhancement of the tendon and/or sheath on the T1-weighted images following IV gadolinium. Tenosynovitis of the foot and ankle may be seen in JRA as well as the seronegative spondyloarthropathies.

In neuroarthropathy, MR imaging shows bone fragmentation and osseous, cartilage, and synovial debris associated with a joint effusion and joint disorganization as well as synovial enhancement following IV gadolinium. The joint changes are destructive and progressive.[45]

In chronic post-traumatic hemarthrosis, hemophilic arthropathy, and pigmented villonodular synovitis (PVNS), a progressive arthritis develops with hemosiderin deposition in the synovial lining resulting in low signal intensity on all sequences.[46] Synovial biopsy is required to confirm the diagnosis of PVNS.

Inflammation at the site of attachment of a ligament or tendon to bone is termed enthesitis and is an important clinical and radiologic feature of the spondyloarthropathies. In the foot, enthesitis occurs at the insertion of Achilles tendon and plantar fascia to the calcaneus and causes heel pain and local swelling. Bone erosion or spur formation may be seen at these sites on radiographs. On MR imaging, early changes include a bone marrow edema pattern similar to that seen following trauma, with localized, patchy, low signal intensity on T1-weighted images (Figure 10.17), and high signal on T2-weighted and IR sequences. MR imaging also shows early bone erosion and/or bone apposition, as well as thickening or increased signal intensity within the Achilles tendon or plantar fascia. Other causes for painful heel include overuse, a calcaneal stress fracture, foreign body, trauma, subacute or chronic infection, cysts, tumors and tumorlike lesions, Sever disease, tarsal tunnel syndrome, plantar heel fat pad inflammation, or plantar fascial tears which are usually secondary to local steroid injection.[47] Heel pain is a relatively frequent complaint in children and adolescents.

INFECTION

Osteomyelitis in children is generally hematogenous and metaphyseal. In the ankle and foot, the distal tibia, distal fibula, or posterior calcaneus are most commonly involved although any bone

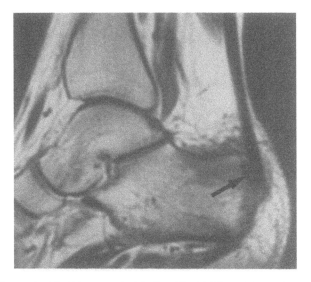

FIGURE 10.17 Achilles enthesitis (13-year-old girl). This HLA B27–positive patient presented with left heel pain and swelling and no history of trauma. Sagittal T1-weighted SE image (TR 600/TE 11) shows patchy low-signal areas in the posterior calcaneus consistent with bone marrow edema. An erosion is evident at the site of attachment of the Achilles tendon (arrow). Both findings relate to an active Achilles enthesitis.

may be affected. Infection in the foot is usually secondary to puncture injuries. The puncture wound may be obvious; however, at times, it may be difficult or impossible to detect.[5] Septic arthritis may be hematogenous or secondary to extension of infection from the metaphysis through the growth plate to the epiphysis and then to the joint space, or from an adjacent soft-tissue infection.

As in other parts of the upper or lower extremities, suspected osteomyelitis or septic arthritis initially needs to be imaged with radiographs.[48] They are helpful for anatomic localization and exclusion of other conditions such as fracture, tumor, or tumorlike condition (e.g., Langerhans cell histiocytosis). In osteomyelitis, MR imaging shows early marrow changes resulting from hyperemia, inflammatory edema, and exudate. These changes are not specific and must be correlated with the findings on clinical examination, laboratory tests (particularly the leukocyte count and the erythrocyte sedimentation rate or ESR), radiographs, and bone and/or gallium scintigraphy. Noninfectious causes of marrow edema can also be seen following trauma or associated with infarction, reactive inflammation from enthesitis, and nonpyogenic arthritic conditions. On T1-weighted images, low signal replaces the normal high signal intensity of fatty marrow. On T2-weighted images, the same areas demonstrate high signal intensity in the bone marrow and adjacent soft tissues[49] and are most conspicuous on fat-suppressed T2-weighted or IR sequences (Figure 10.18). MR imaging may also reveal subperiosteal or soft-tissue fluid collections or abscesses. In children, the cortex is easily permeated and the periosteum is only loosely attached to the cortex and is easily lifted up allowing relatively large subperiosteal abscesses to form, especially in the short tubular bones of the foot. A subperiosteal abscess may rupture, allowing extension of infection into the nearby soft tissues. Soft-tissue abscesses with or without adjacent osteomyelitis of the foot may

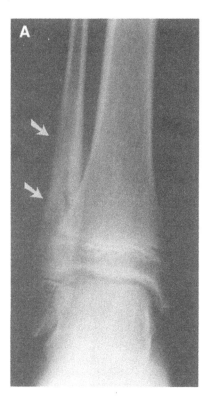 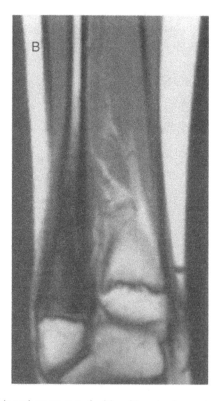

FIGURE 10.18 Fibular osteomyelitis (10-year-old girl). This patient presented with ankle pain, fever, elevated erythrocyte sedimentation rate, and leukocytosis. (A) Anteroposterior radiograph shows a mixed sclerotic and lytic lesion in the distal diaphysis and metaphysis of the fibula down to the growth plate (arrows). Periosteal reaction is also seen. (B) Coronal oblique T1-weighted SE image (TR 450/TE 10) shows extensive low signal intensity in the distal diaphysis and metaphysis of the fibula with sparing of the epiphysis.   (*continued*)

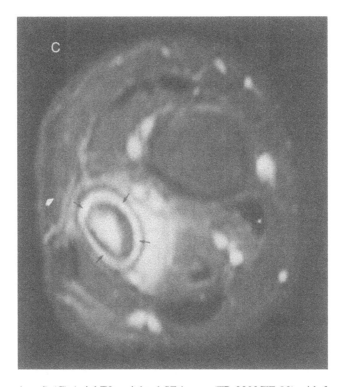

FIGURE 10.18 (continued) (C) Axial T2-weighted SE image (TR 2000/TE 90) with fat suppression reveals the pronounced edema in the fibular bone marrow and adjacent soft tissues. A circumferential subperiosteal fluid (pus) accumulation is also seen (small arrows). The normal tibial fatty marrow is low signal intensity on this image.

also occur. These abscesses may show rim enhancement of vascularized, inflamed connective tissue on T1-weighted sequences with fat suppression following IV gadolinium. Abscess identification and localization are required for planning therapeutic options.

In septic arthritis, ultrasound or MR imaging may demonstrate the nonspecific findings of a joint effusion, associated with internal debris and irregular synovial thickening. In this setting, MR imaging following IV gadolinium optimally delineates the abnormal synovium. In the acute phase, aspiration and culture of the joint fluid to identify the offending organism are necessary. Early diagnosis and rapid treatment are imperative to avoid complications as the proteolytic enzymes in the purulent effusion rapidly destroy the articular cartilage. MR imaging can provide a detailed assessment of the articular cartilage and adjacent bone marrow and soft tissue in this situation.

A Brodie abscess most commonly occurs in the distal tibia or posterior calcaneus, manifested as a localized round or oval intraosseous metaphyseal lesion of low signal on T1-weighted images and high signal on T2-weighted images, with surrounding bone marrow edema. There is usually marked rim enhancement after IV gadolinium enhancement. A sequestrum, or fragment of dead bone, may be present within the bone abscess and can be suspected on MR imaging when an amorphous fragment of low signal intensity is present that does not enhance after IV gadolinium. Rarely, a primary epiphyseal bone abscess (without metaphyseal involvement) may be seen in the foot or ankle.

MASSES

The multiplanar capability of MR imaging is a feature that offers a distinct advantage over other imaging modalities in the assessment of vascular masses, cysts, tumors, and tumor-like conditions

This capability enables more accurate assessment of the relation of a lesion to the surrounding soft-tissue structures. In some cases, MR imaging allows a specific diagnosis to be made and facilitates surgical planning in all lesions.

Familiarity with signal characteristics on various imaging sequences is helpful in rendering specific diagnoses.[50,51] Signal characteristics in conjunction with the age of the patient and a knowledge of tumor prevalence in particular age categories frequently are of assistance in narrowing the differential diagnosis of a lesion.

While MR imaging is an excellent technique to assess the relationship of a lesion to surrounding structures and to suggest the histologic origin of a lesion, it does not accurately predict benignity or malignancy. Such features as the tumor margins and the homogeneity of the lesion do not prove to be useful in differentiating benign and malignant pathologies.[51,52] Both benign and malignant lesions may have heterogeneous signal characteristics. Poorly defined margins have been seen in lesions such as osteoid osteoma, intramuscular capillary hemangioma, and aggressive fibromatosis,[52,53] all of which are benign in histology and behavior. With respect to signal characteristics, low signal intensity on T2-weighted images is suggestive of benignity; however, both benign and malignant lesions may demonstrate high signal intensity on T2-weighted images.

HEMANGIOMAS AND VASCULAR ANOMALIES

Several classification systems have been proposed for this group of lesions.[54-56] Some systems consider only the size of the vessel comprising the lesion, with four categories of hemangiomas described — capillary, cavernous, mixed (capillary and cavernous), and venous, with a separate category for arteriovenous malformations.[55,56] Others divide the lesions based on the velocity of flow within the lesion, further subdividing the categories of fast flow and slow flow lesions according to the size of the component vessels.[54] The remainder of this discussion, however, employs the classification originally proposed by Mulliken et al.[54a] in which the anomalies are described utilizing the characteristics of cellular turnover, histology, natural history, and physical findings.[57,58] Hemangiomas are considered to be separate from vascular malformations; the latter may be further divided based on the type of vessel contained within.

Hemangiomas are the most common tumors of infancy and, in the pediatric age group, are located in the head, neck, and chest.[53] While rarely identifiable at birth, they may be present in as many as 10 to 12% of Caucasian children by 1 year of age. Their natural history is rapid growth during infancy and involution by age 5 to 10 years. Although numerous mitoses may be detected in these lesions on light microscopy, this feature is not felt to be an indication of malignancy.[59] MR imaging is especially valuable in detecting the margins of a vascular mass when the border of the lesion is difficult to appreciate on physical examination. The signal characteristics must take into account the size of the vessels and the phase of the lesion (proliferating, involuting, or involuted).

Classically, hemangiomas are isointense to or slightly hyperintense to skeletal muscle on T1-weighted images and markedly hyperintense to muscle on T2-weighted images.[56,58,60] The masses are usually heterogeneous in signal characteristics, a feature that is more common in larger lesions. The heterogeneity is a reflection of nonvascular tissues contained in the lesion and is often manifested as a serpentine or lacelike pattern of high signal on T1-weighted images and low signal intensity on T2-weighted images. In addition to fat, which accounts for the foci of high signal intensity on T1-weighted images, hemangiomas may also contain smooth muscle, thrombus, and hemosiderin. Another hemangiomatous element responsible for increased signal on T1-weighted images is slow-flowing blood pooled in cavernous spaces, while a variety of features including fast-flowing blood, fibrous septa, calcification, and hemosiderin contribute to decreased signal on T1-weighted images. Intravenous contrast is not routinely utilized in imaging vascular lesions, but has been shown in some examples to increase the conspicuity of the serpentine pattern of

inhomogeneity.[60] Intravenous administration of gadolinium can allow differentiation of proliferating and involuting hemangiomas from involuted hemangiomas as the former will enhance
intensely, whereas the latter will not.[58] The borders of a hemangioma are considerably better
defined on T2-weighted images compared with T1-weighted images.[56]

The signal characteristics of a particular hemangioma will be influenced by its phase of
development. Proliferating hemangiomas will be isointense or hypointense to muscle on T1-
weighted images and hyperintense to muscle on T2-weighted images; on both sequences, flow
voids representing feeding arteries and draining veins will be seen. The signal characteristics
in the involuting phase are influenced greatly by the percentage of fat comprising the lesion.
In the involuted phase, signal is largely influenced by the increased amount of fat present,
such that hemangiomas in this phase will be of high signal on T1- and low signal on T2-
weighted images.[58]

Vascular anomalies can be considered malformations of capillary, lymphatic, venous, arterial, and combined types. While hemangiomas are considered to be tumors, vascular malformations are considered developmental anomalies.[4] Capillary, venous, and capillary–venous
malformations are low-flow anomalies, while arterial and arteriovenous malformations represent
high-flow anomalies.

Unlike hemangiomas, which grow rapidly while a child is young and then involute, the growth
of a vascular malformation parallels that of the child.[53] Venous malformations exhibit isointensity
to muscle on T1-weighted images and high signal on T2-weighted images (Figure 10.19A and B).
Thrombi show high signal foci on T1-weighted images and flow voids on T2-weighted images.
The enhancement pattern of a venous malformation may be either homogeneous or heterogeneous.[58]
MR venography has been proved to compensate for some of the shortfalls of traditional angiography
(poor opacification of veins due to slow filling on arteriography, nonfilling of deep veins due to
preferential filling of dilated superficial veins on venography, lack of venous access in an edematous
extremity) in imaging these malformations.[4] Direct injection, MR imaging, and MR venography
can be utilized to assess the response of vascular malformations to a variety of therapies including
embolization and sclerosis (Figure 10.19C and D).

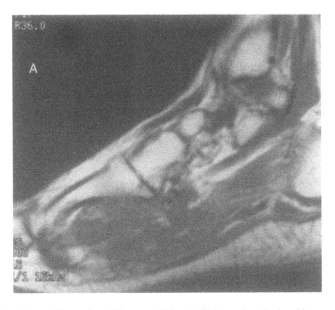

FIGURE 10.19 Vascular malformation (18-year-old boy). This patient had a history of an unsuccessful
attempt to resect a "hemangioma" from the plantar soft tissues. The recurrent vascular malformation was
partially treated with ethanol embolization. (A) Sagittal SE T1-weighted (TR 500/TE 18) image demonstrates
a mass in the plantar soft tissues that is isointense to muscle.   (*continued*)

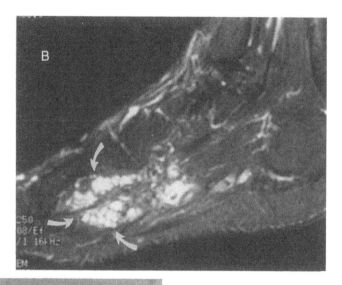

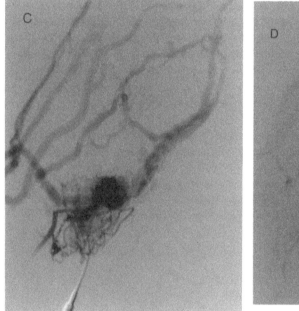
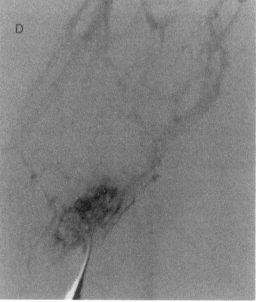

FIGURE 10.19 (continued) (B) Sagittal fat-suppressed SE T2-weighted (TR 4250/TE 108) image demonstrates heterogeneous increased signal (arrows). Linear low-signal fibrous septations separate the high-signal lobules. (C) Prior to embolization, multiple dilated vascular channels are demonstrated. (D) Utilizing ultrasound guidance, two separate vascular spaces were cannulated, and embolization was performed resulting in a significant decrease in size and number of vessels.

CYSTS

The ganglion cyst is the most frequently encountered cystic structure in the ankle and foot, although this lesion is considerably more common on the dorsum of the wrist.[53] Ganglia arise from a capsule of a joint or from a tendon sheath and often fluctuate in size. Classically, ganglia are tender and because they are readily diagnosed clinically, it is rarely necessary to image them. On MR imaging, ganglia are usually well defined and show low signal on T1-weighted images and high signal intensity on T2-weighted images due to their fluid content (Figure 10.20).[52]

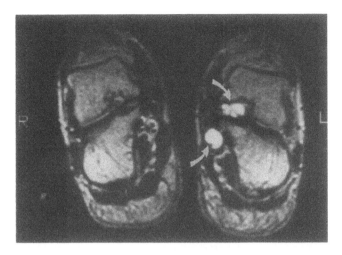

FIGURE 10.20 Soft tissue ganglion (11-year-old boy). Coronal SE T2-weighted (TR 3000/TE 80) image demonstrates increased signal intensity in a lobulated lesion on the medial side of the left hind foot (arrows). A few low-signal-intensity septations are present. No fluid–fluid levels are identified and the adjacent bones are unaffected.

TUMOR-LIKE CONDITIONS

The prototypical tumor-like condition affecting the foot and ankle is plantar fibromatosis, a lesion of benign histology which behaves aggressively. It does not metastasize systemically, but can involve adjacent bone, muscle, and skin.[61] This lesion does, however, respect muscle and fascial planes so that joint motion is not affected. Plantar fibromatosis is usually asymptomatic but may be more painful in cases of recurrent lesions. Nonsurgical therapy, such as corticosteroid injections, is favored since surgical therapy results in a high rate of recurrence, necessitating wider margins of resection with each additional surgery.[53,61] Subtotal fasciectomy has been reported to be effective in preventing recurrent fibromatosis, even in those patients who had recurrent disease despite previous wide excision.[61] Other investigators have recommended radiation as an adjunct to more limited surgery. In some cases of fibromatosis in which estrogen receptors are present, tamoxifen may be administered as adjuvant chemotherapy.[53]

Aggressive fibromatosis generally presents after the age of 10 years, most commonly between puberty and age 40. Under the age of 10 years, the risk of local recurrence is felt to be greater.

The challenge with fibromatosis, when attempting surgical treatment, is to determine the local extent of the lesion. Not only is this difficult surgically, but it is also difficult on imaging (both CT and MR imaging) and histologically. It is usually fairly simple to distinguish fibromatosis from fibrosarcoma histologically, however, if an adequate sample has been biopsied.[53]

On MR imaging, fibromatosis is usually low signal intensity on both T1- and T2-weighted sequences (Figure 10.21).

TUMORS

There is scant literature regarding tumors of the foot and ankle, reflecting the infrequency of involvement of the bones and soft tissues in this region, both in adults and in children. Most tumors of the foot and ankle are benign and arise from the soft tissues.[62] Tumors that arise from bone are also overwhelmingly benign (83.5% benign).[63]

A study of nearly 19,000 benign mesenchymal tumors culled from the nearly 40,000 soft-tissue lesions seen at the Armed Forces Institute of Pathology between 1980 and 1989 was undertaken to categorize them according to the diagnosis, location within the body, and age of the patient. A mere 147 occurred in the foot and ankle of children less than 16 years old. The most frequent

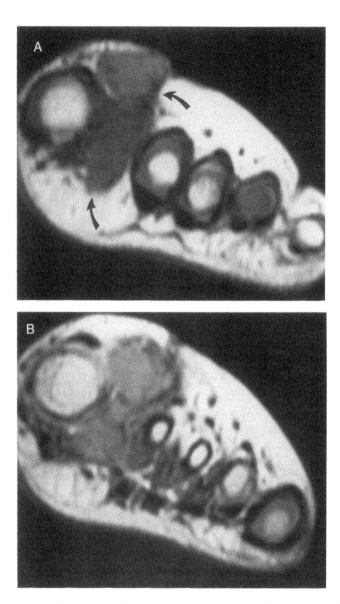

FIGURE 10.21 Aggressive fibromatosis (3-year-old girl). (A) Coronal T1-weighted (TR 600/TE 15) SE image of the foot demonstrates a mass isointense to muscle between the first and second toes (arrows). No osseous involvement is evident. (B) Coronal proton density (TR 2000/TE 20) SE image of the foot reveals slight increased signal intensity in the lesion compared with adjacent muscle, which is less intense than fat. The mass recurred following initial resection necessitating below-the-ankle amputation. The lesion recurred 4 years later at the distal portion of the stump and the ipsilateral knee regions.

lesions were fibromatosis, hemangioma, and granuloma annulare.[26] The MR imaging appearances of the first two have been described above.

Bone tumors also occur infrequently in the foot and ankle. In a Mayo Clinic review of 6034 bone tumors, 1.7% of all lesions were located within the foot. To emphasize further the rarity of these lesions, of the 29 types of bone tumor, 12 types were not reported to occur in the foot. The most common tumor seen in this series was Ewing sarcoma.

In most published series, the frequency of osteosarcomas affecting the bones of the foot is between 0.17 and 2.08% of all osteosarcomas.[64] A review of 1929 cases of osteosarcoma seen at the Rizzoli Orthopedic Institute in Bologna, Italy between 1911 and 1992 revealed 12 tumors in the foot, representing 0.6% of all cases.[64]

Benign Tumors

Only 6% of aneurysmal bone cysts (ABC) occur in the tarsal bones (6% of all ABC) whereas 19% of giant cell tumors (GCT) of bone occur in this anatomic region.[65] The distinction between the two lesions may be difficult, but is important because the therapy is different. ABC typically occurs in the pediatric population and the tubular bones in the foot are most commonly affected compared with the small tarsal bones. MR imaging has been useful for assessing features such as septations, cortical integrity, pathologic fracture, soft-tissue mass, spread to the adjacent joint, and fluid–fluid levels. ABC and GCT in the foot can be differentiated on MR imaging by the greater frequency of fluid–fluid levels in ABC (47% in ABC, 20% in GCT), and the higher frequency of both pathologic fractures (67% in GCT, 20% in ABC) and articular extension (83% in GCT, 33% in ABC) in GCT.[65] ABC may be primary or associated with other bone lesions such as GCT, fibrous dysplasia, unicameral bone cyst, chondroblastoma, and nonossifying fibroma (Figure 10.22).

GCT of the tendon sheath or capsule is rare and is usually painless at presentation. Soft-tissue GCT requires surgical treatment and has the potential for recurrence if incompletely excised. There is little experience with MR imaging of these lesions; in one published report, the lesion was isointense to muscle on T1-weighted images and did not appear as a discrete mass that was clearly separable from muscle.[66]

Chondroblastoma, a lesion often localized to the epiphyses, may also occur in the tarsal bones, especially the talus and calcaneus.[67] In a series of 332 chondroblastomas reviewed at the Armed Forces Institute of Pathology between 1960 and 1990, the mean age of those in the foot was 25.5 years, significantly greater than the mean age of those in the extremities, which was 17.3 years. Therefore, chondroblastoma of the foot is more of an adult entity.

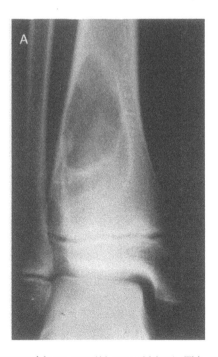

FIGURE 10.22 Secondary aneurysmal bone cyst (11-year-old boy). This patient had a histopathologically proven ABC complicating a nonossifying fibroma of the distal tibia. (A) Anteroposterior radiograph shows a large, eccentric, oval, lucent lesion in the distal tibial metaphysis without periosteal reaction.   (*continued*)

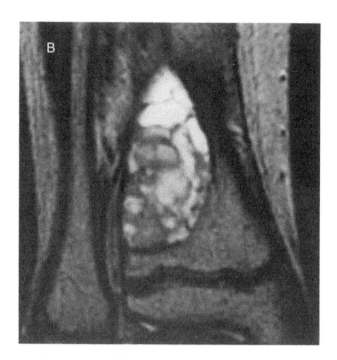

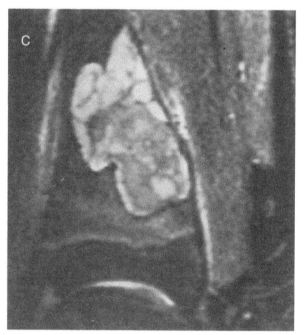

FIGURE 10.22 (continued) (B) Coronal SE T2-weighted image (TR 3000/TE 100), with fat suppression reveals multiple loculations and high signal in the upper part of the lesion consistent with the ABC component of the lesion. (C) Sagittal IR image (TR 4000/TE 36/TI 160) shows similar findings as seen on (B), with an intact cortex and no fluid–fluid levels.

Chondromyxoid fibromas are rare lesions, accounting for only 1% of all primary bone tumors. They typically occur in the second decade of life. The knee is the most common site, followed in frequency by the small bones of the foot which represent 17% of all chondromyxoid fibromas.[68]

Recurrence of these lesions can occur and is generally a reflection of inadequate primary treatment. The radiographic appearances of chondromyxoid fibroma range from benign, resembling an enchondroma, to very aggressive, resembling a sarcoma. The MR imaging findings are nonspecific, revealing low signal on T1-weighted images and high signal intensity on T2-weighted images. Chondromyxoid fibromas enhance with IV gadolinium administration.

Malignant Tumors

Ewing sarcoma is the most common malignant neoplasm of the foot,[69] although fewer than 40 cases have been reported in the literature.[70] There is frequently a delay in the diagnosis, as the lesions are initially misdiagnosed as avascular necrosis and infection. The 5-year survival rate in Ewing sarcoma has increased significantly and currently ranges from 50 to 70%.[69] The treatment of Ewing sarcoma utilizes both surgery and chemotherapy. Tumors of the foot are particularly amenable to surgical extirpation with either a below-knee amputation or ray resection. Published reports indicate that surgical resection of the tumor has led to a significantly increased 5-year survival (75%) compared with radiation therapy (34%).[69] Additionally, radiation has its attendant risks of physeal damage and resultant limb length discrepancy. MR imaging of the primary lesion is only one part of the imaging workup of a patient with Ewing sarcoma. The features on MR imaging do not distinguish it from other malignant tumors. Since 25% of patients with Ewing sarcoma have metastases at time of diagnosis,[70] a CT scan of the chest and a radionuclide bone scan are an important part of the complete workup of the patient to search for distant metastases prior to treatment.

Osteosarcoma is the second most common malignant bone tumor; however, it rarely involves the bones of the foot and ankle. Involvement of the ankle is more frequent than the foot, and in the foot a tarsal or metatarsal bone is usually affected. In contrast to osteosarcomas located elsewhere in the body which have a peak age of 15 to 20 years, those in the feet affect an older population with a mean age of 33 years in one published report.[64] Also, in contrast to osteosarcomas in general, lesions in the feet are frequently low grade histologically and therefore have a better prognosis, despite their frequent late diagnosis. As with osteosarcomas in any location, MR imaging can define the extent of the lesion in bone and soft tissue, the presence of skip metastases, and intra-articular extension, but cannot offer a specific diagnosis (Figure 10.23).

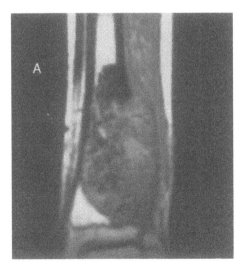

FIGURE 10.23 Osteosarcoma of the distal tibia (11-year-old boy). (A) Coronal SE T1-weighted (TR 600/TE 20) image demonstrates a predominantly low-signal-intensity lesion replacing the normal high-signal-intensity marrow of the diametaphysis. *(continued)*

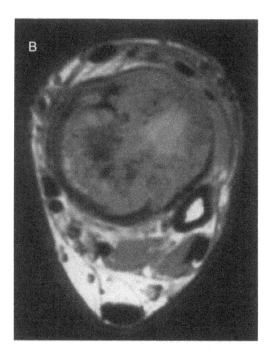

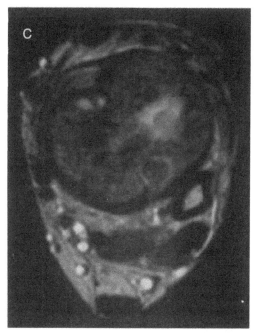

FIGURE 10.23 (continued) (B and C) Axial first and second echoes of an SE dual-echo sequence (TR 1800/TE 20 and 80) of the distal tibia demonstrate mild heterogeneity of marrow signal. Although the findings of heterogeneity and expansion of the marrow cavity with loss of definition of the cortex suggest malignancy, the diagnosis is nonspecific.

The vast majority of soft-tissue malignancies of the foot including clear cell sarcoma, malignant fibrous histiocytoma, and synovial sarcoma occur in adults,[71] but have been reported in children.[72] They are not discussed here because of their rarity.

SUMMARY

In summary, a knowledge of the relative prevalence of specific mass lesions in a given age group can be extremely helpful when assessing the MR imaging signal characteristics of a particular lesion and attempting to render a well-ordered differential diagnosis. When considering the foot and ankle, more lesions involve the soft tissues than bone and considerably more lesions are benign than malignant, such that the most commonly encountered masses are either vascular lesions or fibromatosis. An understanding of the change in signal characteristics of hemangiomas as they involute and of the difficulty in assessing the margins of fibromatosis will be most beneficial to the consulting clinician.

REFERENCES

1. Mosca, V. S., The child's foot: principles in management, *J. Pediatr. Orthop.*, 18, 281, 1998.
2. Barnewolt, C. E. and Chung, T., Techniques, coils, pulse sequences, and contrast enhancement in pediatric musculoskeletal MR imaging, *MRI Clin. North Am.*, 6, 441, 1998.
3. American Society of Anesthesiologists task force on sedation and analgesia by nonanesthesiologists: practice guidelines for sedation and analgesia by nonanesthesiologists, *Anesthesiology*, 84, 459, 1996.
4. Laor, T., Burrows, P. E., and Hoffer, F. A., Magnetic resonance venography of congenital vascular malformations of the extremities, *Pediatr. Radiol.*, 26, 371, 1996.
5. Stazzone, M. M. and Hubbard, A.M., The pediatric foot and ankle, *MRI Clin. North Am.*, 6, 661, 1998.
6. Hubbard, A. M., Meyer, J. S., Davidson, R. S. et al., Relationship between the ossification center and cartilaginous anlage in the normal hind foot in children: study with MR imaging, *AJR*, 161, 849, 1993.
7. Barnewolt, C. E., Shapiro, F., and Jaramillo, D., Normal gadolinium-enhanced MR images of the developing appendicular skeleton. Part 1: cartilaginous epiphysis and physis, *AJR*, 169, 183, 1997.
8. Chung, T. and Jaramillo, D., Normal maturing distal tibia and fibula: changes with age at MR imaging, *Radiology*, 194, 227, 1995.
9. Dwek, J. R., Shapiro, F., Laor, T. et al., Normal gadolinium enhanced MR images of the developing appendicular skeleton. Part 2: epiphyseal and metaphyseal marrow, *AJR*, 169, 191, 1997.
10. Miller, T. T., Staron, R. B., Feldman, F., Parisien, M., Glucksman, W. J., and Gandolfo, L. H., The symptomatic accessory tarsal navicular bone: assessment with MR imaging, *Radiology*, 195, 849, 1995.
11. Link, S. C., Erickson, S. J., and Timins, M. E., MR imaging of the ankle and foot: normal structures and anatomic variants that may simulate disease, *AJR*, 161, 607, 1993.
12. Hoffinger, S. A., Evaluation and management of pediatric foot deformities, *Pediatr. Clin. North Am.*, 43, 1091, 1996.
13. Tolat, V., Bothroyd, A., Carty, H. et al., Ultrasound: a helpful guide in the treatment of congental talipes equinovarus, *J. Pediatr. Orthop.*, 4, 65, 1995.
14. Drennan, J., Ed., *The Child's Foot and Ankle*. Raven Press, New York, 1992.
15. Johnston, C. E., Hobatho, M. C., Baker, K. J. et al., Three-dimensional analysis of club foot deformity by computed tomography, *J. Pediatr. Orthop.*, 4, 39, 1995.
16. Simons, G. W., Calcaneocuboid joint deformity in talipes equinovarus: an overview and update, *J. Pediatr. Orthop.*, 4, 25, 1995.
17. Grayhack, J. J., Zawin, J. K., Shore, R. M. et al., Assessment of calcaneocuboid joint deformity by magnetic resonance imaging in talipes equinovarus, *J. Pediatr. Orthop.*, 4, 36, 1995.
18. Wang, C., Petursdottir, I., Leifsdottir, I., Rehnberg, L., and Ahlström, H., MRI multiplanar reconstruction in the assessment of congenital talipes equinovarus, *Pediatr. Radiol.*, 29, 262, 1999.
19. Cahuzac, J. P., Baunin, C., Luu, S. et al., Assessment of hind foot deformity by three dimensional MRI in infant club foot, *J. Bone Joint Surg.*, 81(B), 97, 1999.
20. Hubbard, A. M., Davidson, R. S., Meyer, J. S. et al., Magnetic resonance imaging of skew foot, *J. Bone Joint Surg.*, 78(A), 389, 1996.
21. Lateur, L., Van Hoe, L., Banghillewe, K. et al., Subtalar coalition. Diagnosis with the C sign on lateral radiographs of the ankle, *Radiology*, 193, 847, 1994.

22. Wechsler, R. J., Schweitzer, M. E., Deely, D. M. et al., Tarsal coalition: depiction and characterization with CT and MR imaging, *Radiology*, 193, 447, 1994.
23. Mahboubi, S. and Davidson, R., MR imaging in longitudinal epiphyseal bracket in children, *Pediatr. Radiol.*, 29, 259, 1999.
24. Laor, T., Jaramillo, D., Hoffer, F. A. et al., MR imaging in congenital lower limb anomalies, *Pediatr. Radiol.*, 26, 381, 1996.
25. Azouz, E. M., Slomic, A. M., Marton, D., Rigault, P., and Finidori, G., The variable manifestations of dysplasia epiphysealis hemimelica, *Pediatr. Radiol.*, 15, 44, 1985.
26. Azouz, E. M., Costa, T., and Fitch, N., Radiologic findings in the Proteus syndrome, *Pediatr. Radiol.*, 17, 481, 1987.
27. Hollister, M. C. and DeSmet, A. A., MR imaging of the foot and ankle in sports injuries, *Semin. Musculoskeletal Radiol.*, 1, 105, 1997.
28. Greenspan, A. and Anderson, M. W., Imaging of the foot and ankle, *Curr. Opin. Orthop.*, 7, 61, 1996.
29. Rubin, D. A., Towers, J. D., and Britton, C. A., MR imaging of the foot: utility of complex oblique imaging planes, *AJR*, 166, 1079, 1996.
30. Jaramillo, D., Hoffer, F.A., Shapiro, F., and Rand., F., MR imaging of fractures of the growth plate, *AJR*, 155, 1261, 1990.
31. Smith, B.G., Rand, F., Jaramillo, D., and Shapiro, F., Early MR imaging of lower extremity physeal fracture-separation. A preliminary report, *J. Pediatr. Orthop.*, 14, 526, 1994.
32. Petit, P., Panuel, M., Fauré, F., Jouve, J. L., Bourlière-Najean, B., Bollini, G., and Devred, P., Acute fracture of the distal tibial physis: role of gradient-echo MR imaging versus plain film examination, *AJR*, 166, 1203, 1996.
33. Rogers, L. F. and Poznanski, A. K., Imaging of epiphyseal injuries. State of the art, *Radiology*, 191, 297, 1994.
34. Jaramillo, D. and Shapiro, F., Musculoskeletal trauma in children, *MRI Clin. North Am.*, 6, 521, 1998.
35. Jaramillo, D. and Shapiro, F., Growth cartilage. Normal appearance, variants and abnormalities, *MRI Clin. North Am.*, 6, 455, 1998.
36. DeSmet, A. A., Ilahi, O. A., and Graf, B. K., Reassessment of the MR criteria for stability of osteochondritis dissecans in the knee and ankle, *Skeletal Radiol.*, 25, 159, 1996.
37. DeSmet, A. A., Fisher, D. R., Burnstein, M. I., Graf, B. K., and Lange, R. H., Value of MR imaging in staging osteochondral lesions of the talus (osteochondritis dissecans): results in 14 patients, *AJR*, 154, 555, 1990.
38. Bohndorf, K., Osteochondritis (osteochondrosis) dissecans: a review and new MRI classification, *Eur. Radiol.*, 8, 103, 1998.
39. Abrahim-zadeh, R., Klein, R.M., Leslie, D., and Norman, A., Characteristics of calcaneal bone infarction: an MR imaging investigation, *Skeletal Radiol.*, 27, 321, 1998.
40. Mubarak, S. J., Osteochondrosis of the lateral cuneiform: another cause of a limp in a child, *J. Bone Joint Surg.*, 74(A), 285, 1992.
41. Feldman, F., Staron, R. B., and Haramati, N., Magnetic resonance imaging of the foot and ankle, *Rheum. Dis. Clin. North Am.*, 17, 617, 1991.
42. Munk, P. L., Vellet, A. D., Levin, M. F., and Helms, C. A., Current status of magnetic resonance imaging of the ankle and the hindfoot, *Can. Assoc. Radiol. J.*, 43, 19, 1992.
43. Azouz, E. M. and Duffy C. M., Juvenile spondyloarthropathies: clinical manifestations and medical imaging, *Skeletal Radiol.*, 24, 399, 1995.
44. Gylys-Morin, V. M., MR imaging of pediatric musculoskeletal inflammatory and infectious disorders, *MRI Clin. North Am.*, 6, 537, 1998.
45. Whitten, C. G., Moore, T. E., Yuh, W. T. C., Kathol, M. H., Renfrew, D. L., and Walker, C. W., The use of intravenous gadopentate dimeglumine in magnetic resonance imaging of synovial lesions, *Skeletal Radiol.*, 21, 215, 1992.
46. Lin, J., Jacobson, J. A., Jamadar, D. A., and Ellis, J. H., Pigmented villonodular synovitis and related lesions: the spectrum of imaging findings, *AJR*, 172, 191, 1999.
47. Erickson, S. J. and Johnson, J. E., MR imaging of the ankle and foot, *Radiol. Clin. North Am.*, 35, 163, 1997.
48. Azouz, E. M. and Oudjhane, K., Disorders of the upper extremity in children, *MRI Clin. North Am.*, 6, 677, 1998.

49. Greenspan, A., Advanced imaging of the foot and ankle, *Curr. Opin. Orthop.*, 9, 18, 1998.
50. Kransdorf, M. J., Benign soft tissue tumors in a large referral population: distribution of specific diagnoses by age, sex, and location, *AJR*, 164, 395, 1995.
51. Wetzel, L. H. and Levine, E., Soft-tissue tumors of the foot: value of MR imaging for specific diagnosis, *AJR*, 155, 1025, 1990.
52. Kier, R., MR imaging of foot and ankle tumors, *Magn. Reson. Imaging*, 11, 149, 1993.
53. Smith, J. T. and Yandow, S. M., Benign soft-tissue lesions in children, *Orthop. Clin. North Am.*, 27, 645, 1996.
54. Upton, J. and Coombs, C., Vascular tumors in children, *Hand Clin.*, 11, 307, 1995.
55. Nelson, M. C. et al., Magnetic resonance imaging of peripheral soft tissue hemangiomas, *Skeletal Radiol.*, 19, 477, 1990.
56. Buetow, P. C., Kransdorf, M. J., Moser, R. P. et al., Radiologic appearance of intramuscular hemangioma with emphasis on MR imaging, *AJR*, 154, 563, 1990.
57. Meyer, J. S., Hoffer, F. A., Barnes, P. D. et al., Biological classification of soft-tissue vascular anomalies: MR correlation, *AJR*, 157, 559, 1991.
58. Burrows, P. E., Robertson, R. L., and Barnes, P. D., Angiography and the evaluation of cerebrovascular disease in childhood, *Neuroimaging Clin. North Am.*, 6, 561, 1996.
59. Greenspan, A., McGahan, J. P., Vogelsang, P. et al., Imaging strategies in the evaluation of soft-tissue hemangioma of the extremities: correlation of the findings of plain radiography, angiography, CT, MRI, and ultrasonography in 12 histologically proven cases, *Skeletal Radiol.*, 21, 11, 1992.
60. Memis, A., Arkun, R., Ustun, E. E. et al., Magnetic resonance imaging of intramuscular hemangiomas with emphasis on contrast enhancement patterns, *Clin. Radiol.*, 51, 198, 1996.
61. Aluisio, F. V., Mair, S. D., and Hall, R. L., Plantar fibromatosis: treatment of primary and recurrent lesions and factors associated with recurrence, *Foot Ankle Int.*, 17, 672, 1996.
62. Ozdemir, H. M. and Yildiz, Y., Tumors of the foot and ankle: analysis of 196 cases, *J. Foot Ankle Surg.*, 36, 403, 1997.
63. Murari, T. M., Callaghan, J. J., Berrey, B. H. et al., Primary benign and malignant osseous neoplasms of the foot, *Foot Ankle Int.*, 10, 69, 1989.
64. Biscaglia, R., Gasbarrini, A., Bohling, T. et al., Osteosarcoma of the bones of the foot — an easily misdiagnosed malignant tumor, *Mayo Clin. Proc.*, 73, 842, 1998.
65. Casadei, R., Ruggieri, P., Mascato, M. et al., Aneurysmal bone cyst and giant cell tumor ot the foot, *Foot Ankle Int.*, 17, 487,1996.
66. Butler, B. W., McCarty, J. M., and Danforth, R. D., Benign giant cell tumor of the foot, *J. Foot Ankle Surg.*, 32, 299, 1993.
67. Fink, B. R., Temple, H. T., Chiricosta, F. M. et al., Chondroblastoma of the foot, *Foot Ankle Int.*, 18, 236, 1997.
68. O'Connor, P. J., Gibbon, W. W., Hardy, G. et al., Chondromyxoid fibroma of the foot, *Skeletal Radiol.*, 25, 143, 1996.
69. Adkins, C. D., Kitaoka, H. B., Seidl, R. K. et al., Ewing's sarcoma of the foot, *Clin. Orthop.*, 343, 173, 1997.
70. Leeson, M. C. and Smith, M. J., Ewing's sarcoma of the foot, *Foot Ankle Int.*, 10, 147, 1989.
71. Seale, K. S., Lange, T. A., Monson, D. et al., Soft tissue tumors of the foot and ankle, *Foot Ankle Int.*, 9, 19, 1988.
72. Azouz, E. M., Vickar, D. B., and Brown, K. L. B., Computed tomogaphy of synovial sarcoma of the foot, *J. Can. Assoc. Radiol.*, 35, 85, 1984.

11 MR Imaging of the Foot and Ankle: The Orthopedic Surgeon's Perspective

David F. Sitler and Annunziato Amendola

CONTENTS

INTRODUCTION

The complex anatomy, biomechanics, and associated diagnoses affecting the foot and ankle can be intimidating to the clinician. A systematic and logical approach is necessary to use the diagnostic tools available efficiently to investigate and treat these problems. In most instances, the symptomatic foot can be evaluated with a good history, physical exam, and routine imaging studies. Radiographic examination, including computed tomography (CT), remains the preferred and basic method of evaluating bony anatomy. Magnetic resonance (MR) imaging, as discussed in previous chapters, offers the best imaging of soft-tissue, joint, and bone marrow pathology. In addition, it is a multiplanar technique, which facilitates the evaluation and depicts the relationship of complex anatomic structures in various oblique planes. Using thin-slices, oblique angles, and dedicated surface coils, many authors have illustrated the utility of MR imaging in a foot and ankle orthopedic practice.[1-4]

As these modern imaging technologies have advanced, so has the ability to diagnose pathology that previously was only suspected or missed. However, MR imaging is expensive and not routinely available in all health-care facilities. No single imaging modality, even MR imaging, is omniscient.[5] Effective communication outlining the clinical problem to radiologist is essential in developing a logical approach to a diagnosis. The clinician should have a clear rationale of how the information provided by the study will alter the management of the patient. The purpose of this chapter is to discuss the use of MR imaging from an orthopedic viewpoint focusing on common clinical problems.

TENDON DISORDERS

Nine tendons cross the ankle joint to control the movement of the foot and ankle. Anteriorly, the tibialis anterior, extensor hallucis longus, extensor digitorum longus, and peroneus tertius muscles are responsible for dorsiflexion of the ankle and extension of the toes. Posterolaterally, the peroneus longus and brevis muscles are evertors of the foot and weak plantar flexors of the ankle. Posteromedially, the tendons of the tibialis posterior, flexor digitorum longus, and flexor hallucis longus muscles act as invertors of the foot, flexors of the toes, and weak ankle plantar flexors. Posteriorly, the Achilles tendon provides plantar flexion force for the ankle. All but the Achilles tendon make a significant bend as they cross the ankle to insert on the bones of the foot, predisposing them to overload at this point. These tendons are susceptible to injuries, which include inflammatory overuse conditions, partial tears, complete tears, and subluxation. The term *tendonitis* is misleading when discussing inflammation involving tendons since inflammation of the tendon itself does not occur. More appropriately, tenosynovitis describes inflammation and hypertrophy of the synovial tissue lining the tendon sheath. Paratendinitis is inflammation and thickening of the paratenon surrounding the tendon. Finally, tendinosis refers to degeneration of the collagen bundles within the tendon itself. Tendon rupture is the terminal stage of tendon degeneration These different entities can be clearly visualized on MR imaging. Conditions involving the posterior tibial, Achilles, flexor hallucis longus, and the peroneal tendons will be discussed.

POSTERIOR TIBIAL TENDON

Among the tendons that curve around the ankle, one of the most frequently affected with inflammation and dysfunction is the posterior tibial tendon (PTT). The PTT passes posterior to the axis of the ankle and medial to the axis of the subtalar joint. It inserts onto the navicular, cuneiforms, and the base of metatarsals two through four.[4] The PTT acts to plantarflex and invert the foot primarily through the transverse tarsal joint. This action functions to invert the mid-foot and elevate the medial longitudinal arch, which locks the transverse tarsal joint. This allows the foot to be in a rigid position facilitating push off at the end of the stance phase of gait.

The acquired flat-foot deformity caused by PTT dysfunction or rupture was described by several authors in the 1970s and 1980s.[6-10] Typically the medial longitudinal arch collapses, the forefoot abducts and assumes a varus position through the talonavicular joint, and the hind foot everts assuming a valgus position. As the condition progresses, there is a loss of the secondary soft-tissue supportive structures, which includes the deltoid ligament, the talonavicular capsule, and the spring ligament. With the hind foot in a valgus position the Achilles tendon everts the calcaneus since it is now lateral to the axis of the subtalar joint.

The etiology of PTT dysfunction varies from degenerative rupture to inflammatory synovitis and occasionally acute trauma.[11,12] Preexisting pes planus deformity predisposes the PTT to chronic overload leading to gradual intrinsic failure.[13] Risk factors include hypertension, obesity, diabetes, prior surgery or trauma about the medial aspect of the foot, and treatment with steroids.[11] Ruptures of the PTT are most often due to intrinsic failure rather than extrinsic trauma. Surgical exploration of the PTT has consistently revealed the site of injury posterior and distal to the medial malleolus. Frey et al. demonstrated a zone of hypovascularity, which starts about 1.5 cm distal to the medial malleolus and extends proximally about 1.5 cm, which corresponds to the injury zone.[14] A combination of the mechanical forces applied to the tendon as it bends around the medial malleolus and the vascular watershed area predisposes this tendon to injury.

A careful history and examination are important to diagnose and stage the disease. In the early stage of PTT dysfunction, patients complain of discomfort located medially along the course of the tendon. They have fatigue and aching on the medial arch with activity. As the condition progresses, patients notice a change in the shape of their foot to a flat-foot deformity. With increasing deformity, the pain shifts to the lateral side because of impingement on the fibula by the calcaneus.

The physical examination should assess alignment of the foot from above, behind and during gait. Johnson and Storm[15] described being able to visualize more of the lesser toes past the lateral side of the foot when viewed from behind because of the forefoot abduction. He called this the "too many toes" sign.[15] The foot should be palpated to find the areas of swelling and tenderness. A single-limb heel-rise test determines the function of the PTT. Normally, the PTT inverts and stabilizes the hind foot to allow the gastrocnemius–soleus complex to elevate the heel. If the PTT is dysfunctioning, the patient will either not be able to perform the test or the heel will remain in a valgus position. The deformity should then be manipulated. In the early stages the foot is supple and the deformities are easily corrected and typically consist of forefoot varus with the hind foot in neutral. As the condition progresses, the foot becomes stiff and the deformities fixed.

The clinical stages of PTT dysfunction were described by Johnson and Strom in 1989.[15] Stage I is characterized by medial pain and swelling with an intact tendon of normal length. Inflammation is present and degeneration of the tendon may also be present. In stage II the PTT is elongated. The deformity, however, is mild and the hind foot is correctable. The limb is weak and the patient is unable to do a single-heel rise. In stage III the tendon has degenerated and the deformity is more severe and fixed. Some authors also describe a stage IV that is characterized by valgus angulation of the talus and degeneration of the ankle joint.[16] Most foot and ankle surgeons alter their treatment plans according to the clinical stages (Table 11.1).

The diagnosis of PTT dysfunction can usually be made by a good history and physical exam. A good understanding of the characteristic symptoms, risk factors, and physical findings will usually suggest the diagnosis with a high degree of certainty. Standing radiographs of the feet and ankles are recommended to evaluate alignment and the possible presence of subtalar and ankle degenerative arthritis.[16] However, not every patient presents with the classic signs and symptoms. In the early

TABLE 11.1
Treatment of PTT Dysfunction

Stage	Nonsurgical	Surgical
Stage I	Anti-inflammatory medication	Tenosynovectomy +/–
	Immobilization for 6 to 8 weeks	Calcaneal osteotomy +/–
	Orthotic arch supports with medial posting	Tenodesis of FDL to PTT or FDL transfer
Stage II	Orthotic arch support with medial posting	FDL transfer +
	Hinged ankle foot orthosis	Calcaneal osteotomy +/–
	Sinus tarsi injections	Medial column stabilization
Stage III	Rigid ankle-foot orthosis	Triple arthrodesis
Stage IV	Rigid ankle-foot orthosis	Tibiotalocalcaneal arthrodesis

Note: FDL = flexor digitorum longus, PTT = posterior tibial tendon.

stages of the disease the "too many toes" sign and single-heel test may not yet be positive and in these cases further imaging studies such as MR imaging are recommended.[17] In the younger athletic population, this entity is less common and more often associated with trauma.[18] Differentiation from ligamentous and bone injuries involves a careful clinical evaluation incorporating sophisticated diagnostic testing such as MR imaging. Early recognition of the injury and appropriate orthopedic referral is needed to avoid prolonged disability.[18]

Several authors have investigated the use of MR imaging in preoperative grading of PTT dysfunction.[19-21] Rosenberg et al.[19] studied PTT injuries in 22 patients with CT and MR imaging in which they compared the imaging findings to surgical observation. A staging system that compared the surgical findings was described as follows. A type 1 injury is a partially torn bulbous tendon with vertical splits and defects. A type 2 injury is a partially torn attenuated (i.e., reduced circumference) tendon. A complete rupture with a tendon gap is a type 3 injury. Their results suggested that MR imaging provided greater definition of tendon pathology and correlation with the surgical findings. Implicit in Rosenberg's study is that surgical grading should be considered the gold standard. Conti et al.[20] looked at 20 feet in their study with MR imaging. They found that MR imaging usually indicated more extensive disease than was apparent at surgery. However, the MR imaging staging correlated better than intraoperative staging in terms of success or failure of reconstructive surgery at an average 2-year follow-up. They concluded that MR imaging might be helpful in preoperative planning when considering surgical reconstruction. Other authors feel strongly that MR imaging is rarely needed. Myerson[16] states that MR imaging is not required to make a diagnosis and does not assist in the planning of treatment for PTT dysfunction.

In general, when the diagnosis of PTT dysfunction is suspected but cannot be confirmed by examination, MR imaging is useful. This is especially true in the younger population where early diagnosis and intervention is important. Also, when surgery is considered and the surgeon is unsure of the clinical stage of PTT dysfunction, MR imaging may be helpful in preoperative planning.

ACHILLES TENDON

The anatomy of the Achilles tendon and therefore its pathology differs from other tendons about the ankle. The Achilles tendon inserts on the posterior aspect of the calcaneus and does not curve past the ankle. It is composed of tendinous fibers from the gastrocnemius and soleus muscles that merge together and spiral toward their insertion on the calcaneal tuberosity. The gastrocnemius and soleus complex is a powerful plantar flexor of the foot. Unlike the PTT, it does not have a synovial sheath but is surrounded by a layer of fatty connective tissue called a paratenon. The blood supply of the Achilles tendon arises from three sources: the musculotendinous junction, the osseous insertion, and multiple mesotenal vessels that enter the tendon from the ventral surface. Carr and Norris[22] demonstrated a watershed area of hypovascularity in the midsection of the tendon using cadaveric injection techniques. This is the portion of the tendon most-often injured. The tendon structure also changes with age and in response to physical activity. The tendon fibers lose their "wavy" configuration and collagen fibril bundles thicken reducing the cell/matrix ratio both with age and inactivity.[23] These changes also may contribute to tendon failure.

Pathologic conditions affecting the Achilles tendon include inflammation, degeneration, and rupture. The term *tenosynovitis* and *tendonitis* are often used to describe a painful Achilles tendon. These terms, however, are misleading and ambiguous. Puddu et al.[24] proposed a more useful description of the pathologic conditions of the Achilles tendon as follows: 1. Paratenonitis involves inflammation and thickening of the paratenon; 2. Tendinosis is the degeneration of the tendon; 3. Paratenonitis with tendinosis includes both processes.[24] All of these conditions can be imaged and differentiated on MR imaging.[25] MR imaging is also superior in detection of incomplete tendon ruptures and the evaluation of various stages of chronic degenerative changes.[26]

Most Achilles tendon problems are related to overuse syndromes. The primary risk factors are advancing age and mechanical malalignment of the lower extremity.[26] The typical patient with

Achilles tendon problems is between 35 and 45 years of age and participates in weekend or occasional sports activities. There is also a high incidence of paratenonitis and tendinosis in competitive runners.[27]

Paratenonitis and tendinosis usually respond to conservative measures consisting of activity modification, static stretching, physiotherapy, and nonsteroidal medication.[26,27] However, if symptoms persist, surgical excision of the hypertrophic paratenon and the degenerative portion of the tendon is recommended.[26,28,29] MR imaging is useful in identifying and locating the area of tendon degeneration if present and therefore aids in preoperative planning.

Ruptures of the Achilles tendon usually occur 2 to 6 cm from its insertion, corresponding to the area of experimentally proven hypovascularity previously noted. A history of a recent change in a training regimen or previous posterior ankle pain may be elicited. Patients frequently describe the sensation of being kicked in the back of their ankle with subsequent inability to run or finish the sporting event. The patient should be examined in the prone position with the feet over the end of the table. Swelling and ecchymosis along the posterior aspect of the leg may be present. Usually a defect in the tendon can be palpated, unless a hematoma obscures this finding. The failure of the foot to plantarflex passively when the calf is squeezed was described by Thompson and Doherty[30] in 1962 as a way to diagnose the tear clinically.

The diagnosis of an Achilles tendon tear should be accomplished with a history and physical examination. However, it is too often missed or misdiagnosed as an ankle sprain. In a study by Inglis et al.,[31] 23% of 167 Achilles tendon ruptures were initially misdiagnosed by the primary treating physician. Ultrasound can be used to visualize the tendon when in doubt. This modality, although more user dependent, is less expensive than MR imaging and is becoming increasingly available. MR imaging, on the other hand, is superior in diagnosing partial tears and evaluating the condition and orientation of the torn fibers.[26,32]

The treatment of an acute rupture is basically divided into operative or nonoperative intervention. Adequate clinical results have been obtained with a period of casting followed by a course of physiotherapy. Surgical treatment, however, provides a slight increase in strength recovery and a lower rerupture rate.[31,33] Some authors have proposed using imaging studies to evaluate the diastasis of the torn tendon at 20° of plantar flexion to predict the outcome with casting.[26] If a diastasis persists in plantar flexion, surgical treatment is recommended. To accomplish this, either ultrasound or MR imaging could be used, depending on the expense, reliability, and availability of these modalities at a given site.

Treatment of neglected tendon ruptures is a challenging problem, as the results are less favorable than treatment obtained during the acute phase. When there is a significant gap present, a good result can only be obtained by surgically approximating the musculotendinous unit near its normal resting length. It is important to diagnose an Achilles tendon rupture in the acute phase. If there is any difficulty in establishing an accurate diagnosis, further investigation by means of MR imaging may be useful.

PERONEAL TENDONS

The peroneal muscles occupy the lateral compartment of the leg. The peroneus longus muscle lies lateral and posterior to the peroneus brevis, and both usually become tendinous structures before reaching the ankle joint. The peroneus brevis, however, has a long musculotendinous junction and may have muscle fibers extending beyond the lateral malleolus for 2 to 3 cm. A common synovial sheath begins about 4 cm above the lateral malleolus, then bisects into separate sheaths at the level of the calcaneocuboid joint. The synovial sheath and the surrounding structures form a fibro-osseous tunnel for the tendons. The tunnel is bordered medially by the posterior talofibular and calcaneofibular ligaments, laterally by the superior peroneal retinaculum, and anteriorly by the posterior aspect of the fibula. The posterior surface of the lateral malleolus has a shallow sulcus or peroneal groove for the tendons that is variable in depth and width.[34–37] The superior peroneal retinaculum extends from the lateral aspect of the fibula and the lateral retromalleolar groove, crosses the peroneal tendons posteriorly, and inserts into the calcaneus and the Achilles tendon. It is the primary stabilizing structure for the tendons.[38]

The peroneus longus tendon continues under the peroneal process of the calcaneus and heads toward the cuboid. Finally, the tendon bends around the tubercle of the cuboid and passes obliquely across the plantar aspect of the foot. It inserts on the base of the first metatarsal and medial cuneiform. The longus usually has a sesamoid bone in the area of the cuboid tubercle called the os peroneum. The peroneus longus muscle plantarflexes the first metatarsal, pronates, abducts, and everts the foot and plantarflexes the ankle. It contributes to lateral ankle stability and participates in the midstance phase of gait and push off.

The peroneus brevis tendon lies in the retromalleaolar sulcus where the longus tendon presses it against the fibula. It turns anteriorly over the lateral surface of the calcaneofibular ligament to insert on the base of the fifth metatarsal. The brevis muscle is a strong abductor of the foot. It is also a secondary flexor of the ankle and a foot evertor. It also contributes to lateral ankle stability.

Injuries to the peroneal tendons involve tenosynovitis, entrapment, dislocation, and rupture. Tenosynovitis and tendonitis occur when an athlete resumes play after a period of decreased activity. Symptoms of pain develop behind the lateral malleolus and around the lateral heel with toe-off when sprinting, cutting, or jogging. Tenderness and swelling is present along the tendon sheaths. For acute conditions, treatment consists of rest, ice, compressive dressing, and elevation. If symptoms subside, the athlete is to resume gentle motion followed by a gradual increase in activities.

Chronic tendonitis presents after several weeks or months and represents an overuse syndrome. There may be minimal swelling with this condition. If pain, swelling, and tenderness occur without associated increase in activity, then rhuematoid arthritis and other seronegative arthritides must be considered. Hypertrophy of peroneus brevis muscle tissue or a peroneus quartus muscle within the tendon sheaths is also associated with chronic tendon disorders.[39] Treatment of chronic tendonitis includes physiotherapy, bracing, orthotics, and nonsteroidal anti-inflammatory agents (NSAIDs). In recalcitrant cases, surgical debridement is indicated.

MR imaging is useful in cases that are difficult to diagnose or those that must be differentiated from lateral ligament injuries.[40] In cases resistant to conservative treatment MR imaging is indicated for preoperative evaluation. Anatomic anomalies causing impingement of the tendons and intratendinous pathology are best assessed with MR imaging and should be addressed in the operating room.[37,40-43]

Subluxation and dislocation of the peroneal tendons is well documented in the literature and, although first associated with skiing accidents, has been reported in many sport activities.[36] As noted above, these tendons lie in a shallow groove behind the lateral malleolus. This sulcus can vary greatly, ranging in width from 5 to 10 mm. The depth can be as much as 3 mm. However, Edwards[35] found the groove was either flat or convex in 18% of specimens. A shallow groove combined with reflexive contraction of the peroneal tendons during injury results in disruption of their fibro-osseous sheath. The tendons displace laterally and anteriorly in front of the lateral malleolus and the superior peroneal retinaculum is stripped from the posterolateral border of the fibula.

The diagnosis of peroneal tendon subluxation or dislocation is based on clinical examination, but in the acute phase it is often difficult to differentiate this condition from an ankle sprain. Pain along the tendon sheath with ankle dorsiflexion and eversion is common. The subluxation can also be observed when the tendons snap over the fibula. Occasionally, the tendons may be irreducible and lie on the malleolus. Radiographs are useful in excluding associated pathology including a "rim fracture" off the posterolateral border of the malleolus. MR imaging can demonstrate an enlarged tendon tunnel posterior to the fibula along with a deficiency in the attachment of the superior peroneal retinaculum but is seldom needed in the management of the problem. In symptomatic patients, surgical deepening of the fibular groove and reconstruction of the superior peroneal retinaculum is indicated to prevent chronic redislocation because this injury can be disabling and can lead to additional peroneal tendon pathology.[34]

Partial tears of the peroneal tendons are commonly encountered. They are longitudinal in orientation, can occur in either tendon, and may consist of a single or multiple tears within the same tendon. Lateral ankle instability, tendon subluxation/dislocation, and calcaneal fractures have been associated with these tears. The symptoms and clinical findings are the same as noted for acute and chronic tenosynovitis. There is evidence, however, that some partial tears remain asymptomatic throughout life. Sobel et al.[44,45] noted a high incidence of partial tears in mostly elderly cadaveric specimens without evidence of trauma or ligamentous injury.

Typically, the peroneus brevis tendon develops tears within the fibular groove as a result of a dynamic mechanical insult. Laxity of the superior peroneal retinaculum combined with mechanical compression by peroneus longus causes the peroneus brevis to splay out and eventually split over the sharp posterior edge of the fibula.[44] Schweitzer et al.[37] looked at 20 ankles with surgically confirmed peroneal splits on MR imaging. They demonstrated a high frequency of bisected peroneus brevis tendons, a convex or flat fibular groove, and a posterolateral marrow-containing fibular spur associated with this injury.[37] If symptoms are persistent, surgical debridement and tenosynovectomy are suggested. MR imaging can both diagnose and evaluate the status of the tendon and is indicated in these cases.[37,39,41,42,44,45]

The peroneus longus tendon tears in a different region, but the principle of high stress over a localized area overloading the tendon is the same as with other tendon injuries. The lesion occurs where the tendon bends beneath the cuboid in the area of the os peroneum when present. The treatment and evaluation is the same as for the peroneus brevis tendon.

Complete rupture of the peroneal tendons is rare. The most common injury is a rupture of the longus tendon in the area of the os peroneum. Displacement of the os can be seen on radiographs. This accessory bone, however, is only ossified in 20% of the population. In these cases, MR imaging reveals increased fluid within the tendon sheath along the lateral calcaneus and loss of tendon continuity. Pain, swelling, and weakness are the usual clinical findings. Direct repair of the tendon is recommended and MR imaging is helpful in evaluating the gap between the tendon ends so the surgeon can prepare for the possibility of tendon grafting or tenodesis to the calcaneus if necessary.

FLEXOR HALLUCIS LONGUS AND OS TRIGONUM SYNDROME

There is an extensive differential diagnosis for pain related to the back of the heel or "posterior triangle" pain. Two common causes of heel pain are flexor hallucis longus (FHL) tendonitis and the os trigonum syndrome, and both entities often exist together.

FHL tendonitis is common in dancers, gymnasts, soccer players, and those who practice other sports that require excessive plantar flexion. Hamilton[46] describes the FHL as the "Achilles tendon of the dancer's foot." It is strained as it passes posterior to the talus between the medial and lateral posterior processes where it enters a fibro-osseous tunnel. Progressive inflammation can lead to stenosing tenosynovitis which can cause triggering of the great toe or, in severe cases, the tendon may become frozen in the sheath causing a "pseudo hallux rigidus."[46]

Symptoms of FHL tendonitis consist of recurrent pain, tenderness, and swelling behind the medial malleolus of the ankle. The tendon sheath is painful to palpation and on passive hallux dorsiflexion there is posterior ankle pain and decreased motion.

Conservative treatment as described for other tendon inflammatory conditions can usually reverse the symptoms. Efforts should be made to alter dance techniques to decrease contributing factors. In severe cases that do not respond to conservative measures, tenolysis is indicated.

The os trigonum syndrome relates to pathology of the posterolateral process of the talus. The os trigonum is an ossified body within the posterolateral process of the talus connected to the talus by an intervening bridge of cartilage. It represents either a secondary ossification center or a fracture. The underlying pathologies resulting in this syndrome include (1) an acute fracture of the trigonal process of the talus, (2) a chronic stress fracture of the trigonal process, (3) impingement of the posterolateral process against the posterior tibial plafond. Brodsky and Khalil[47] use the term "talar compression syndrome" to describe the same entity.

The symptoms of pain and tenderness are located deep to the Achilles tendon on the posterolateral side of the ankle and are exacerbated by forced plantar flexion of the foot.[48] The diagnosis may be further confirmed by injection of local anesthetic into the affected area with temporary relief of their symptoms.

Treatment should be designed to interrupt the chronic cycle of pain and swelling secondary to the impingement. Avoidance of dance positions that exacerbate the symptoms is imperative. Athletes with recurrent or unremitting symptoms may warrant surgical removal of the os trigonum.[49] If there is coexisiting tenosynovitis of the FHL, this problem should be addressed at the same time.

The diagnosis of both of these conditions is usually made by clinical examination. Because of the large number of conditions that can produce posterior triangle pain, some patients may be difficult to diagnose and manage. Wakeley et al.[48] studied three patients with posterior ankle pain in which MR imaging delineated the anatomic site of abnormality and coexisting pathology in all patients. When there is clinical doubt, MR imaging is the technique of choice for investigating FHL tendonitis and os trigonum syndrome. Knowledge of coexisting pathology allows the surgeon to plan an appropriate surgical approach.

ANKLE SPRAINS

Ankle ligament sprains are among the most common musculoskeletal injuries seen by physicians. They constitute up to 10% of all injuries treated in emergency rooms and 15% of all sports injuries.[50] Although most of these injuries heal uneventfully, persistent instability or chronic pain may develop in some patients. Prompt diagnosis and treatment can shorten the recovery time and decrease the prevalence of residual symptoms.

LATERAL LIGAMENTS

The lateral collateral ligament complex consists of the anterior talofibular ligament (ATFL), calcaneofibular ligament (CFL), and posterior talofibular ligament (PTFL). The ATFL and the CFL are the most important lateral ligaments clinically. The ATFL is the most frequently injured lateral ligament followed by the CFL. The CFL is rarely injured without a coexisting injury to the ATFL.

The ATFL is a thickening of the ankle capsule that extends from the anterior edge of the distal part of the fibula to the talar neck. It is oriented horizontally when the foot is in neutral position and more vertically in plantar flexion. The ligament develops increased stress in plantar flexion and is more susceptible to injury in this position.

The CFL is a discrete extra-articular, round ligament that courses obliquely from the tip of the fibula, under the peroneal tendons, to the lateral aspect of the calcaneal tuberosity. Because it is oriented more vertically when the foot is in neutral and dorsal flexion, it is the primary stabilizer against inversion forces in these positions. Since the CFL crosses the subtalar joint, it also has a major role in the stabilization of this joint.

The PTFL arises from the medial aspect of the distal fibula and passes almost horizontally to insert along the posterolateral tubercle of the talus. It separates the tibiotalar joint from the subtalar joint and is an intra-articular ligament.

Typically, injuries to the lateral ankle ligaments occur when an inversion force and/or an internal rotation force is applied to a plantarflexed foot. The ATFL is injured first and is followed in incidence by injury to the CFL. Rarely, a continuation of the applied force ruptures the PTFL.

The patient's history is important to determine the mechanism of injury, identify any previous ankle trauma, and establish the performance level of the individual. Although the majority of ankle sprains are inversion injuries, it is important to identify injuries that occurred from either an eversion or external rotation force during ankle dorsiflexion. These other mechanisms of injury should alert the examiner to consider damage to other structures such as the syndesmotic complex, deltoid ligament, or peroneal tendons.

Inspection of the injured ankle reveals swelling and ecchymosis distal to the fibula with pain on palpation over the injured structures. Assessing the anterior displacement of the talus in relation to the tibia (anterior drawer), tests the integrity of the ATFL. Talar instability is also tested with the talar tilt test, performed by applying an inversion force to the heel while stabilizing the tibia. The talar tilt is useful in assessing combined injuries of the ATFL and the CFL; however, the amount of talar tilt within the mortise of the ankle is difficult to determine clinically because of subtalar motion.

Injuries of individual ligaments are traditionally graded as first, second, or third degree, depending on the severity. A grade I sprain is a mild injury limited to microtears and stretching of the ligament. The athlete is able to bear weight and usually is able to finish the sporting event. Grade II sprains are partial macroscopic tears. The athlete can usually bear weight but is unable to continue the sporting activity. A grade III sprain involves a complete disruption of the ligament in which the athlete is usually unable to bear weight or to continue the sport. Because the lateral ankle ligament complex is made up of several ligaments, some authors try to distinguish between a single, double, or triple ligament injury.[51] Gaebler et al.[52] developed a grading system based on MR imaging findings as follows: grade 0 represents ankle sprains without ligament lesions, grade I consists of lesions of the ATFL, grade II consists of lesions of the ATFL and CFL, and grade III is a triple ligament injury. The injuries are further subdivided into incomplete or complete ruptures.

There is general agreement that grade I and II sprains heal uneventfully and are best treated with nonoperative therapy. The treatment of grade III, double or triple ligament sprains, is more controversial. Some surgeons prefer acute operative repair, especially for high-level athletes.[52] In 1991, Kannus and Renstrom[53] reviewed 12 studies analyzing operation, casting, or early controlled mobilization for grade II and III ankle sprains and concluded that there was no advantage to acute operative repair for lateral ligament injuries. However, persistent disability after an acute rupture of the lateral ligaments of the ankle has been reported in about 20% of patients.[54] Late surgical reconstruction is effective for patients with chronic, symptomatic instability, and many surgical procedures have been described to address this problem. An imbrication of the ATFL and CFL reinforced with the inferior extensor retinaculum as described by Brostrom[54] with the modifications described by Gould et al.[57] and Karlsson et al.[56] is recommended.

In general, all severe joint injuries should be examined radiographically. Additional imaging investigations are controversial for ankle sprains. Stress views of the ankle are the most economical and readily available type of imaging after standard radiographs. There is a wide range of normal values reported in the literature, ranging from an absolute value of 10° to a side-to-side difference of 5 to 15° for talar tilt and an anterior translation of 3 to 6 mm for the anterior stress test.[52,55,58,59] This variability makes the stress tests difficult to interpret when evaluating ankle instability.

MR imaging can demonstrate the normal and torn ATFL and CFL accurately.[1] Frey and associates[50] studied 15 acute ankle sprains with MR imaging. They compared the MR imaging findings with clinical examination and found that the examination was only 25% accurate in the diagnosis of grade II injuries but was 100% accurate for grade III injuries.[50] Chandnani and associates[60] compared MR arthrography, MR imaging, and stress radiography in 17 patients who underwent surgery for chronic ankle instability. They found MR arthrography was the most accurate of the three modalities with 100% sensitivity for ATFL ruptures and 90% sensitivity for CFL ruptures.[60] Gaebler and associates[52] studied 112 athletes with acute ankle sprains using the talar tilt test and MR imaging. The surgical findings were compared in 25 of the athletes who were treated operatively. Their results suggested that MR imaging is a reliable method for diagnosing and confirming "triple ligament" injuries, which are surgically treated at their institution.[52] MR imaging also revealed concurrent injuries of the talar dome, peroneal tendons, posterior tibial tendon, and other structures around the ankle in all the above studies.

MR imaging is not recommended for all acute ankle sprains, but is very helpful for the few patients who do not respond to initial conservative treatment or have associated periarticular injuries. In the author's experience, MR imaging is more useful to diagnose occult joint injuries such as osteochondral lesions, subchondral contusions, and joint arthrosis. The decision to repair the lateral ligaments surgically for chronic instability is based on clinical findings.

SYNDESMOTIC COMPLEX

The syndesmotic complex consists of the anterior tibiofibular ligament, the posterior tibiofibular ligament, and the interosseous ligament and membrane. An intact syndesmosis is essential to maintain the normal function of the ankle joint. It allows motion of the fibula with respect to the tibia that is needed for normal ankle articulation while contributing to the stability of the ankle. Studies have also shown that one sixth of the body weight transmitted to the knee is borne by the fibula.[61] This force is transferred through the syndesmotic complex.[62]

Injury to the syndesmotic complex is usually associated with an ankle fracture and is included in the most commonly used ankle fracture classification systems.[63,64] The Lauge–Hansen system was derived from cadaveric experiments and surgical observations. In this classification, syndesmosis injury occurs in pronation–abduction and pronation–eversion (external rotation) injuries.[63] The diagnosis is made by looking at the pattern of the fracture and observing medial joint space widening. These classification systems, however, do not address injury to the complex without fracture.

Injury to the syndesmotic complex without fracture has been reported as a cause of recurrent ankle sprains and sprains associated with a prolonged recovery.[65] This injury consists of a simple distal sprain without instability or a complete disruption of the syndesmotic complex with diastasis of the tibiotalar joint. Hopkinson et al.[65] looked at 1344 ankle sprains and reported an incidence of clinically detectable syndesmosis injuries of 1%. They described a clinical test, "the squeeze test," to help diagnose the injury. The test is positive when squeezing the fibula and tibia together above the midpoint of the calf causes pain in the ankle. This maneuver actually causes separation of the distal fibula and tibia, stressing the torn complex.[66] Of the 10 patients followed-up with syndesmotic sprains, only two showed widening of the mortise on plain or stress radiographs. Of the 10 patients, 9 had calcification in the area of the syndesmosis on follow-up radiographs. This calcification has also been described in professional football injuries and is occasionally symptomatic.[67]

The treatment goal for syndesmotic injuries is to obtain and maintain an anatomic reduction and allow appropriate healing. Eliminating the lateral shift of the talus in the mortise is important. Ramsey and Hamilton[68] illustrated that a lateral talar shift of 1 mm reduces the joint contact area by 42%. For injuries without diastasis, a prolonged healing time and return to sport is expected. For those injuries with a diastasis, a trans-syndesmotic screw may be indicated.

Radiographic diagnosis of a syndesmotic injury is important and several parameters have been described in the literature. The easiest technique is to evaluate the symmetry of the superior, medial, and lateral aspects of the ankle joint space on the mortise view.[69] This assessment is inaccurate, however, if the mortise view is not exact. Harper and Keller[70] found that the space between the lateral border of the tibia and the medial border of the fibula, measured 1 cm above the tibial plafond, should be less than 6 mm on the AP view. Another radiographic parameter described is that the overlap between the distal fibula and the anterior tibial tubercle should be >6 mm on the AP view and >1 mm on the mortise view.[69] If no diastasis of the distal tibiofibular joint is demonstrated on standard views, stress radiographs may be required, which are performed by applying an external rotation force to the foot with resultant widening of the mortise when positive.[17]

Injury to the syndesmosis without gross diastasis of the distal tibiofibular joint in the absence of a fibular fracture does occur. Further investigations are indicated in the situation of a severe ligamentous ankle sprain refractory to treatment. Vogl et al.[72] looked at 38 patients with acute ankle trauma and a clinical suspicion of a syndesmotic tear with radiographs and MR imaging in which they concluded that MR imaging of the syndesmotic complex is highly sensitive and specific in the evaluation of syndesmotic injuries. In those patients whom physical examination and conventional radiographs suggest a syndesmotic injury, MR imaging may be useful although our experience is that this area is not always well visualized on MR imaging.

ANTERIOR IMPINGEMENT

Chronic anterior ankle pain, after an inversion injury, can cause functional disability for some patients. This pain is thought to be caused by both bone and soft-tissue impingement of the talotibial joint. The early reports of impingement syndromes described osseous causes and were generally noted in athletes whose sports require sudden acceleration, jumping, and extremes of dorsiflexion or plantar flexion. Osseous exostoses from the anterior tibia and talar neck were described by Morris[73] and subsequently reported by McMurray[74] who termed this condition "footballer's ankle." These lesions are thought to be caused by repetitive traction of the joint capsule on the anterior aspect of the ankle. The clinical examination and the presence of the exostoses on radiographs establish the diagnosis of footballer's ankle and MR imaging is rarely indicated.

Anterolateral ankle impingement caused by soft-tissue entrapment is also a common cause of residual ankle pain after an injury. Wolin et al.[75] described a meniscoid mass of hyalinized fibrous tissue between the talus and fibula in the lateral gutter of symptomatic patients. Bassett et al.[76] described a separate distal fasicle of the anterioinferior tibiofibular ligament that can cause talar impingement and pain in the anterior aspect of the ankle after inversion injuries. Ferkel and colleagues[77] attributed the soft-tissue impingement to chronic hypertrophy of the synovium without involvement of the ligamentous tissues. It appears that the impingement process begins with an injury to the anterior talofibular ligament and synovial tissue that starts a scarring process, producing the different lesions described above. Initial management of the impingement syndrome should consist of modalities designed to reduce the inflammation and strengthen the injured soft tissues and secondary muscular stabilizers of the ankle. When conservative treatment fails, arthroscopic treatment consisting of debridement of the offending soft tissue and/or bone spurs provides good results.[77]

Although there is much discussion in the literature about the pathologic process and arthroscopic evaluation and treatment of anterolateral ankle impingement, little has been written about the most effective way to diagnose this entity without an invasive procedure. Liu et al.[78] compared the clinical examination and MR imaging findings in 22 patients who had preoperative MR imaging and arthroscopic evaluation of their ankles because of chronic anterolateral pain. A positive clinical evaluation required five of the following findings: (1) anterolateral ankle joint tenderness, (2) anterolateral ankle joint swelling, (3) pain with forced dorsiflexion, (4) pain with single-leg squat test, (5) pain with activities, and (6) absence of ankle instability. They found the clinical examination was 94% sensitive and 75% specific compared with MR imaging, which was 39% sensitive and 50% specific in predicting the presence of impingement syndrome.[78] MR imaging is not beneficial or cost-effective in the evaluation of anterolateral ankle impingement based on currently reported techniques and experience.

OCCULT OSSEOUS INJURIES

Occult osseous injuries, primarily "bruises" or contusions, may be seen on MR imaging investigations of ankle sprains. The clinical significance of these findings is uncertain and not adequately discussed in the literature. Occult osseous injuries in the knee, however, have been shown to occur in characteristic patterns associated with ligamentous injuries.[79–82]

Mink and Deutsch[79] retrospectively found a 72% incidence of bone bruises in 25 anterior cruciate ligament (ACL) injured knees and concluded that bone bruises had a high association with ACL tears. They followed two of these patients and noted complete resolution of the lesion.[79] Vellet and associates[81] prospectively studied 120 consecutive patients who presented with an acute post-traumatic knee hemarthrosis with MR imaging and arthroscopy and found a 72% incidence of occult osseous lesions. These lesions occurred in a predictable pattern consistent with the mechanism of injury. A small cohort of 21 patients in this study was investigated 6 to 12 months after their injury with MR imaging and osteochondral sequelae were found in 66% of patients in this group.

This information cannot be directly applied to the ankle as the incidence, significance, and pattern of similar findings in ankle sprains are not as well documented as in the knee. In the study by Gaebler and associates[52] that evaluated MR imaging and the talar tilt method for diagnosing lateral ankle ligament injuries, they noted an increasing incidence of bone bruises on the MR imaging with increasing talar tilt. Their incidence ranged from 48 to 68%. They had no comment on the injury pattern of these bone contusions.

In a retrospective study of 109 MR imaging studies on patients with ankle sprains, Labovitz and Schweitzer[83] found occult bone injury in 39% of patients. A higher frequency of bone bruises were present in patients with multiple ligament injuries. The pattern of bruising corresponded to rotational instability, impaction of the contralateral side of the joint from the ligament injury, and/or microalvusion injury from soft-tissue attachments. The amount of time after the injury that the bone bruise was noted ranged from 3 weeks to 1 year.

In summary, MR imaging should not be routinely used to evaluate acute ankle sprains. However, chronic ankle pain can complicate the recovery from an apparent benign injury and MR imaging can identify occult osseous injuries. These injuries may explain the patient's symptoms and help to direct treatment but their long-term outcome is yet to be determined.

OSTEOCHONDRAL LESIONS OF THE TALUS

Osteochondral lesions of the talus (OLT), otherwise known as osteochondral defects, osteochondritis dissecans, flake fracture, or transchondral fractures, were first reported in the knee and later in the ankle in the late 1800s and early 1900s. The prevalence of OLT is said to be 0.002/1000 persons; however, this number may be low because many cases go undiagnosed.[84] Bosien et al.[85] also noted in 1955 that OLT occur at a rate of 6.5/100 ankle sprains.

Early reports suggested that the etiology of OLT was from ischemic necrosis of the subchondral bone followed by separation of the fragment and its attached articular cartilage.[86] Although these early investigators suggested a primary vascular cause for the development of OLT, more recent reports suggest a traumatic cause.

In 1959 Berndt and Harty[87] analyzed 54 reports of 191 transchondral fractures of the talar dome and added 24 of their own cases. They also presented data on 15 cadaveric ankles, which were subjected to various forces. They found that lateral OLT lesions were shallow and located in the anterior third of the talus and were produced by inversion and dorsiflexion forces in the cadaveric specimens. The medial OLT lesions, on the other hand, were deeper, broader, and located in the middle and posterior third of the talus and were produced in cadaver ankles with inversion, plantar flexion, and rotational forces.

Other investigations also support a traumatic etiology. Canale and Belding[88] reported on 31 lesions and found that all of the lateral, but only 64% of the medial, lesions related a significant traumatic event. In another study, 25 patients from the U.S. military were presented by Alexander and Lichtman,[89] who noted all lateral lesions were associated with a sprain or trauma, while only 82% of the patients with medial lesions reported a history of trauma. Finally, Flick and Gould[90] reviewed the literature reported before 1985 and found that 98% of lateral talar dome and 70% of medial talar dome lesions were associated with a history of trauma. These key studies illustrate that almost all of the lateral lesions and most of the medial lesions are associated with trauma and represent transchondral fractures, whereas patients without a clear-cut history of trauma are more likely to have a medial lesion.

Diagnosing and staging of OLT is important for treatment and prognosis but unfortunately the diagnosis is often missed or delayed.[91] Symptoms may be subtle but include pain swelling, occasional catching, and recurrent sprains or giving way of the ankle. There may be tenderness and limited range of motion on examination. Radiographs may appear normal or show very subtle findings, further delaying the diagnosis.

The usefulness of bone scanning, CT, and MR imaging in diagnosing OLT in 24 patients with ankle injury was studied by Anderson et al.[92] in 1989. Of these patients, 14 presented with persistent ankle symptoms and normal radiographs. All 14 patients had abnormal bone scans and an OLT demonstrated on MR imaging. Four of the CTs in this group were interpreted as normal. They concluded that scintigraphy should be used to assess patients with negative radiographs when there is a high clinical suspicion of an OLT. In patients whose bone scan shows talar pathology, an MR examination is warranted. In patients with abnormal radiographs, MR imaging did not provide more information than CT.

The delay in diagnosis and treatment of OLT has been addressed by several authors. Alexander and Lichtman[89] reported that a delay of nearly 15 months for surgical excision did not have an adverse effect on the outcome. Pettine and Morrey,[93] however, looked at 71 OLT 7.5 years after the onset of symptoms to determine which factors influenced the final result and found that a delay in treatment adversely affected the outcome. Pritsch et al.[94] also noted a progression in the severity of lesions while under observation.

Treatment of OLT ranges from activity modification and physiotherapy for stable lesions to excision and curettage of unstable lesions and loose bodies. If the fragment is large enough, then open reduction and internal fixation is indicated. Both open and arthroscopic treatment has been reported to have good results. Recently, arthroscopic drilling or excision has been recommended for symptomatic lesions failing nonoperative therapy.[94–97]

Staging and grading systems for OLT should guide the treatment and correlate with outcome. Berndt and Harty[87] suggested a staging system in their 1959 article. Although they did not state whether this system was based on radiographic observations or inspection of the lesion at surgery, their criteria have been applied in most studies as a radiographic staging system. The stages are as follows: stage I, a small compression fracture; stage II, incomplete avulsion of the fragment; stage III, complete avulsion without displacement; and stage IV, avulsed fragment displaced into the joint. Canale and Belding[88] used this system to correlate the radiographic findings, treatment, and outcome of 31 lesions. They concluded that stage I and II lesions should be treated nonoperatively, stage IV lesions should be treated with early excision, and stage III lesions should be treated nonoperatively initially but if symptoms persist then surgical excision is indicated.

Pritsch et al.[94] studied radiographs using the above criteria and correlated them with arthroscopic findings in 24 patients. They used an arthroscopic grading system of grade I, intact cartilage; grade II, intact but soft cartilage; and grade III, frayed cartilage, and found a lack of correlation between the radiographic appearance and the findings at arthroscopy. They recommended that arthroscopic findings should guide the treatment of these lesions.

Stetson and Ferkel[91] developed a CT classification and arthroscopic grading system to guide their treatment of OLT. They recommended CT in the case of a known diagnosis of an osteochondral lesion of the talus and MR imaging for patients with ankle pain of unknown etiology.

The use of MR imaging to analyze the mechanical stability of an osteochondral lesion was first investigated by Mesgarzadeh et al.[98] in 1987. They studied 21 knees with osteochondritis dissecans and found that MR imaging permitted direct visualization of loosening and fragment displacement, and assessment of *in situ* loosening from grossly unstable lesions. De Smet et al.[99] also evaluated the value of MR imaging in staging OLT in which they accurately predicted the presence and extent of attachment of the fragment to the talus in 13 of 14 lesions.

A staging system based on MR imaging findings of OLT was developed by Dipaola et al.[100] In a double-blinded prospective study of 12 patients with osteochondral lesions of either the knee or talus, 11 of 12 lesions were accurately staged on MR imaging compared with arthroscopy. Their staging system was as follows: stage I, thickening of articular cartilage and low-signal changes; stage II, articular cartilage breached with low-signal rim behind the fragment; stage III, articular cartilage breached with high-signal changes behind the fragment; stage IV, loose body. They did not discuss treatments or outcomes based on the staging system.

A logical diagnostic approach is needed for evaluation of OTL. Patients who present with an acute ankle injury accompanied by hemarthrosis or significant tenderness over an osseous structure should be initially assessed with standard radiographs. If an OLT is present, then either CT or MR imaging should be obtained to delineate the size, location, stability, and degree of displacement. If there is persistent pain without a demonstrable radiographic abnormality, MR imaging should be obtained to assess for both bone and soft-tissue injuries that might contribute to the symptoms.

ENTRAPMENT NEUROPATHIES

Nerve dysfunction is a frequent unrecognized cause of foot pain. Familiarity with nerve disorders in combination with an accurate knowledge of nerve anatomy greatly facilitates the evaluation of nerve entrapment syndromes.

There are five important nerves that enter the foot at the level of the ankle. Medially, the posterior tibial nerve courses behind the medial malleolus with the posterior tibial artery between the flexor digitorum longus and flexor hallucis longus tendons. It divides into the calcaneal sensory branch and medial and lateral plantar nerves. The plantar nerves provide intrinsic motor function and sensation to the plantar aspect of the foot. Anteromedially, the saphenous nerve parallels the saphenous vein and provides sensation to the dorsomedial ankle and mid-foot. The deep peroneal nerve courses with the anterior tibial artery deep to and between the extensor hallucis longus and extensor digitorum longus tendons beneath the extensor retinaculum. It sends a motor branch to the extensor digitorum brevis and provides sensation to the first web space. The superficial peroneal nerve exits the lateral compartment fascia of the lower leg about 13 cm above the tip of the lateral malleolus to become superficial.[101] It branches into medial and intermediate cutaneous nerves providing sensation to the dorsal aspect of the foot. The sural nerve exits the posterior compartment fascia over the gastrocnemius muscle and swings lateral, passing 2 cm posterior and distal to the tip of the lateral malleolus. It sends branches to supply sensation to the lateral heel, lateral aspect of the foot, and small toe.

Many of these nerves pass through fibrous tunnels under the extensor or flexor retinacula as they course around the ankle. They are susceptible to impingement from footwear, malalignment, space-occupying lesions, and local irritation. Although nerve problems can occur at virtually any location along their course, clinical experience has identified common locations of entrapment and characteristic symptoms that aid in the evaluation and treatment of affected patients.

Nerve pain is often diffuse and poorly defined. Patients present with burning, tingling, numbness, and cramping of their foot. Proximal nerve lesions such as lumbar disk disease are also potential sources of referred pain to the foot and should be evaluated. Nerve dysfunction associated with neuropathy, metabolic disorders, and reflex sympathetic dystrophy should be considered.

TARSAL TUNNEL NERVE ENTRAPMENT

Nerve entrapment within the tarsal tunnel can cause dysfunction of the entire posterior tibial nerve or any of its terminal branches. Symptoms of tarsal tunnel syndrome can be relatively nonspecific, with poorly defined burning pain and parasthesias along the medial aspect of the heel and the plantar aspect of the foot and toes. This syndrome may be caused by bony impingement, fibrosis, tenosynovitis, soft-tissue hypertrophy, or by space-occupying lesions. Space-occupying lesions include ganglia, neurilemmomas and other soft-tissue tumors, accessory or hypertrophic muscles, and vascular lesions.

Examination of the tarsal tunnel should include a general inspection of the foot to assess limb alignment or bone deformities that could affect the posterior tibial nerve. Palpation along the posterior medial ankle may reveal a source of extrinsic compression from tenosynovitis, ganglia, or tumor. Percussion along the course of the nerve may produce pain or parasthesias along the anatomic distribution of the nerve. This maneuver may also help localize the area of impingement. Diagnostic studies should include radiographs to evaluate osseous impingement and electrodiagnostic studies to evaluate other causes of nerve pain.[102]

MR imaging has been shown to be effective in evaluating the tarsal tunnel and its contents and is the preferred modality for assessing space-occupying lesions. Erickson et al.[103] used MR imaging to evaluate six patients with tarsal tunnel syndrome and found mechanical causes of impingement in all six patients including neurilemmomas, tenosynovitis, a ganglion cyst, post-traumatic fibrosis, and a post-traumatic neuroma. The MR imaging findings were confirmed surgically in five cases. Frey and Kerr[104] also found that MR imaging revealed an inflammatory lesion or mass in most patients.

Tarsal tunnel syndrome should initially be treated conservatively. In refractory cases, surgical release of the flexor retinaculum or excision of the space-occupying lesion can provide relief. Pfeiffer and Cracchiolo[105] found that surgical results were more favorable in patients who had a space-occupying lesion identified preoperatively. Therefore, MR imaging plays a key role in the diagnosis and preoperative evaluation of patients with symptoms consistent with tarsal tunnel syndrome.

ANTERIOR TARSAL TUNNEL SYNDROME

Impingement of the deep peroneal nerve is a rare phenomenom that causes neuritic pain on the dorsum of the foot and numbness in the first web space. There are several potential sites of entrapment. The extensor retinaculum is a Y-shaped structure with a superomedial and an inferomedial band. The anterior tarsal tunnel is a fibro-osseous canal between the inferior extensor retinaculum and the talus and navicular. The deep peroneal nerve and the dorsal pedis artery pass through this tunnel between the flexor hallucis longus and extensor digitorum longus tendons.

The causes of deep peroneal nerve entrapment are varied. Trauma such as a direct blow to the anterior ankle or an ankle sprain can be a precipitating factor. Shoe contact pressure, pressure from underlying osteophytes, chronic edema, and space-occupying lesions may also be a source of nerve entrapment.

The evaluation of this syndrome, as with other nerve entrapments, consists of a thorough examination and consideration of more proximal causes of nerve symptoms. Radiographs and electrodiagnostic studies are useful. As with posterior tarsal tunnel syndrome, MR imaging can help to evaluate for space-occupying lesions and may be indicated when nonoperative treatment fails and surgery is being considered.

SUPERFICIAL PERONEAL NERVE ENTRAPMENT

Entrapment of the superficial peroneal nerve is also relatively uncommon. Pain on the anterolateral lower leg that extends across the ankle joint to the dorsum of the foot is a common complaint. This entrapment syndrome has been associated with chronic ankle sprains, muscle herniation, exertional compartment syndrome, direct trauma, fibular fractures, and space-occupying lesions. The usual site of entrapment is where the superficial peroneal nerve exits the fascia of the lateral compartment 3 to 18 cm above the tip of the lateral malleolus.[101]

A careful history and physical will narrow the possible causes. Percussion along the course of the nerve often reproduces symptoms in the distribution of the superficial nerve. Electrodiagnostic studies and MR imaging are less helpful with this entrapment syndrome.

SURAL NERVE ENTRAPMENT

Sural nerve entrapment is an unusual clinical problem. It has been associated with recurrent ankle sprains, fractures of the calcaneus or fifth metatarsal, chronic inflammation of the Achilles tendon, and space-occupying lesions.[106]

The clinical findings are similar to those encountered in other entrapment syndromes around the foot. The site of entrapment is best localized by percussion of the nerve. Passive stretching of the nerve with plantar flexion and inversion of the foot may help localize the problem.[102]

Treatment is directed toward reducing pressure on the nerve and addressing underlying causes such as ankle instability or Achilles tendonitis. Local exploration and decompression may be helpful in rare cases that do not respond to conservative therapy.

MR imaging may be helpful in evaluating soft-tissue impingement of this nerve but is usually not required.

INTERDIGITAL NEUROMA

Morton's metatarsalgia was first described by Thomas G. Morton in 1867 and further clarified by Nissen in 1948.[107] This common clinical syndrome consists of forefoot pain on the sole of the foot, most often in the third web space and rarely in the second or fourth web space. The pain may range from a mild ache to a burning, neuritic pain radiating to the toes, aggravated by walking or standing and relieved by sitting, removing the shoe, and massaging the foot. The onset of symptoms is typically in the fifth and sixth decades of life and women are usually more frequently affected than men. More than one web space may be symptomatic and bilateral involvement is common.

The physical examination typically reveals reproducible pain by compressing the forefoot while applying direct plantar pressure over the affected web space.[108] Occasionally this two-plane compression test will elicit a painful click, thought to be the displacement of the affected digital nerve below the metatarsal heads and transverse metatarsal ligament. Some patients may also demonstrate numbness in the web space and along the toes.

The cause of Morton's metatarsalgia has been debated in the literature. In 1948 Nissen suggested that the nerve lesion is ischemic in origin based on the microscopic examination of specimens taken from 27 patients.[107] However, Guiloff and associates[108a] looked at 16 patients in 1984 with electrophysiological and histological observations and found evidence compatible with an entrapment syndrome of the digital nerve. Shereff and Grande[109] in 1991 used electron microscopic analysis of 10 surgical specimens of interdigital neuroma and concluded that the degeneration and necrosis of the nerve was consistent with damage due to mechanical impingement. Read et al.[110] most recently compared the sonographic findings with histopathology. In 19 of 20 cases, the histopathology confirmed the presence of prominent mucoid degeneration within the loose fibro-fatty web space tissues around the neuroma specimens. They concluded that chronic repetitive trauma to the nerve, bursa, and intervening connective tissues is the likely cause of Morton's neuroma.

The treatment of Morton's metatarsalgia usually starts with simple measures that include activity modification, oral anti-inflamatory agents, and shoe modification. If symptoms persist, then custom orthotics and corticosteroid injections may be used. The response to steroid injection can be both therapeutic and diagnostic. When conservative measures fail, surgical resection of the interdigital nerve and its surrounding abnormal tissue is indicated.

Morton's metatarsalgia is most often a clinical diagnosis. However, a confident diagnosis and/or localization of the affected web space may be difficult when the reported pain is more diffuse and the physical findings are ambiguous. In these cases further imaging may be helpful.

The usefulness of MR imaging to evaluate Morton's metatarsalgia has been discussed by several investigators. Erickson et al.[111] evaluated 17 feet with symptoms suggestive of plantar interdigital neuroma with high-resolution MR imaging using a solenoid coil. Of the 17 feet, 6 were operated on, at which time the MR imaging findings were confirmed and they concluded that MR imaging is a highly accurate, operator-independent modality for detecting Morton's neuromas. Resch et al.,[112] on the other hand, were only able to diagnose five of eight surgically confirmed neuromas with MR imaging using a low-field-strength 0.3 T magnet and they concluded that MR imaging was less useful in this setting.[112]

The prevalence of presumed Morton's neuromas in the asymptomatic population was investigated by Zanetti et al.[113] They obtained MR imaging data on 70 asymptomatic patients and compared the size to 16 symptomatic, surgically proven Morton's neuromas. In all, 24 Morton's neuromas were diagnosed (prevalence, 30%) in which the average size was 4.5 mm in asymptomatic individuals compared with 5.6 mm in symptomatic subjects. They concluded that a diagnosis of Morton's neuroma on MR imaging may only be relevant when the transverse diameter is 5 mm or more and can be correlated to clinical findings. In a different study, Zanetti et al.[114] studied 32 consecutive patients with suspected Morton's neuromas on MR imaging. Of the 32 patients, 16 were evaluated surgically. They found MR imaging had a sensitivy of 87%, specificity of 100%, and an accuracy of 89%. In 6 of 15 proven neuromas, the clinician was unable to identify the correct intermetatarsal space and concluded that MR imaging is accurate in diagnosing Morton's neuroma and may be important for correct localization.

In conclusion, the MR imaging finding alone of Morton's neuroma does not predict clinical symptoms or the outcome from surgical intervention. However, in those few cases where the clinical diagnosis is difficult, MR imaging is useful in locating and diagnosing Morton's metatarsalgia.

INFECTION

Musculoskeletal infections present a diagnostic and therapeutic challenge for the orthopedic surgeon. Early diagnosis allows expedient institution of treatment, which prevents further soft-tissue, bone, and joint destruction. Differentiating soft-tissue infection from involvement of bone is critical in determining the appropriate treatment. Local wound care, limited antibiotic therapy, and minor surgery can commonly manage soft-tissue infection. Osteomyelitis, on the other hand, is more refractory to treatment, often requiring prolonged intravenous antibiotic therapy and more aggressive debridement. Infection in the foot is commonly seen in patients with underlying diabetes. In these patients, infection often occurs in the setting of cellulitis, peripheral ischemia, and neuroarthropathy, making the definitive diagnosis of osseous involvement difficult.[3] The extent of soft-tissue and bone involvement must be determined to assess the type, route, and duration of antibiotic treatment and the need for possible surgical debridement.

Ulceration of the diabetic foot is a common problem. Plantar ulcers are caused by weight-bearing pressure, whereas dorsal ulcers are caused by shoe pressure. A combination of neuropathy, vascular compromise, bony prominence, and foot deformity creates a foot at risk for ulceration and ultimately infection. The treatment of these lesions is based on relieving the pressure insult by altering the shoe and/or the shape of the foot and treating the infection if present.

The prevalence of osteomyelitis associated with diabetic foot ulcers is not well documented in the literature. Newman and colleagues[115] reported a 68% prevalence in 41 foot ulcers studied prospectively using bone biopsy as the diagnostic gold standard. They noted that only 32% of these cases were diagnosed clinically by the referring physicians.

Radiographic examination remains the initial step in the imaging workup of osteomyelitis. In a patient with normal bones, radiographs may be all that is needed to make the diagnosis. The classic radiographic signs of bone resorption depend on vascularity of the bone. Therefore, in patients with diabetic neuropathy, vascular compromise, and neuroarthropathy, radiographs are unreliable.

When the initial radiographs are negative but there is a high clinical suspicion of osteomyelitis, further investigation is needed. MR imaging has been used to diagnosis osteomyelitis with reported sensitivities of 94 to 100% and specificities ranging from 69 to 96%.[3] However, fractures and rapidly progressive neuropathic changes can be associated with nonspecific high-signal changes within bones, and thus be indistinguishable from osteomyelitis.[3] Other modalities also available to help with the diagnosis include the triple-phase bone scan, indium-111 white blood cell scan, and CT.

A selected review of the literature reveals mixed opinions. Weinstein and colleagues[116] in 1993 prospectively evaluated 47 patients with MR imaging, 14 of whom had triple-phase bone scanning, and obtained pathologic confirmation from 32 patients. They found MR imaging was more sensitive but was equal in specificity to the triple-phase bone scan. There were three false-positives in this study and they concluded that MR imaging is indicated when radiographs are negative for osteomyelitis or when the extent and accurate depiction of the infective process will facilitate surgical planning.

In 1994, Levine et al.[117] reported on 27 diabetic patients with clinically suspected osteomyelitis. Of the patients, 11 had technetium bone scans and 12 had indium-labeled leukocyte scintigraphy. They reported the accuracy of MR imaging was 90%, technetium bone scan 45%, and indium-labeled leukocyte scintigraphy 50%. They concluded that MR imaging was a powerful, noninvasive tool for determining the presence or absence of osteomyelitis in the patient with a diabetic foot ulcer.

In 1995, Morrison et al.[118] studied 62 patients, 27 with diabetes and 35 witout diabetes, with suspected osteomyelitis of the foot. Using a combination of bone biopsy and clinical response to treatment to establish the diagnosis, they found the triple-phase bone scan and MR imaging to have comparable sensitivity and specificity. In their institution, MR imaging resulted in a shorter hospital stay and was also comparable in price with the triple-phase bone scan.

Craig et al.,[119] on the other hand, studied 13 patients with 15 MR studies using the anatomic and histologic specimens of the resected tissue as a standard of reference. They concluded that marrow edema cannot be reliably distinguished from osteomyelitis on MR imaging but that MR imaging is useful in planning surgical resections. Morrison and associates[120] looked at this problem in 1998 by retrospectively reviewing the MR examinations of 73 feet. They were able to identify secondary signs that increased the sensitivity of MR imaging to 96%.

Seabold and associates looked at patients with complications who also have neuropathic osteoarthropathy. They studied 14 patients with clinical and/or radiographic evidence of neuropathic osteoarthropathy with combined technetium bone scan and indium-111 white blood cell studies. Seven of these patients also had MR imaging studies. Of 16 indium-111 white blood cell studies, 5 had false-positive uptake at noninfected sites. Three of the seven MR imaging studies were also false positive. They concluded that the findings on indium-111 white blood cell studies and MR imaging of rapidly progressive, noninfected neuropathic osteoarthropathy might be indistinguishable from those of osteomyelitis.

To help evaluate the patient with suspected osteomyelitis who has clinical cellulitis and negative radiographs, either MR imaging or triple-phase bone and indium-111 white blood cell scans are recommended. The choice between these modalities should be made by considering the cost, availability of the studies, and preference of the consulting radiologist. The orthopedic surgeon should understand the ambiguity of both studies and correlate the imaging findings with the clinical presentation.

STRESS FRACTURES

Stress fractures of the lower extremity are common injuries affecting a broad range of individuals from the young to the elderly, from fitness enthusiasts to the medically disabled patient. They can cause persistent pain that interferes with activities of daily living. As the preoccupation with physical fitness increases in our society, the potential for stress fractures may increase.

Bone is a dynamic tissue that remodels in response to forces that strengthen the area being stressed. When bone does not adapt normally to these repetitive forces, stress fractures may occur. Resorption of bone by osteoclastic activity is a more rapid process than the osteoblastic replacement of bone.[121] Therefore, there is a period of time during the remodeling process when the bone is weak and microfractures may develop. This injury can occur in normal bone subject to abnormal stress or in abnormal bone subject to normal stress, the latter referred to as insufficiency fractures.

The most common bones affected in the foot and ankle are the metatarsals, tibia, and calcaneus, and the reported incidence of stress fractures ranges from 1.3 to 31%.[122] Stress fractures have potentially serious sequelae including progression to a displaced fracture, delayed union, nonunion, and chronic pain. Accurate and prompt diagnosis may help prevent these complications.

The clinical presentation of a stress fracture includes localized pain with insidious onset that worsens with impact activities. In the athlete, the symptoms may initially only occur with the sporting activity, but with continued stress the pain may occur with activities of daily living. A history of recent change in the patient's activity, training regimen, or footwear is often found. Examination of the involved area may reveal pain with palpation or percussion and local swelling.

The diagnosis of stress fractures needs to be confirmed by the use of several imaging modalities. Initially, radiographs should be obtained. Findings such as periosteal new bone formation, endosteal thickening, and/or a radiolucent line extending through a cortex are suggestive of a stress fracture in the correct clinical setting. The radiographic findings often lag 2 to 3 weeks behind the onset of symptoms.[122] Prather et al.[123] found radiographic examination alone was only 64% accurate in the diagnosis of a stress fracture. Therefore, further studies are needed.

A bone scan is more sensitive than radiographs in diagnosing stress fractures but is less specific. A false-positive rate of 13 to 24% has been reported in the literature; yet this modality is most often used to confirm the diagnosis.[123,124]

MR imaging can show periosteal reaction and marrow edema which aids in diagnosing stress fractures.[125–127] Steinbronn and associates[122] presented four cases of stress fractures in which MR imaging was used to establish the diagnosis after the appropriate initial studies were inconclusive. They felt that MR imaging was useful in a select group of patients with suspected stress fractures of the foot and ankle.[122] Fredericson and associates[129] studied 18 symptomatic legs in runners with medial tibial pain using MR imaging and scintigraphy. They developed a grading system based on the MR imaging findings and compared their grading system to one developed by Zwas et al.[128] based on bone scan findings. They noted that MR imaging was more accurate in correlating the degree of bone involvement with clinical symptoms, enabling more appropriate recommendations for rehabilitation and return to impact activity.

Most patients with stress fractures respond to treatment ranging from activity modification, protected weight bearing, to casting. With a classic history and examination, treatment can be instituted while the patient is followed with serial radiographic exams. If further diagnostic confirmation is needed, both MR imaging and a bone scan can be helpful. The choice between MR imaging and bone scan should be governed by the cost and availability of these studies.

TUMORS

SOFT-TISSUE TUMORS AND TUMOR-LIKE LESIONS

Soft-tissue tumors and tumor-like lesions are common in the foot and ankle, and the great majority of lesions are benign.[50] They usually present early in their course compared with other areas of the body when the mass is relatively small and can be excised more easily.

MR imaging is highly sensitive for detection and evaluation of the extent of musculoskeletal tumors. Conventional radiographs, however, remain the primary modality for characterization of bone tumors.[3] The main role of MR imaging is in anatomic localization of the tumor, surgical staging, and detection of recurrence.

Some tumors and soft-tissue lesions can be identified on the basis of their location and appearance on MR imaging. Such lesions have been discussed in detail in preceding chapters.[130]

PLANTAR FIBROMATOSIS

Plantar fibromatosis is a benign condition related to Dupuytren's disease of the hand which should be differentiated from other tumors of the foot.[130] It is a disorder of fibrous tissue proliferation, characterized by the replacement of the plantar aponeurosis with abnormal fibrous tissue. Patients with plantar fibromatosis usually present with a painless, slow-growing nodule on the plantar surface of their foot.[3]

The lesions of plantar fibromatosis are not usually demonstrated on radiographs or bone scan. MR imaging is thought to be the most helpful diagnostic tool.[131] Morrison et al.[132] retrospectively evaluated 19 feet with plantar fibromatosis and compared the MR imaging findings to a control group. They reported that plantar fibromatosis is a benign but infiltrative neoplasm with a characteristic location and appearance on MR imaging.[132]

Nonoperative treatment is preferred for this entity because of the potential for local recurrence. Accommodative semi-rigid orthotics and appropriate footwear should be used to alleviate pressure on the lesion. The major indication for operative intervention is failure of optimal nonoperative treatment. In this situation, a wide excision of the plantar fascia is recommended.[131]

CHRONIC FOOT AND ANKLE PAIN OF UNKNOWN ETIOLOGY

This symptom complex is a common presentation in patients with foot and ankle dysfunction. These patients have often undergone numerous consultations and treatments that have failed. A detailed history and examination are essential for a diagnosis. If all routine investigations are normal, the clinician is faced with the decision to investigate the problem further. In the presence of a confusing clinical picture, such investigations will likely have a low yield because of poor clinical correlation.

The author's approach is as follows. If the clinical exam is nonspecific and does not localize the pain to a certain anatomic region, then a bone scan is obtained to exclude bony or occult joint pathology. If the bone scan is negative and the clinical exam is nonspecific, further investigations are probably not useful. If the bone scan is positive, then MR imaging is useful in obtaining more-detailed anatomic information.

When the clinical symptoms localize to a specific antomic area or if a diagnostic local injection of an anesthetic relieves the symptoms, then a bone scan is not needed. In these cases MR imaging can provide information about soft-tissue and osseous pathology at the involved site. The type of occult pathology that may be diagnosed in these cases includes early arthritis with normal radiographs, fibrous tarsal coalition, sinus tarsi syndrome, and benign tumorous conditions.

This approach is summarized in the following flow diagram.

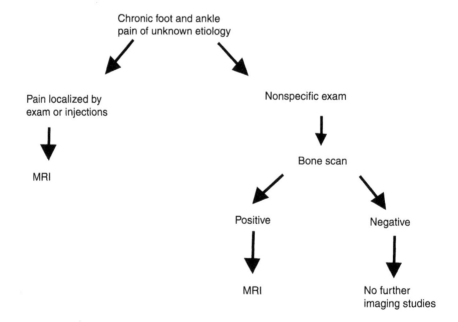

REFERENCES

1. Ferkel, R. D., Flannigan, B. D., and Elkins, B. S., Magnetic resonance imaging of the foot and ankle: correlation of normal anatomy with pathologic conditions, *Foot Ankle*, 11, 289–305, 1991.

2. Haygood, T. M., Magnetic resonance imaging of the musculoskeletal system: Part 7. The ankle, *Clin. Orthop. Relat. Res.*, 336, 318–336, 1997.

3. Hochman, M. G., Min, K. K., and Zilberfarb, J. L., MR imaging of the symptomatic ankle and foot, *Orthop. Clin. North Am.*, 28, 659–683, 1997.

4. Erickson, S. J. and Johnson, J. E., MR imaging of the ankle and foot, *Radiol. Clin. North Am.*, 35, 10(4), 453–460, 1994.

5. Fowler, P. J., Dye, S. F., Herzog, R. J., and Nottage, W. M., Current concepts in orthopaedic imaging: knee and shoulder, paper presented at the 63rd Annual Meeting of the Academy of Orthopedic Surgeons, 1996.

6. Mann, R. A. and Specht, L. H., Posterior tibial tendon ruptures — analysis of eight cases, *Foot Ankle*, 2, 350, 1982.

7. Jahss, M. H., Spontaneous rupture of the tibialis posterior tendon: clinical findings, tenographic studies and a new technique of repair, *Foot Ankle*, 3, 158–166, 1982.

8. Johnson, K. A., Tibialis posterior tendon rupture, *Clin. Orthop. Relat. Res.*, 177, 147, 1983.

9. Goldner, J. L., Keats, P. K., Bassett, F. H. L., and Clippinger, F. W., Progressive talipes equinovalgus due to trauma or degeneration of the posterior tibial tendon and medial plantar ligaments, *Orthop. Clin. North Am.*, 5, 39–51, 1974.

10. Henceroth, W. D. L. and Deyerle, W. M., The acquired unilateral flatfoot in the adult: some causative factors, *Foot Ankle*, 2, 304–308, 1982.

11. Holmes, G. B. and Mann, R. A., Possible epidemiological factors associated with rupture of the posterior tibial tendon, *Foot Ankle*, 13, 70-79, 1992.

12. Funk, D. A., Cass, J. R., and Johnson, K. A., Acquired adult flat foot secondary to posterior tibial-tendon pathology, *J. Bone Joint Surg.*, 68-A, 95–102, 1986.

13. Dyal, C. M., Feder, J., and Deland, J. T., Pes planus in patients with posterior tibial tendon insufficiencey, asymptomatic versus symptomatic foot, *Foot Ankle*, 18, 85–88, 1997.

14. Frey, C., Shereff, M., and Greenidge, N., Vascularity of the posterior tibial tendon, *J. Bone Joint Surg.*, 72-A, 884–887, 1990.

15. Johnson, K. A. and Strom, D. E., Tibialis posterior tendon dysfunction, *Clin. Orthop. Relat. Res.*, 239, 196–206, 1989.

16. Myerson, M. S., Adult acquired flatfoot deformity: treatment of dysfunction of the posterior tibial tendon, in *Instructional Course Lectures,* Vol. 46, D. S. Springfield, Ed., American Academy of Orthopaedic Surgeons, Rosemont, IL, 1997, 393–405.

17. Alexander, I. J., Johnson, K. A., and Berquist, T. H., Magnetic resonance imaging in the diagnosis of disruption of the posterior tibial tendon, *Foot Ankle*, 8, 144–147, 1987.

18. Conti, S. F., Posterior tibial tendon problems in athletes, *Orthop. Clin. North Am.*, 25, 109–121, 1994.

19. Rosenberg, Z. S., Cheung, Y., Jahss, M. H., Noto, A. M., Norman, A., and Leeds, N. E., Rupture of posterior tibial tendon: CT and MR imaging with surgical correlation, *Radiology*, 169, 229–235, 1988.

20. Conti, S. F., Michelson, J., and Jahss, M. H., Clinical significance of magnetic resonance imaging in preoperative planning for reconstruction of posterior tibial tendon ruptures, *Foot Ankle*, 13, 208–214, 1992.

21. Narvaez, J., Narvaez, J. A., Sanchez-Marquez, A., Clavaguera, M. T., Rodriguez-Moreno, J., and Gil, M., Posterior tibial tendon dysfunction as a cause of acquired flatfoot in the adult: value of magnetic resonance imaging, *Br. J. Rheumatol.*, 36, 136–139, 1997.

22. Carr, A. J. and Norris, S. H., The blood supply of the calcaneal tendon, *J. Bone Joint Surg. (Br.)*, 71-B, 100–101, 1989.

23. Strocchi, R., De Pasquale, V., Guizzardi, S., Gavoni, P., Facchini, A., Raspanti, M., Girolami, M., and Giannini, S., Human Achilles tendon: morphological and morphometric variations as a function of age, *Foot Ankle*, 12, 100-104, 1991.

24. Puddu, G., Ippolito, E., and Postacchini, F., A classification of Achilles tendon disease, *Am. J. Sports Med.*, 4, 145–150, 1976.

25. Quinn, S. F., Murray, W. T., Clark, R. A., and Cochran, C. F., Achilles tendon: MR imaging at 1.5T, *Radiology*, 164, 767–770, 1987.
26. Saltzman, C. L. and Tearse, D. S., Achilles tendon injuries, *J. Am. Acad. Orthop. Surg.*, 6, 316–325, 1998.
27. Clement, D. B., Taunton, J. E., and Smart, G. W., Achilles tendinitis and peritendinitis etiology and treatment, *Am. J. Sports Med.*, 12, 179–184, 1984.
28. Schepsis, A. A. and Leach, R. E., Surgical management of Achilles tendinitis, *Am. J. Sports Med.*, 15, 308–315, 1987.
29. Leach, R. E., Schepsis, A. A., and Takai, H., Long-term results of surgical management of Achilles tendinitis in runners, *Clin. Orthop. Relat. Res.*, 282, 208–212, 1992.
30. Thompson, T. C. and Doherty, J. H., Spontaneous rupture of tendon of Achilles: a new clinical diagnostic test, *J. Trauma*, 2, 126–129, 1962.
31. Inglis, A. E., Scott, W. N., Sculco, T. P., and Patterson, A. H., Ruptures of the tendo Achilles: an objective assessment of surgical and nonsurgical treatment, *J. Bone Joint Surg.*, 58A, 990–993, 1976.
32. Keene, J. S., Lash, E. G., Fisher, D. R., and De Smet, A. A., Magnetic resonance imaging of Achilles tendon ruptures, *Am. J. Sports Med.*, 17, 333–337, 1989.
33. Cetti, R., Christensen, S., Ejsted, R., Jensen, N. M., and Jorgensen, U., Operative versus nonoperative treatment of Achilles tendon rupture: a prospective randomized study and review of the literature, *Am. J. Sports Med.*, 21, 791–798, 1993.
34. Kollias, S. L. and Ferkel, R. D., Fibular grooving for recurrent peroneal tendon subluxation, *Am. J. Sports Med.*, 25, 329–335, 1997.
35. Edwards, M. E., The relations of the peroneal tendons to the fibula, calcaneus, and cuboideum, *Am. J. Anat.*, 42, 213–253, 1928.
36. Brage, M. E. and Hansen, S. T., Traumatic subluxatiion/dislocation of the peroneal tendons, *Foot Ankle*, 13, 423–431, 1992.
37. Schweitzer, M. E., Eid, M. E., Deely, D., Wapner, K., and Hecht, P., Using MR imaging to differentiate peroneal splits from other peroneal disorders, *Am. J. Radiol.*, 168, 129–133, 1997.
38. Purnell, M. L., Drummond, D. S., and Engber, W. D., Congentital dislocation of the peroneal tendons in the calcaneovalgus foot, *J. Bone Joint Surg. (Br.)*, 65-B, 316–319, 1983.
39. Rosenberg, Z. S., Beltran, J., Cheung, Y. Y., Colon, E., and Herraiz, F., MR features of longitudinal tears of the peroneus brevis tendon, *Am. J. Radiol.*, 168, 141–147, 1997.
40. Sammarco, G. J., Peroneal tendon injuries, *Orthop. Clin. North Am.*, 25, 135–145, 1994.
41. Khoury, N. J., El-Khoury, G. Y., Saltzman, C. L., and Kathol, M. H., Peroneus longus and brevis tendon tears. MR imaging evaluation, *Radiology*, 200, 833–841, 1996.
42. Tjin A Ton, E. R., Schweitzer, M. E., and Karasick, D., MR imging of peroneal tendon disorders, *Am. J. Radiol.*, 168, 135–140, 1997.
43. Buschmann, W. R., Cheung, Y., and Jahss, M. H., Magnetic resonance imaging of anomalous leg muscles, accessory soleus, peroneus quartus and the flexor digitorum longus accessorius, *Foot Ankle*, 12, 109–116, 1991.
44. Sobel, M., Geppert, M. J., Olson, E. J., Bohne, W. H. O., and Arnoczky, S. P., The dynamics of peroneus brevis tendon splits: a proposed mechanism, technique of diagnosis, and classification of injury, *Foot Ankle*, 13, 413–422, 1992.
45. Sobel, M., Bohne, W. H. O., and Markisz, J. A., Cadaver correlation of peroneal tendon changes with magnetic resonance imaging, *Foot Ankle*, 11, 384–388, 1991.
46. Hamilton, W. G., Stenosing tenosynovitis of the flexor hallucis longus tendon and posterior impingement upon the os trigonum in ballet dancers, *Foot Ankle*, 3, 74–80, 1982.
47. Brodsky, A. E. and Khalil, M. A., Talar compression syndrome, *Foot Ankle*, 8, 82–83, 1987.
48. Wakeley, C. J., Johnson, D. P., and Watt, I., The value of MR imaging in the diagnosis of the os trigonum syndrome, *Skeletal Radiol.*, 25, 133–136, 1996.
49. Marotta, J. J. and Micheli, L. J., Os trigonum impingement in dancers, *Am. J. Sports Med.*, 20, 533–536, 1992.
50. Frey, C., Bell, J., Teresi, L., Kerr, R., and Feder, K., A Comparison of MRI and clincal examination of acute lateral ankle sprains, *Foot Ankle*, 17, 533–537, 1996.
51. Black, H. M., Brand, R. L., and Eichelberger, M. R., An improved technique for the evaluation of ligamentous injury in severe ankle sprains, *Am. J. Sports Med.*, 6, 276–282, 1978.

52. Gaebler, C., Kukla, C., Breitenseher, M. J., Nellas, Z. J., Mittlboeck, M., Trattnig, S., and Vecsei, V., Diagnosis of lateral ankle ligament injuries, comparison between talar tilt, MRI and operative findings in 112 athletes, *Acta Orthop. Scand.*, 68, 286–290, 1997.
53. Kannus, P. and Renstrom, P., Treatment of acute tears of the lateral ligaments of the ankle: operation, cast, or early controlled mobilization, *J. Bone Joint Surg.*, 73-A, 305–312, 1991.
54. Brostrom, L., Sprained ankles: VI. Surgical treatment of "chronic" ligament ruptures, *Acta Chir. Scand.*, 132, 551–565, 1966.
54a. Mulliken, J. B. and Glowacki, J., Hemangiomas and vascular malformations in infants and children: a classification based on endothelial characteristics, *Plast. Reconstr. Surg.*, 69, 412, 1982.
55. Colville, M. R., Surgical treatment of the unstable ankle, *J. Am. Acad. Orthop. Surg.*, 6, 368–377, 1998.
56. Karlsson, J., Bergsten, T., Lansinger, O., and Peterson, L., Reconstruction of the lateral ligaments of the ankle for chronic lateral instability, *J. Bone Joint Surg.*, 70-A, 581–588, 1988.
57. Gould, N., Seligson, D., and Gassman, J., Early and late repair of lateral ligments of the ankle, *Foot Ankle*, 1, 84–89, 1980.
58. Cox, J. S. and Hewes, T. F., "Normal" talar tilt angle, *Clin. Orthop. Relat. Res.*, 140, 37–41, 1979.
59. Grace, D. L., Lateral ankle ligament injuries, *Clin. Orthop. Relat. Res.*, 183, 153–159, 1984.
60. Chandnani, V. P., Harper, M. T., Ficke, J. R., Gagliardi, J. A., Rolling, L., Christensen, K. P., and Hansen, M. F., Chronic ankle instability: evaluation with MR arthrography, MR imaging, and stress radiography, *Radiology*, 192, 189–194, 1994.
61. Lambert, K., The weight-bearing function of the fibula, *J. Bone Joint Surg.*, 53-A, 507, 1971.
62. Scranton, P. E., McMasters, J. H., and Delley, E., Dynamic fibular function, *Clin. Orthop. Relat. Res.*, 156, 76–81, 1976.
63. Lauge-Hansen, N., Fracture of the ankle II: combined experimental-surgical and experimental-roentgonologic investigations, *Arch. Surg.*, 60, 957–985, 1950.
64. Muller, M. E., Allgower, M., Schneider, R., and Willenegger, H., *Manual of Internal Fixation*, Springer-Verlag, Berlin, 1991.
65. Hopkinson, W. J., St. Pierre, P., Ryan, J. B., and Wheeler, J. H., Syndesmosis sprains of the ankle, *Foot Ankle*, 10, 325–330, 1990.
66. Teitz, C. C. and Harrington, R. M., A biomechanical analysis of the squeeze test for sprains of the syndesmotic ligaments of the ankle, *Foot Ankle*, 19, 489–492, 1998.
67. Veltri, D. M., Pagnani, M. J., O'Brien, S. J., Warren, R. F., Ryan, M. D., and Barnes, R. P., Symptomatic ossification of the tibiofibular syndesmosis in professional footbal players: a sequela of the syndesmotic ankle sprain, *Foot Ankle*, 16, 285–290, 1995.
68. Ramsey, P. L. and Hamilton, W., Changes in tibiotalar area of contact caused by lateral talar shift, *J. Bone Joint Surg.*, 58-A, 356–357, 1976.
69. Amendola, A., Controversies in diagnosis and management of syndesmosis injuries of the ankle, *Foot Ankle*, 13, 44–50, 1992.
70. Harper, M. C. and Keller, T. S., A radiographic evaluation of the tibiofibular syndesmosis, *Foot Ankle*, 10, 156–160, 1989.
71. Xenos, J., Hopkinson, W. J., Mulligan, M. E., Olson, E. J., and Popovic, N. A., The tibiofibula syndesmosis, evaluation of the ligamentous structures, methods of fixation, and radiographic assessment, *J. Bone Joint Surg.*, 77-A, 847–856, 1995.
72. Vogl, T. J., Hochmuth, K., Diebold, T., Lubrich, J., Hofmann, R., Ullrich, S., Sollner, O., Bisson, S., Sudkamp, N., Maeurer, J., Haas, N., and Rolank, F., Magnetic resonance imaging in the diagnosis of acute injured distal tibiofibular syndesmosis, *Invest. Radiol.*, 32, 401–409, 1997.
73. Morris, L. H., Athlete's ankle, *J. Bone Joint Surg. (Br.)*, 25-B, 220, 1943.
74. McMurray, T. P., Footballer's ankle, *J. Bone Joint Surg.*, 32-B, 68–69, 1950.
75. Wolin, I., Glassman, F., Sideman, S., and Levinthal, D. H., Internal derangement of the talofibular component of the ankle, *Surg. Gynecol. Obstet.*, 19, 193–200, 1950.
76. Bassett, F. H., III, Gates, H. S., III, Billys, J. B., Orris, H. B., and Nikolaou, P. K., Talar impingement by the anteroinferior tibiofibular ligament, *J. Bone Joint Surg.*, 72-A, 55–59, 1990.
77. Ferkel, R. D., Karzel, R. P., Delpizzo, W., Friedan, M. J., and Fischer, S. P., Arthroscopic treatment of anterolateral impingement of the ankle, *Am. J. Sports Med.*, 19, 440–446, 1991.
78. Liu, S. H., Nuccion, S. L., and Inerman, G., Diagnosis of anterolateral ankle impingement: comparison between magnetic resonance imaging and clinical examination, *Am. J. Sports Med.*, 25, 389–393, 1997.

79. Mink, J. H. and Deutsch, A. L., Occult cartilage and bone injuries of the knee: detection, classification, and assessment with MR imaging, *Radiology*, 170, 823–829, 1989.

80. Kaplan, P. A., Walker, C. W., Kilcoyne, R. F., Brown, D. E., Tusek, D., and Dussault, R. G., Occult fracture patterns of the knee associated with anterior cruciate ligament tears: assessment with MR imaging, *Radiology*, 183, 835–838, 1992.

81. Vellet, A. D., Marks, P. H., Fowler, P. J., and Munro, T. G., Occult post-traumatic osteochondral lesions of the knee: prevalence, classification, and short-term sequelae evaluated with MR imaging, *Radiology*, 178, 271–276, 1991.

82. Marks, P. H., Goldenberg, J. A., Vezina, W. C., Camberlain, M. J., Vellet, A. D., and Fowler, P. J., Subchrondral bone infractions in acute ligamentous knee injuries demonstrated on bone scintigraphy and magnetic resonance imaging, *J. Nucl. Med.*, 33, 516–520, 1992.

83. Labovitz, J. M. and Schweitzer, M. E., Occult osseous injuries after ankle sprains: incidence, location, pattern and age, *Foot Ankle*, 19, 661–667, 1998.

84. Bauer, M., Jonsson, K., and Linden, B., Osteochondritis dissecans of the ankle, *J. Bone Joint Surg.*, 69-B, 93–96, 1987.

85. Bosien, J. K., Stables, O. S., and Russell, S. W., Residual disability following acute ankle sprains, *J. Bone Joint Surg.*, 37-A, 1237–1243, 1955.

86. Stone, J. W., Osteochondral lesions of the talar dome, *J. Am. Acad. Orthop. Surg.*, 4, 63–73, 1996.

87. Berndt, A. L. and Harty, M., Transchondral fractures (osteochondritis dissecans) of the talus, *J. Bone Joint Surg.*, 41-A, 988–1019, 1959.

88. Canale, S. T. and Belding, R. H., Osteochondral lesions of the talus, *J. Bone Joint Surg.*, 62-A, 97–102, 1980.

89. Alexander, A. H. and Lichtman, D. M., Surgical treatment of transchondral talar-dome fractures (ostechondritis dissecans), *J. Bone Joint Surg.*, 62-A, 646–652, 1980.

90. Flick, A. B. and Gould, N., Osteochondritis dissecans of the talus (transchondral fractures of the talus): review of the literature and new surgical approach for medial dome lesions, *Foot Ankle*, 5, 165–185, 1985.

91. Stetson, W. B. and Ferkel, R. D., Ankle arthroscopy: II. Indications and results, *J. Am. Acad. Orthop. Surg.*, 4, 24–34, 1996.

92. Anderson, I. F., Crichton, K. J., Grattan-Smith, T., Cooper, R. A., and Brazier, D., Osteochondral fractures of the dome of the talus, *J. Bone Joint Surg.*, 71-A, 1143–1152, 1989.

93. Pettine, K. A. and Morrey, B. F., Osteochondral fractures of the talus, *J. Bone Joint Surg. (Br.)*, 69-B, 89–92, 1987.

94. Pritsch, M., Horoshovski, H., and Farine, I., Arthroscopic treatment of osteochondral lesions of the talus, *J. Bone Joint Surg.*, 68-A, 862–865, 1986.

95. Amendola, A., Petrick, J., and Webster-Bogaert, S., Ankle arthroscopy: outcome in 79 consecutive patients, *J. Arthrosc. Relat. Surg.*, 12, 565–573, 1996.

96. Bryant, O. D. and Siegel, M. G., Osteochondritis dissecans of the talus: a new technique for arthroscopic drilling, *Arthrosc., J. Arthrosc. Relat. Surg.*, 9, 238–241, 1993.

97. Buecken, K. V., Barrack, R. L., Alexander, A. H., and Ertl, J. P., Arthroscopic treatment of transchondral talar dome fractures, *Am. J. Sports Med.*, 17, 350–356, 1989.

98. Mesgarzadeh, M., Sapega, A. A., Bonakdarpour, A., Revesz, G., Moyer, R. A., Maurer, A. H., and Alburger, P. D., Osteochondritis dissecans: analysis of mechanical stability with radiography scintigraphy, and MR imaging, *Radiology*, 165, 775–780, 1987.

99. De Smet, A. A., Fisher, D. R., Burnstein, M. I., Graf, B. K., and Lange, R. H., Value of MR imaging in staging osteochondral lesions of the talus (osteochondritis dissecans): results in 14 patients, *Am. J. Radiol.*, 154, 555–558, 1990.

100. Dipaola, J. D., Nelson, D. W., and Colville, M. R., Characterizing osteochondral lesions by magnetic resonance imaging, *J. Arthrosc. Relat. Surg.*, 7, 101–104, 1991.

101. Adkison, D. P., Bosse, M. J., Gaccione, D. R., and Gabriel, K. R., Anatomical variations in the course of the superficial peroneal nerve, *J. Bone Joint Surg.*, 73-A, 112–114, 1991.

102. Beskin, J. L., Nerve entrapment syndromes of the foot and ankle, *J. Am. Acad. Orthop. Surg.*, 5, 261–269, 1997.

103. Erickson, S. J., Quinn, S. F., Keeland, J. B., Smith, J. W., Johnson, J. E., Carrera, G. J., Shereff, M. J., Hyde, J. S., and Jesmanowicz, A., MR imaging of the tarsal tunnel and related spaces: normal and abnormal findings with anatomic correlation, *Am. J. Radiol.*, 155, 328, 1990.

104. Frey, C. and Kerr, R., Magnetic resonance imaging and the evaluation of tarsal tunnel syndrome, *Foot Ankle*, 14, 159–164, 1993.

105. Pfeiffer, W. H. and Cracchiolo, A., Clinical results after tarsal tunnel decompression, *J. Bone Joint Surg.*, 76-A, 1222–1230, 1994.

106. Pringle, R. M., Protheroe, K., and Mukherjee, S. K., Entrapment neuropathy of the sural nerve, *J. Bone Joint Surg. (Br.)*, 56-B, 465–468, 1974.

107. Nissen, K. I., Plantar digital neuritis: Morton's metatarsalgia, *J. Bone Joint Surg. (Br.)*, 30-B, 84–94, 1948.

108. Mulder, J. D., The causative mechanism in Morton's metatarsalgia, *J. Bone Joint Surg. (Br.)*, 33-B, 94–95, 1951.

108a. Guiloff, R. J., Scadding, J. W., and Klenerman, L., Morton's metatarsalgia: clinical, electrophysiological and historical observations, *J. Bone Joint Surg. Br.*, 66(B), 586–591, 1984.

109. Shereff, M. J. and Grande, D. A., Electron microscopic analysis of the interdigital neuroma, *Clin. Orthop. Relat. Res.*, 271, 296–299, 1991.

110. Read, J. W., Noakes, J. B., Derr, D., Crichton, K. J., Slater, H. K., and Bonar, F., Morton's metatarsalgia: sonographic findings and correlated histopathology, *Foot Ankle*, 20, 153–161, 1999.

111. Erickson, S. J., Canale, P. B., Carrera, G. F., Johnson, J. E., Shereff, M. J., Gould, J. S., Hyde, J. S., and Jesmanowicz, A., Interdigital (Morton) neuroma: high-resolution MR imaging with a solenoid coil, *Radiology*, 181, 833–836, 1991.

112. Resch, S., Stenstrom, A., Jonsson, A., and Jonsson, K., The diagnostic efficacy of magnetic resonance imaging and ultrasonography in Morton's neuroma: a radiological-surgical correlation, *Foot Ankle*, 15, 88–92, 1994.

113. Zanetti, M., Strehle, J. K., Zollinger, H., and Hodler, J., Morton neuroma and fluid in the intermetatarsal bursae on MR images of 70 asymptomatic volunteers, *Radiology*, 203, 516–520, 1997.

114. Zanetti, M., Ledermann, T., Zollinger, H., and Odler, J., Efficacy of MR imaging in patients suspected of having Morton's neuroma, *AJR*, 168, 529–532, 1997.

115. Newman, L. G., Waller, J., Palestro, C. J., Schwartz, M., Klein, M. J., Hermann, G., Harrington, E., Roman, S. H., and Stagnaro-Green, A., Unsuspected osteomyelitis in diabetic foot ulcers: diagnosis and monitoring by leukocyte scanning with indium in 111 oxyquinoline, *J. Am. Med. Assoc.*, 266, 1246–1251, 1991.

116. Weinstein, D., Wang, A., Chambers, R., Stewart, C. A., and Motz, H. A., Evaluation of magnetic resonance imaging in the diagnosis of osteomyelitis in diabetic foot infections, *Foot Ankle*, 14, 18–22, 1993.

117. Levine, S. E., Neagle, C. E., Esterhai, J. L., Wright, D. G., and Dalinka, M. K., Magnetic resonance imaging for the diagnosis of osteomyelitis in the diabetic patient with a foot ulcer, *Foot Ankle*, 15, 151–156, 1994.

118. Morrison, W. B., Schweitzer, M. E., Wapner, K. L., Hecht, P. J., Gannon, F. H., and Behm, W. R., Osteomyelitis in feet of diabetics: clinical accuracy, surgical utility, and cost-effectiveness of MR imaging, *Radiology*, 196, 557–564, 1995.

119. Craig, J. G., Amin, M. B., Wu, K., Eyler, W. R., Holsbeeck, M. T., Bouffard, J. A., and Shirazi, K., Osteomyelitis of the diabetic foot: MR imaging-pathologic correlation, *Radiology*, 203, 849–855, 1997.

120. Morrison, W. B., Schweitzer, M. E., Batte, W. G., Radack, D. P., and Russel, K. M., Osteomyelitis of the foot: relative importace of primary and secondary MR imaging signs, *Radiology*, 207, 625–632, 1998.

121. Santi, M., Sartoris, D. J., and Resnick, D., Diagnostic imaging of tarsal and metatarsal stress fractures, *Orthop. Rev.*, 18, 178–185, 1989.

122. Steinbronn, D. J., Bennett, G. L., and Kay, D. B., The use of magnetic resonance imaging in the diagnosis of stress fractures of the foot and ankle: four case reports, *Foot Ankle*, 15, 80–83, 1994.

123. Prather, J. L., Nusynowitz, M. L., Snowdy, H. A., Hughes, A. D., McCartney, W. H., and Bagg, R. J., Scintigraphic findings in stress fractures, *J. Bone Joint Surg.*, 56-A, 869–874, 1977.

124. Geslien, G. E., Thrall, J. H., and Espinosa, J. L., Early detection of stress fracture using 99mTc-polyphosphate, *Radiology*, 121, 683–687, 1976.
125. Lee, J. K. and Yao, L., Stress fractures: MR imaging, *Radiology*, 169, 217–220, 1988.
126. Martin, S. D., Healey, J. H., and Horowitz, S., Stress fracture MRI, *Orthop.*, 16, 75–78, 1993.
127. Stafford, S. A., Ronsenthal, D. I., and Gebhardt, M. C., MRI in stress fracture, *Am. J. Radiol.*, 147, 553–556, 1986.
128. Zwas, S. T., Elkanovitch, R., and Frank, G., Interpretation and classification of bone scintigraphic findings in stress fractures, *J. Nucl. Med.*, 28, 452–457, 1987.
129. Fredericson, M., Bergman, A. G., Hoffman, K. L., and Dillingham, M. S., Tibial stress reaction in runners: correlation of clinical symptoms and scintigraphy with a new magnetic resonance imaging grading system, *Am. J. Sports Med.*, 23, 472–481, 1995.
130. Palma, L., Santucci, A., Gigante, A., Digiulio, A., and Carloni, S., Plantar fibromatosis: an immuno-histochemical and ultrastructural study, *Foot Ankle*, 20, 253–257, 1999.
131. Lee, T. H., Wapner, K. L., and Hecht, P. J., Current concepts review, plantar fibromatosis, *J. Bone Joint Surg.*, 75A, 1080–1084, 1993.
132. Morrison, W. B., Schweitzer, M. E., Wapner, K. L., and Lackman, R. D., Plantar fibromatosis: a benign aggressive neoplasm with a characteristic appearance on MR images, *Radiology*, 193, 841–845, 1994.

Index

F

Fast low-angle shot (FLASH) sequence, 23
Fast-spin-echo (FSE), 98
  imaging, 23, 180
  sequences, 23, 55
Fatigue-type stress fractures, 247
Fat suppression
  approaches used to achieve, 25
  heterogeneous, 26
  images, 17, 25
  inversion recovery, 124
  on low-field systems, 26
  phase-contrast method of, 26
  spectral, 24
  techniques, 237
FDL, *see* Flexor digitorum longus
FHL, *see* Flexor hallucis longus
Fibromas, chondromyxoid, 264, 265
Fibromatosis, 262, 267
Fibrous coalition, 242
Fibula
  growth and development of, 236
  osteomyelitis, 256
Field of view (FOV), 4
  imaging whole foot, 159
  increasing of, 5
  rectangular, 24
FLASH sequence, *see* Fast low-angle shot sequence
Flat-foot deformity, 273
Flexor digitorum longus (FDL), 102
Flexor hallucis brevis, 47
Flexor hallucis longus (FHL), 102, 277
Flexor tendons, 100
Fluid–fluid levels, 80
Foot
  deformities, 233, 240, 242
  pain, of unknown etiology, 290
  segments of, 38
Foot and ankle disease, 210
FOV, *see* Field of view
Fracture(s)
  compression, 56
  Type I, 54
Freiberg disease, 248, 250
Frequency encoding, 4
FSE, *see* Fast-spin-echo

G

Gadolinium
  contrast administration, 211
  diffusion of, 253
  enhancement, 170, 200, 235, 237
  infusion of intravenous, 130
  soft-tissue abscess, 161
Ganglion, 129
  cyst, 260, 285
  intraosseous, 64, 68
  soft tissue, 220, 261

tarsal tunnel syndrome caused by, 222, 223
GCT, *see* Giant cell tumor
GCTTS, *see* Giant cell tumor of tendon sheath
Genu valgum, 245
Giant cell tumor (GCT), 69, 71, 73, 263
Giant cell tumor of tendon sheath (GCTTS), 126, 201, 208, 209
Gigantism, localized, 244
Gout, 189, 191
Gradient coils, 2
Gradient-echo
  MR imaging, 247
  sequences, 29, 114
    pulse, 21
    sequences blooming if, 142
Gradient-recalled-echo (GRE) images, 235
Grainy image, 7
GRE images, *see* Gradient-recalled-echo images

H

HADD, *see* Hydroxyapatite deposition disease
Hallux bursitis, 225
Hammer toe, 224
Heel varus malalignment, 220
Hemagioma(s), 135, 204, 258
  epithelioid, 136
  signal characteristics of, 259
Hemangiomatosis, 244
Hematogeneous osteomyelitis, 170, 172
Hemophilia, 204
High-field MR systems, 6
Hind foot deformity, 245
Histiocytoma, malignant fibrous, 266
Hydroxyapatite deposition disease (HADD), 189, 193
Hyperparathyroidism, 98
Hypertension, 273

I

Image(s)
  coronal postgadolinium fat-suppressed T1-weighted, 163
  coronal spin-echo T2-weighted, 206
  fat-suppressed, 25
  gradient-recalled-echo, 235
  grainy, 7
  PDW, 40
  proton-density-weighted, 77
  sagittal spin-echo T1-weighted, 212
Imaging
  coronal plane, 28
  dual-echo FSE, 23
  FSE, 23
  gadolinium-enhanced, 200
  multiplanar, 20
  options, 19
  plane
    for metatarsals, 16